Clinical Scenarios in Vascular Surgery

CLINICAL SCENARIOS IN SURGERY SERIES

Clinical Scenarios in Vascular Surgery

Editors

Gilbert R. Upchurch, Jr., MD

Associate Professor
Vascular Surgery Section
University of Michigan Healthcare System
Ann Arbor, Michigan

Peter K. Henke, MD

Assistant Professor
Vascular Surgery Section
University of Michigan Healthcare System
Ann Arbor, Michigan

LIPPINCOTT WILLIAMS & WILKINS
A **Wolters Kluwer** Company

Philadelphia • Baltimore • New York • London
Buenos Aires • Hong Kong • Sydney • Tokyo

Acquisitions Editor: Brian Brown
Developmental Editor: Dovetail Content Solutions and Michelle LaPlante
Production Manager: Bridgett Dougherty
Manufacturing Manager: Ben Rivera
Marketing Manager: Adam Glazer
Production Services: Nesbitt Graphics, Inc.
Printer: Maple Press

Library of Congress Cataloging-in-Publication Data
Clinical scenarios in vascular surgery / editors, Gilbert R. Upchurch, Jr., Peter K. Henke.
    p. ; cm. — (Clinical scenarios in surgery series)
 Includes bibliographical references and index.
 ISBN 0-7817-5262-0
 1. Blood-vessels—Surgery—Case studies. I. Upchurch, Gilbert R. II. Henke, Peter K. III. Series.
 [DNLM: 1. Vascular Surgical Procedures—methods—Case Reports. 2. Diagnostic Techniques, Surgical—Case Reports. 3. Vascular Diseases—diagnosis—Case Reports. WG 170 C6415 2005]
 RD598.5.C586 2005
 617.4'13—dc22

                                                              2004023425

                         10 9 8 7 6 5 4 3 2 1

contents

Section I.   Cerebrovascular Disease

Section II. Upper Extremity Arterial Disease

Section III. Aortic Aneurysm

contributing authors

Gorav Ailawadi, MD
Vascular Surgery Section
University of Michigan
Ann Arbor, Michigan

Ahsan T. Ali, MD
Assistant Professor
Department of Vascular Surgery
University of Arkansas for Medical Sciences
Faculty
University Hospital (UAMS)
Little Rock, Arkansas

Omar Araim, MD
Chief Resident
Department of Surgery
St. Joseph Mercy Hospital
Ann Arbor, Michigan

Michel A. Bartoli, MD
Department of Surgery
Section of Vascular Surgery
Washington University School of Medicine
St. Louis, Missouri

Michael Belkin, MD
Associate Professor
Department of Surgery
Harvard Medical School
Chief, Division of Vascular Surgery
Brigham and Womens Hospital
Boston, Massachusetts

Scott A. Berceli, MD, PhD
Assistant Professor of Surgery
Department of Surgery
University of Florida
Gainesville, Florida

Joshua Bernheim, MD
Cornell University, Weill Medical College
Columbia University, College of Physicians and Surgeons
New York Presbyterian Hospital
New York, New York

Robert D. Brook, MD
Assistant Professor of Medicine
Department of Internal Medicine
University of Michigan
Department of Internal Medicine
University of Michigan Hospital
Ann Arbor, Michigan

Ruth L. Bush, MD
Assistant Professor of Surgery
Division of Vascular Surgery and Endovascular Therapy
Michael E. DeBakey Department of Surgery
Baylor College of Medicine
Houston, Texas

David K.W. Chew, MBBS, FRCSEd, FACS
Division of Vascular Surgery
Brigham and Women's Hospital
VA Boston Healthcare System
Boston, Massachusetts

Michael S. Conte, MD
Associate Surgeon
Division of Vascular Surgery
Brigham and Women's Hospital
Boston, Massachusetts

Matthew A. Corriere, MD
Vanderbilt University
Nashville, Tennessee

John A. Cowan, Jr., MD
Neurosurgery Resident
Department of Neurosurgery
University of Michigan
Ann Arbor, Michigan

Leslie D. Cunningham, MD, PhD
Brigham and Women's Hospital
Boston, Massachusetts

Alan Dardik, MD
Department of Vascular Surgery
Yale University School of Med
New Haven, Connecticut

R. Clement Darling III, MD
Professor of Surgery
Albany Medical Center
Albany, New York

Narasimham L. Dasika, MD
Department of Radiology
University of Michigan
Ann Arbor, Michigan

Mark G. Davies, MD, PhD

Associate Professor
Department of Surgery
University of Rochester
Associate Professor
Vascular Surgery and Endovascular Surgery
Department of Surgery
Strong Memorial Hospital
Rochester, New York

Rajeev Dayal, MD

Cornell University, Weill Medical College
Columbia University, College of Physicians and Surgeons
New York Presbyterian Hospital
New York, New York

Kristopher Deatrick, BS

Medical Student
University of Michigan
Ann Arbor, Michigan

Matthew J. Eagleton, MD

Assistant Professor
Department of Surgery
University of Michigan
Ann Arbor, Michigan

John Eidt, MD

Professor of Surgery
Division of Vascular Surgery
University of Arkansas for Medical Sciences
Chief of Vascular Surgery
Department of Surgery
University Hospital (UAMS)
Little Rock, Arkansas

Jonathan L. Eliason, MD

Section of Vascular Surgery
Department of Surgery
University of Michigan Hospital
Ann Arbor, Michigan

Jennifer S. Engle, MD

Assistant Professor
Section of Vascular Surgery
Department of Surgery
University of Michigan
Ann Arbor, Michigan

James M. Estes, MD

Assistant Professor of Surgery
Tufts University School of Medicine
Attending Surgeon
Division of Vascular Surgery
New England Medical Center
Boston, Massachusetts

Mark Farber, MD

University of North Carolina
Chapel Hill, North Carolina

Peter Faries, MD

Associate Professor
Department of Surgery
Cornell University and Columbia University
Chief of Endovascular Surgery
New York Presbyterian Hospital
New York, New York

Joss D. Fernandez, MD

General Surgery Resident
Department of Surgery
Vanderbilt University Medical Center
Nashville, Tennessee

Dennis R. Gable, MD

Attending Staff
Department of Surgery
Division of Vascular Surgery
Baylor University Medical Center
Dallas, Texas

Hemal G. Gada, BA

Section of Vascular Surgery
Department of Surgery
University of Michigan Medical Center
Ann Arbor, Michigan

Jonathan D. Gates, MD

Assistant Professor of Surgery
Harvard Medical School
Vascular Surgeon, Trauma Surgeon Director
Trauma Center Surgery
Brigham and Women's Hospital
Boston, Massachusetts

Vladimir Grigoryants, MD

Section of Vascular Surgery
Department of Surgery
University of Michigan
Ann Arbor, Michigan

Ajay Gupta, MD

St. Joseph Mercy Hospital
Ypsilanti, Michigan

Raul J. Guzman, MD

Vanderbilt University
Nashville, Tennessee

Brian G. Halloran, MD

St. Joseph Mercy Hospital
Ypsilanti, Michigan

Randall Harada, MD

Section of Vascular Medicine
Department of Internal Medicine
University of Michigan School of Medicine
Ann Arbor, Michigan

Mark R. Hemmila, MD
Assistant Professor
Department of Surgery
University of Michigan School of Medicine
Attending Surgeon
Department of Surgery
University of Michigan Health System
Ann Arbor, Michigan

Peter K. Henke, MD
Assistant Professor
Vascular Surgery Section
University of Michigan School of Medicine
Ann Arbor, Michigan

Susan Hickenbottom, MD
Clinical Associate Professor
Department of Neurology
University of Michigan Health System
Ann Arbor, Michigan

Scott Hollenbeck, MD
Cornell University, Weill Medical College
Columbia University, College of Physicians and Surgeons
New York Presbyterian Hospital
New York, New York

Thomas S. Huber, MD, PhD
Associate Professor
Department of Surgery
University of Florida College of Medicine
Staff Surgeon Department of Surgery
Shands Hospital at the University of Florida
Gainesville, Florida

Mark Iafrati, MD
Associate Professor of Surgery
Department of Surgery
Tufts University
Director of Vascular Surgery Research
Department of Surgery
Tufts New England Medical Center
Boston, Massachusetts

Kamran Idrees, MD
Vascular Laboratory
Beaumont Hospital
Royal Oak, Michigan

K. Craig Kent, MD
Cornell University, Weill Medical College
Columbia University, College of Physicians and Surgeons
New York Presbyterian Hospital
New York, NY 10021

Larry W. Kraiss, MD
Associate Professor
Division of Vascular Surgery
Department of Surgery
University of Utah School of Medicine
Chief Attending Surgeon
University of Utah Hospitals and Clinics
Salt Lake City, Utah

W. Anthony Lee, MD
Assistant Professor of Surgery and Radiology
Division of Vascular Surgery and Endovascular Therapy
University of Florida
Gainesville, Florida

Peter H. Lin, MD
Assistant Professor of Surgery
Division of Vascular Surgery & Endovascular Therapy
Michael E. DeBakey Department of Surgery
Baylor College of Medicine
Houston, Texas

Alan B. Lumsden, MD
Professor of Surgery
Division of Vascular Surgery & Endovascular Therapy
Michael E. DeBakey Department of Surgery
Baylor College of Medicine,
Houston, Texas

William A. Marston, MD
Associate Professor
Division of Vascular Surgery
Department of Surgery
University of North Carolina
Chapel Hill, North Carolina

Jon S. Matsumura, MD
Associate Professor of Surgery
Division of Vascular Surgery
Department of Surgery
Northwestern University
Active Staff
Northwestern Memorial Hospital
Chicago, Illinois

David J. Meier, MD
Section of Vascular Medicine
Department of Internal Medicine
University of Michigan School of Medicine
Ann Arbor, Michigan

Robert Mendes, MD
Division of Vascular Surgery
University of North Carolina, Chapel Hill
Chapel Hill, North Carolina

Ruchi Mishra, BA
Section of Vascular Surgery
University of Michigan School of Medicine
Ann Arbor, Michigan

J. Gregory Modrall, MD
Associate Professor
Division of Vascular and Endovascular Surgery
Department of Surgery
University of Texas Southwestern Medical School
Chief, Vascular Surgery Section
Dallas Veterans Affairs Medical Center
Dallas, Texas

Mohammed M. Moursi, MD
Associate Professor
Department of Surgery
University of Arkansas for Medical Sciences
Chief, Vascular Surgery
Central Arkansas Veterans Healthcare System
Little Rock, Arkansas

Albeir Mousa, MD
Cornell University, Weill Medical College
Columbia University, College of Physicians and Surgeons
New York Presbyterian Hospital
New York, New York

Michelle T. Mueller, MD
Instructor
Division of Vascular Surgery
University of Utah School of Medicine
Salt Lake City, Utah

Debabrata Mukherjee, MD
Director, Peripheral Vascular Interventions
Tyler Gill Professsor of Interventional Cardiology
Department of Internal Medicine, Division of Cardiology
University of Kentucky
Lexington, Kentucky

Thomas C. Naslund, MD
Associate Professor of Surgery
Chief, Division of Vascular Surgery
Vanderbilt University Medical Center
Nashville, Tennessee

Michael J. Naylor, MD
New England Medical Center
Boston, Massachusetts

Audra S. Noel, MD
Assistant Professor of Surgery
Mayo Clinic
Rochester, Minnesota

Christopher D. Owens, MD
Division of Vascular Surgery
Brigham and Women's Hospital
Boston, Massachusetts

C. Keith Ozaki, MD
Associate Professor of Surgery
Department of Surgery
University of Florida College of Medicine
Gainesville, Florida

Federico E. Parodi, MD
Department of Surgery
Section of Vascular Surgery
Washington University School of Medicine
St. Louis, Missouri

Marc A. Passman, MD
Assistant Professor of Surgery
Division of Vascular Surgery
Vanderbilt University Medical Center
Nashville, Tennessee

Philip S.K. Paty, MD
Associate Professor of Surgery
Albany Medical Center
Albany, New York

John Pfeifer, MD
Professor of Surgery
Section of Vascular Surgery
Department of Surgery
University of Michigan
Livonia, Michigan

Joseph D. Raffetto, MD
Boston Medical Center
Boston, Massachusetts

Sanjay Rajagopalan, MD
The Zena and Michael A. Wiener Cardiovascular Institute
Mount Sinai School of Medicine
New York, New York

John E. Rectenwald, MD
Vascular Surgery Fellow
Section of Vascular Surgery
Department of Surgery
University of Michigan
Ann Arbor, Michigan

Amy B. Reed, MD
Department of Surgery
Division of Vascular Surgery
University of Cincinnati Medical Center
Cincinnati, Ohio

Steven D. Rimar, MD
William Beaumont Hospital
Royal Oak, Michigan

Sean P. Roddy, MD
Assistant Professor of Surgery
Albany Medical Center
Albany, New York

Mark R Sarfati, MD
Assistant Professor
Division of Vascular Surgery
University of Utah School of Medicine
Attending Surgeon
Department of Surgery
University of Utah Hospitals and Clinics
Salt Lake City, Utah

Rajabrata Sarkar, MD
Department of Vascular Surgery
University of California—San Francisco
San Francisco, California

Timothy A. Schaub, MD
Section of Vascular Surgery
Department of Surgery
University of Michigan School of Medicine
Ann Arbor, Michigan

Marc L. Schermerhorn, MD

Assistant Professor
Department of Surgery
Harvard Medical School
Chief, Section of Interventional and Endovascular
Surgery
Division of Vascular and Endovascular Surgery
Beth Israel Deaconess Medical Center
Boston, Massachusetts

Mark W. Sebastian, MD

Associate Professor
Duke University
Duke University Medical Center
Durham, North Carolina

Raymond M. Shaheen, MD

Vascular Surgery Fellow
Division of Vascular Surgery
Department of Surgery
Chicago, Illinois

Charles J. Shanley, MD

Associate Chair, Department of Surgery
Research and Education
Beaumont Hospital
Royal Oak, Michigan

James C. Stanley, MD

Professor
Department of Surgery
University of Michigan
Co-Director, Cardiovascular Center
University Hospital
Ann Arbor, Michigan

Majid Tayyarah, MD

Division of Vascular Surgery and Endovascular Therapy
University of Florida
Gainesville, Florida

B. Gregory Thompson, MD

Associate Professor
Department of Neurosurgery
University of Michigan
Ann Arbor, Michigan

Robert W Thompson, MD

Department of Surgery
Section of Vascular Surgery
Washington University School of Medicine
St. Louis, Missouri

Gilbert R. Upchurch, Jr, MD

Associate Professor
Vascular Surgery Section
University of Michigan School of Medicine
Ann Arbor, Michigan

Omaida Velazquez, MD

Assistant Professor
Department of Surgery, Vascular Division
Hospital of the University of Pennsylvania
Philadelphia, Pennsylvania

Wendy L. Wahl, MD

Clinical Associate Professor of Surgery
Director of Trauma Burn Critical Care Services
University of Michigan Health System
Ann Arbor, Michigan

Thomas W. Wakefield, MD

S. Martin Lindenauer Professor and
Chief Section of Vascular Surgery
Department of Surgery
University of Michigan Medical Center and
Ann Arbor Veterans Administration Medical Center
Ann Arbor, Michigan

Margaret H. Walkup, MD

General Surgery Resident
Department of Surgery
University of North Carolina
Chapel Hill, North Carolina

Harry Wasvary, MD

William Beaumont Hospital
Royal Oak, Michigan

David R. Whittaker, MD

Fellow
Dartmouth-Hitchcock Medical Center
Section of Vascular Surgery
Lebanon, New Hampshire

David M. Williams, MD

Department of Radiology
University of Michigan
Ann Arbor, Michigan

Candace Y. Williams, BS

University of Michigan Medical Center
Ann Arbor, Michigan

Seth W. Wolk, MD

Clinical Assistant Professor of Surgery
University of Michigan Medical School
Attending Surgeon
St. Joseph Mercy Hospital
Ann Arbor, Michigan

Derek T. Woodrum, MD

Vascular Surgery Section
University of Michigan Medical School
Ann Arbor, Michigan

Lal P. K. Yilmaz, MD

Department of Surgery
University of California, San Francisco
VA Medical Center
San Francisco, California

Gerald Zelenock, MD

William Beaumont Hospital
Royal Oak, Michigan

Vascular diseases of the peripheral circulation are often complex and challenging to the clinician. This textbook addresses the entirety of common peripheral vascular diseases and will be an important resource to the practicing physician. Encounters with these patients will become increasingly common, given our successful prolongation of life in industrial society and the aging of the baby boomers born between 1946 and 1964. It is incumbent on physicians in training and established clinicians to understand the basics of a patient's presentation, appropriate diagnostic testing, and therapy for vascular diseases.

The most common learning by physicians is with rote memory after repetitive exposure to new words, new tests, and new procedures. However, the best learning comes from experience, especially after successfully evaluating and managing a patient's illness. The case studies presented in this textbook expose the reader to problem solving in a real-world context. It is surprising that medical education has been slow in adapting the learning paradigms of other professions, such as case studies in the business world and case law of our judicial system. Drs. Upchurch and Henke have identified an energetic and engaged group of contributors, and they have organized this textbook in an organ- and disease-specific manner that will facilitate the reader's focus on a given illness. This textbook fulfills a need to reeducate practicing physicians in a changing world of high technology. Its clear approach to vascular disease will be valuable to both primary care physicians and specialists, be they trainees in their early learning stages or seasoned practitioners. There is little question that *Clinical Scenarios in Vascular Surgery* belongs in the offices of busy clinicians and will be used frequently to enhance their knowledge, improve their practice, and benefit their patients.

James C. Stanley, MD
Professor of Surgery
Section of Vascular Surgery
University of Michigan

preface

Clinical Scenarios in Vascular Surgery is a first edition focusing on vascular disease in a series of clinical, case-based texts aimed at the medical student, trainee, and young vascular specialists including surgeons, vascular medicine physicians, and interventionalists. The field of vascular care is rapidly changing, primarily because of faster and more accurate diagnostic tools, as well as better therapies. Surgeons and non-surgeons treat vascular disease in the arterial, venous, and lymphatic systems, and these entities will only become more commonplace as the population ages. However, satisfactory treatment outcomes rely on proper decision making at all steps in the vascular patient's care.

The decision making begins with the proper diagnosis, which is still primarily based on a good history and physical examination. The goal of this text is to describe the typical presentation, describe diagnostic and therapeutic algorithms, and provide succinct supporting data at how these therapeutic decisions were made. Typical complicated disease courses, surgical outcomes, and pitfalls to avoid are described in many of these case scenarios. Selected references are included for the reader interested in more in-depth information about a particular topic.

The chapters are original and have been written primarily by young, practicing, academic vascular specialists who are well-versed in the problems described on a day-to-day basis. The structure of each chapter follows the same basic format that "walks" the reader through the given vascular disease entity. This format allows a focused and directed approach to clinically oriented management that is supported by the current literature. It is not the goal of this text to be all-inclusive. We also anticipate this book to be of particular appeal to vascular trainees studying for oral specialty board examinations.

This book would not have been possible without the hard work of the contributing authors. Their effort and knowledge conveyed on these pages is greatly appreciated by the editors. The persistence and excellent efforts of our publisher, Lippincott Williams & Wilkins, is acknowledged, and Acquisitions Editor Brian Brown deserves special thanks from us. Lastly, we sincerely appreciate the patience and support of our families, in particular our wives Nancy and Barbara. To the readers of this book, we hope it provides succinct and clear information that can be used in daily care of the patient with vascular disease for their benefit.

Gilbert R. Upchurch, Jr., MD
Peter K. Henke, MD

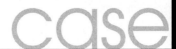

case **1**

John A. Cowan, Jr., MD, and B. Gregory Thompson, MD

Presentation

A 53-year-old right-handed woman with a history of tobacco use and hypertension is rushed to the emergency department after complaining of a severe, sudden headache followed by a momentary loss of consciousness. On examination, the patient is extremely lethargic with photophobia and right-sided hemiparesis.

▨ Noncontrast CT Scan of the Head

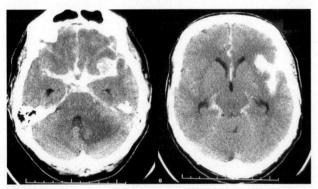

Figure 1-1

CT Scan Report

A noncontrast CT scan of the head reveals diffuse subarachnoid hemorrhage (SAH). A 1x1-cm calcified lesion is noted near the left anterior temporal lobe. A preponderance of the subarachnoid blood is filling the left insula and Sylvian fissure.

Differential Diagnosis

The patient's symptoms suggest a primary central nervous system event. Although headache is generally a nonspecific condition, the acuteness and severity of this patient's headache cause concern for intracerebral hemorrhage (ICH). Ischemic stroke and primary seizure disorder are common neurologic disorders and are nearly always nonpainful events. Intracerebral hemorrhage is generally due to trauma, tumor (primary or metastatic), hypertension, amyloid angiopathy, arteriovenous malformations, or aneurysms. The pattern of blood seen on the presenting CT scan (ie, blood layering in the sulci and extraparenchymal vascular territories, or subarachnoid spaces) is consistent with aneurysm rupture in the left middle cerebral artery (MCA).

Recommendation

Immediate stabilization of the patient's airway, breathing, and circulation (ABCs) is of prime importance. Patients who present with altered sensorium are at high risk for developing respiratory distress and aspiration. Furthermore, control of the patient's serum carbon dioxide levels will help in the management of elevated intracranial pressure. Therefore, the patient is intubated and mechanically ventilated to achieve adequate oxygenation and a partial pressure of carbon dioxide (PCO_2) between 32 and 36 mm Hg. An arterial line is placed and the patient is medicated to achieve systolic blood pressures less than 140 mm Hg. A central venous line is placed for intravenous access and to assess blood volume status. The patient is given loading and maintenance doses of an anticonvulsant and is started on a histamine (H_2) blocker or proton pump inhibitor for gastric protection. Nimodipine, a calcium channel blocker, is begun to lessen vasospasm. An electrocardiogram, serum sodium level, and coagulation studies are also performed. An external ventricular drainage catheter is placed in the right frontal horn of the lateral ventricle at the bedside. This provides immediate assessment of intracranial pressure and allows for drainage of cerebral spinal fluid as needed. The patient is then emergently taken to interventional radiology for a diagnostic angiogram.

Angiogram

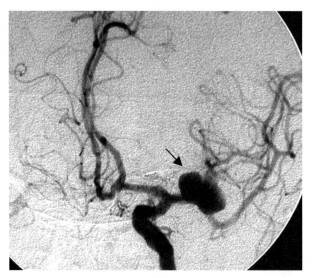

Figure 1-2

Angiogram Report

The angiogram reveals an abnormal bilobed dilation at the bifurcation of the left MCA consistent with an aneurysm.

Diagnosis and Recommendation

Ruptured left MCA aneurysm, amenable to open surgery.

Discussion

Two options exist for the management of a ruptured cerebral artery aneurysm. The newer procedure, endovascular coiling, involves inserting electrolytic detachable metal (usually platinum) coils into the lumen of the aneurysm via the femoral artery. This provides a nidus for thrombosis and essentially seals the aneurysm from normal circulation. The traditional approach is to perform a pterional craniotomy and expose the body of the aneurysm so that a surgical clip can be placed across the neck of the aneurysm. This excludes the aneurysm from normal circulation and reconstructs the lumen of the vessel.

In most cases, the angiographic characteristics of an aneurysm are useful in determining the most appropriate treatment modality. A patient's comorbid conditions and clinical grade are also considered. In this case, the wide neck of the aneurysm lessens the likelihood of successful coiling. Furthermore, the location of the aneurysm is amenable to an open surgical approach. Open surgery is, therefore, recommended.

▮ Surgical Approach

The patient is emergently taken to the operating room. She is placed in a supine position with a shoulder bump placed under her left side. A Mayfield headholder is applied, and her head is turned to the right to facilitate a left pterional approach. Using microsurgical techniques, the body of the aneurysm is dissected free and a titanium clip is applied across the neck of the aneurysm, excluding it from the normal circulation. An intraoperative angiogram is performed to demonstrate complete aneurysm occlusion and normal perfusion of distal MCA branches (Figure 1-3).

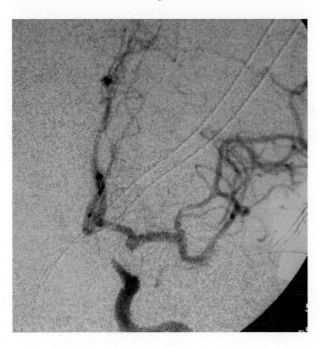

Figure 1-3 An intraoperative angiogram reveals normal blood flow through the left MCA and no residual aneurysm.

Discussion

Cerebral artery aneurysms are thought to be present in 2% to 3% of the population. The peak incidence of rupture is between 40 and 50 years of age with a female predominance (3:2; female:male). The overall mortality after SAH is 43%

to 55% with 20% to 30% morbidity in surviving patients. The risk of re-rupture is highest within the first 2 weeks (approximately 25%) with a 50% re-bleed rate at 6 months. The annual risk of rupture of a known cerebral artery aneurysm is controversial, but is thought to be approximately 1.4% per year. Smoking, hypertension, aneurysms larger than 7 mm, positive family history, aneurysm lobulation, multiple aneurysms, and prior SAH increase the risk of aneurysm rupture. Other medical conditions that predispose patients to cerebral aneurysm formation are autosomal dominant polycystic kidney disease, fibrous dysplasia, and coarctation of the aorta.

Future advances in catheter-based technologies will allow more cerebral aneurysms to be treated without needing open surgery. To date, one randomized controlled trial has compared an endovascular approach to traditional surgery in a limited population with SAH. These investigators found a small morbidity and mortality advantage to endovascular therapy in short-term follow-up. Comparisons of long-term outcomes are currently not available, but are needed.

Suggested Readings

Douglas C, Porterfield R. Nuances of middle cerebral artery aneurysm microsurgery. *Neurosurg.* 2001;48(2):339-346.

International Study of Unruptured Intracranial Aneurysms Investigators. Unruptured intracranial aneurysms—risk of rupture and risks of surgical intervention. *N Engl J Med.* 1998;339(24):1725-1733.

Kassell NF, Torner JC, Haley EC Jr, et al. The International Cooperative Study on the Timing of Aneurysm Surgery. Part 1: Overall management results. *J Neurosurg.* 1990;73(1): 18-36.

Molyneux A, Kerr R, Stratton I, et al. International Subarachnoid Aneurysm Trial (ISAT) Collaborative Group. *Lancet.* 2002;360(9342): 1267-1274.

Stein S. Brief history of surgical timing: surgery for ruptured intracranial aneurysms. *Neurosurg Focus.* 2001;11:1-5. Available at: http://www.neurosurgery.org/focus/aug01/1 1-2-3.pdf.

John E. Rectenwald, MD, and Gilbert R. Upchurch, Jr., MD

Presentation

A 55-year-old male smoker is referred to you for evaluation of right hemispheric transient ischemic attacks. He reports that on multiple occasions he has experienced self-limited left hand and arm weakness and numbness that resolves spontaneously over several hours. In addition to these episodes, his medical history is remarkable for one episode of right-sided monocular blindness. He has mild hypertension and has no history of previous stroke. He denies any previous operations and takes no medications. Physical examination reveals only fullness of the right carotid artery and a right carotid bruit. The contralateral carotid appears normal on physical examination. He has no palpable pulsatile midline abdominal masses or evidence of peripheral vascular disease on examination. He is referred to you for work-up.

Differential Diagnosis

The differential diagnosis of transient ischemic attack (TIA) and amaurosis fugax is broad and somewhat vague, with up to 30% of causes of TIA symptoms being "nonvascular" in origin. The ability to elicit a good history from the patient is essential to accurate diagnosis of TIAs. Careful consideration should be given to cerebrovascular disease (common, internal and rarely external carotid artery atherosclerosis) as the cause of symptoms. Carotid artery aneurysm (CAA) or dissection, thromboembolism from cardiac sources, arteritis (due to medications, irradiation, infection, or trauma), sympathomimetic drugs (eg, cocaine), and fibromuscular dysplasia are less likely, but should be included in the differential diagnosis. Other medical illnesses (eg, a hypercoagulable state or Marfan's syndrome) should be considered in selected cases.

Duplex scanning is the most simple and available modality to investigate suspected carotid artery lesions. It is a noninvasive and proven modality, with the caveats that it may fail to identify a lesion high in the carotid artery (especially if the patient has a short neck) and may overestimate the degree of carotid stenosis in the presence of a contralateral carotid artery occlusion.

Case Continued

A duplex ultrasound scan of the bilateral carotid arteries is ordered. On examination, the left carotid artery is normal; an ultrasound image of the right carotid artery is shown in Figure 2-1.

▓ Carotid Duplex Ultrasound Scan

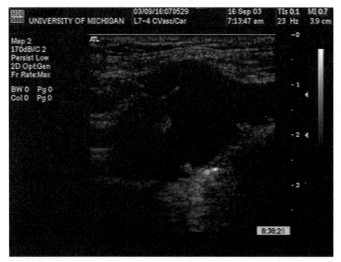

Figure 2-1

Carotid Duplex Ultrasound Scan Report

The duplex ultrasound examination of the right carotid artery demonstrates an aneurysmal common carotid artery and bulb approximately 3 cm in diameter. The proximal right internal carotid artery also appears aneurysmal. There is minimal intraluminal thrombus within the CAA.

Discussion

Although invasive (and associated with a stroke risk of approximately 1%), arteriography is the gold standard for CAAs. It remains a necessary preoperative study for CAAs, even if the diagnosis is first indicated by some other means. Arteriography most often provides the diagnosis and exact location of CAAs. It also detects associated lesions, stenosis, and wall irregularity including carotid fibrodysplasia. Newer technologies, such as magnetic resonance arteriography (MRA) and computed tomography angiogram, may be applicable to this disease, but their availability may be limited. An example of the MRA for this patient is included as an illustration of this imaging technique.

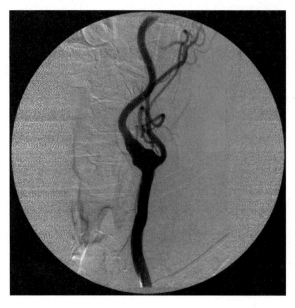

Figure 2-2 Aortic arch and carotid artery angiogram.

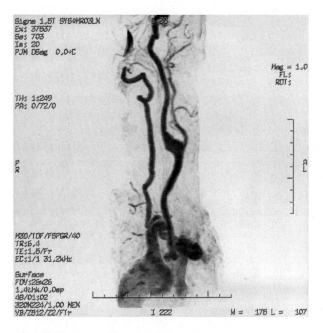

Figure 2-3 MRA image.

Carotid Artery Angiogram Report

The arteriogram above confirms the diagnosis and demonstrates a right CAA involving the right carotid bulb and proximal internal carotid artery. In addition, the arteriogram also demonstrates that the lesion is well removed from the petrous portion of the internal carotid artery (ICA), and that there is no evidence of a pseudoaneurysm or fibrodysplasia. As illustrated above, MRA also can provide quality images and valuable information concerning CAAs. In the future, MRA may have a more definitive role in the diagnosis and management of this disease.

Diagnosis and Recommendation

Even today, untreated CAAs are associated with poor outcomes (21% to 50% mortality rate due to stroke); therefore, surgical therapy is the preferred manner of treatment. At this time, open repair is preferable, because data for an endovascular approach and placement of covered stents for treatment of a CAA are lacking.

In general, the presence of a CAA is an indication for operative repair. However, if the aneurysm was discovered incidentally, is small in size, and the patient is completely asymptomatic or is a poor operative candidate due to comorbid conditions, an argument could be made to treat the patient nonoperatively with close observation, biannual carotid duplex examinations, and antiplatelet therapy. If such a patient demonstrates growth in the size of the aneurysm or develops symptoms, then surgical repair is indicated.

Discussion

Extracranial carotid aneurysms are defined by localized increases of carotid artery caliber of more than 50% of reference values (0.55 cm:0.49 cm, male:female at the level of the ICA; 0.99 cm:0.92 cm, male:female at the carotid bulb). They are relatively rare: recent clinical series spanning decades report only 20 to 50 cases. Most tertiary care hospitals encounter less than one per year. It is estimated that extracranial aneurysms represent 0.4% to 4.0% of all peripheral aneurysms. As opposed to aneurysms in the femoral and popliteal locations, CAAs are infrequently associated with other peripheral arterial aneurysms. CAAs may occur bilaterally approximately 15% to 20% of the time, and therefore necessitate thoughtful evaluation of the contralateral carotid artery. They are more common in males than females (2.5:1), occur at an earlier age (53 to 56 years of age) than atherosclerotic disease, and are frequently associated with hypertension (62%).

Presenting symptoms are most commonly caused by thromboemboli, as rupture of a carotid aneurysm is rare. Approximately two thirds of patients with CAAs present with TIAs. In addition, 33% complain of symptoms of amaurosis fugax and 21% have nonhemispheric symptoms, such as equilibrium disturbances or blurred vision; 8% will present with frank stroke. The remaining one third of patients are asymptomatic, although some may complain of dysphagia. These patients commonly present with an asymptomatic pulsatile neck mass or an incidental finding of CAA on computed tomography scan.

Historically, CAAs were most commonly due to peritonsillar infection. Although one recent clinical series cited postoperative pseudoaneurysm as a common cause, most series report atherosclerosis as the most common etiology. Other causes include carotid artery dysplasia, dissection, trauma, and infection. Regardless of cause, CAA is most often located at the carotid bulb (95%) with extension into the proximal internal carotid artery. It may extend to the carotid siphon in some cases, necessitating arteriography as part of the preoperative work-up.

Until the 1970s, CAAs were operatively managed by carotid artery ligation and were associated with an operative mortality of approximately 30%. More recent data suggest a lower mortality rate (11% to 12%) with ligation. Operative management has evolved since that time, but untreated disease is still associated with an unacceptable stroke rate of 21% to 50%.

Absolute indications for operative repair include symptomatic disease and aneurysm size greater than 2 cm. Current operative strategies range from direct arterial reconstruction with autogenous vein or synthetic grafts to simple aneurysmorrhaphy with patch angioplasty for selected saccular aneurysms. Combined major stroke and mortality rates for these procedures are generally accepted as 9% (range 3% to 20%, depending on the series).

Case Continued

The patient's risk factors for anesthesia and surgery are minimal. Informed consent is obtained. He is started on antiplatelet therapy with aspirin, and is scheduled for open repair of his CAA the following day.

Intraoperatively, the patient is found to have a 2.5-cm aneurysm of the right carotid bulb and proximal right internal carotid artery. The external carotid artery is ligated and the CAA is fully exposed.

■ Surgical Approach

The goal of surgical treatment is resection of the aneurysm with restoration of arterial continuity, while simultaneously avoiding neurologic complications due to thrombosis or thromboembolism. The operative approach to CAA is similar to that of elective carotid endarterectomy. General (rather than regional) endotracheal anesthesia is usually recommended because these procedures may be complex and have a protracted duration. The patient is positioned on a shoulder roll with adequate neck extension and rotation. The neck, upper chest, and groin (if the saphenous vein is to be used as a conduit) are prepared and draped in standard fashion. A cervical incision is made parallel and slightly anterior to the sternocleidomastoid muscle over the carotid bifurcation. The platysma muscle is divided using electrocautery and the carotid sheath is entered. The internal jugular vein is reflected laterally and the facial vein is ligated. The CAA is then exposed with minimal manipulation to avoid embolic complications. The posterior belly of the digastric muscle or the omohyoid muscle can be divided without hesitation to facilitate atraumatic dissection of the carotid. Care is taken to preserve the vagus and hypoglossal nerves, which may adhere to the aneurysm and are frequently injured. Once dissection is satisfactory, systemic heparin is administered intravenously. The common carotid artery below and the internal carotid artery above the aneurysm are controlled with vascular clamps. If the distal extent of the aneurysm is high and does not allow clamping, intraluminal balloon occlusion devices may be used. The external carotid artery is routinely ligated at this point, with the potential to be reimplanted later if collateral circulation is a concern. Intraluminal shunts may be used selectively if there are signs of impaired intracranial collateral blood flow, if the patient has had a prior stroke, or universally depending on surgeon preference. The aneurysm is then resected, and an end-to-end carotid-carotid interposition graft with spatulation of the distal ICA anastomosis is created. Reversed saphenous vein is generally the preferred conduit, but synthetic conduit may be used with good results if autogenous conduit is limited.

Markedly tortuous carotid arteries with limited aneurysmal involvement occasionally may be treated by simple aneurysm resection and primary reanastomosis or reimplantation of the carotid artery. Simple open aneurysmorrhaphy with patch angioplasty can be performed in selected patients with saccular aneurysmal disease, although the long-term success of this operation has not been established definitively. Internal carotid artery ligation is rarely necessary, but if such an approach is required, then postoperative anticoagulation should be considered to prevent stroke from cephalad propagation of thrombos in the ligated distal internal carotid stump.

Once repair is accomplished, the incision should be closed in layers with absorbable suture material according to the surgeon's preference. Closed-suction drainage is generally not necessary. If general anesthesia was used, the patient should be awakened and a thorough neurological assessment performed to assess for any deficits. Acute neurological events within hours of surgery should prompt emergent operative exploration to evaluate for technical failure of the repair and operative correction of any problems discovered.

Case Continued

The CAA is resected and replaced with a saphenous vein interposition graft sewn end to end with the common carotid artery distally and to the internal carotid artery proximally. The distal anastomosis is generously spatulated to avoid later anastomotic stenosis. The external carotid artery is not reimplanted. Postoperatively, the patient does well with no evidence of stroke, but his tongue now deviates to the right on protrusion.

Discussion

Cranial nerve injury after resection for CAA is common because of the presence of the aneurysm and distortion of the anatomy. The vagus and hypoglossal nerves are most often injured. Recent literature reports cite a broad range of incidence (0% to 66%) of cranial nerve injury. The majority of clinical papers report a cranial nerve injury rate of approximately 25%. Most injuries resolve with little morbidity after a few months.

Suggested Readings

El-Sabrout R, Cooley DA. Extracranial carotid artery aneurysms: Texas Heart Institute experience. *J Vasc Surg.* 2000;31:702-712.

Hertzer NR. Extracranial carotid aneurysms: a new look at an old problem. *J Vasc Surg.* 2000;31:823-825.

Painter TA, Hertzer NR, Beven EG, et al. Extracranial carotid aneurysms: report of six cases and review of the literature. *J Vasc Surg.* 1985;2:312-318.

Rosset E, Albertini JN, Magnan PE, et al. Surgical treatment of extracranial internal artery aneurysms. *J Vasc Surg.* 2000;31:713-723.

Stanley JC. Extracranial carotid artery aneurysms. In: Ernst CB, Stanley JC, eds. *Current Therapy in Vascular Disease.* 4th ed. St Louis: Mosby; 2001:104-108.

Zwolack RM, Whitehouse WM, Knake JE, et al. Atherosclerotic extracranial carotid artery aneurysms. *J Vasc Surg.* 1984;1:415-422.

James C. Stanley, MD

Presentation

A 28-year-old woman presents to your office with a classic history of amaurosis fugax on the right that has occurred 3 times in the past month. The last episode was associated with weakness of her left upper extremity lasting 10 minutes. Her past medical history is unremarkable. She has experienced no head or neck trauma. She is a nonsmoker, and there is no family history of cardiovascular disease, including stroke. Physical examination, including retinoscopy, is normal except for a grade III/VI high cervical bruit in the right neck.

Differential Diagnosis

Although a demyelinating or other destructive central nervous system (CNS) disease might cause visual aberrations and motor-sensory changes, this patient's last episode suggests an embolic event affecting the retinal circulation and ipsilateral middle cerebral vessels. Microemboli from a cardiac source with valvular vegetations, or an ulcerated arteriosclerotic plaque in the innominate-carotid vessels deserves consideration. However, in an otherwise healthy young woman, such is unlikely. Nevertheless, a transesophageal echocardiogram did not reveal any abnormalities within the heart. Duplex ultrasonography of the carotid arteries did not reveal any arteriosclerotic changes, although the contour of the uppermost internal carotid artery appeared somewhat irregular. In this setting, fibrodysplasia of the extracranial internal carotid artery (ECICA) is the most likely diagnosis.

Discussion

The precise incidence of carotid artery fibrodysplasia is unknown, although lesions of the ECICA affected 0.42% of 3600 patients undergoing cerebral arteriographic examinations at the University of Michigan. This finding was nearly identical to the 0.4% incidence encountered at the Mayo Clinic. Nevertheless, many of these former examinations were performed for suspected cerebrovascular disease, and thus the true frequency of ECICA fibrodysplasia in the general population would be expected to be lower. Medial fibrodysplasia of the ECICA invariably affects women, with most individuals being premenopausal in their third and fourth decades of life when diagnosed. If previous definitions of medial fibrodysplasia are rigidly applied, this particular dysplastic disease has rarely been described in men.

Complications occurring with medial fibrodysplasia of the ECICA appear to be related to (1) chronic encroachment on the lumen that causes flow reductions, (2) collection of thrombi within the dysplastic cul-de-sacs with distal embolization, and (3) acute occlusive dissections. The precise incidence of these complications has not been determined, but appear to occur in fewer than 5% of cases. The natural history of this disease is ill defined, but is less onerous than previously thought. Progression of ECICA fibrodysplasia may approach 30%, but the exact rate of change has yet to be defined.

The pathogenesis of ECICA fibrodysplasia is poorly understood, but it appears to parallel that occurring in the renal vessels. Three factors have been hypothesized to be important. First, estrogen effects on vascular smooth muscle during the reproductive years are believed to cause smooth muscle transformation to myofibroblasts. Second, very few muscular branches originate from the extracranial portion of the internal carotid artery, thus reducing the source of intrinsic vasa vasorum in this vessel. Such may contribute to mural ischemia in this vessel. Third, unusual traction or stretch stresses that occur with hyperextension and rotation of the neck also appear to contribute to smooth muscle changes in the affected vessels. All three factors—hormones, mural ischemia, and physical stresses—appear to play a role in causing dysplastic changes in the ECICA.

Non-cerebrovascular medial fibrodysplasia affects many patients who present with ECICA lesions. Renal artery involvement affects as many as 25% of these individuals. The frequency of ECICA lesions in patients presenting with renal artery dysplasia may be even higher, and it has been reported to be 50% in patients who underwent arteriographic assessments of both vessels.

Diagnostic Test

Carotid arteriography is essential to confirm the diagnosis of internal carotid artery fibrodysplasia. Such a study should include bilateral carotid artery studies, as well as an evaluation of the intracranial circulation. Conventional arteriography, because of its greater detail, is favored over magnetic resonance arteriography (MRA) or reformatted axial computed tomography (CT) studies.

▊ Carotid Arteriography

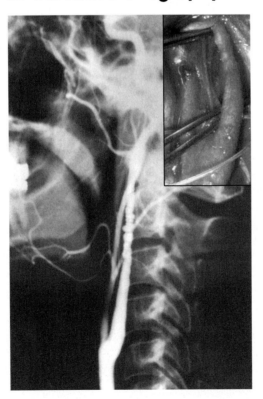

Figure 3-1

Carotid Arteriography Report

Carotid arteriography demonstrates medial fibrodysplasia of the ECICA adjacent to the second and third cervical vertebrae, with characteristic serial stenoses alternating with mural aneurysms. The beaded appearance of dysplastic upper cervical internal carotid artery is evident at operation (*insert*).

Discussion

Medial fibrodysplasia of the ECICA typically involves a 2-cm to 6-cm segment of the internal carotid artery adjacent to the second and third cervical vertebrae. The serial stenoses are usually evident on direct examination of the artery (see Fig. 3-1, *insert*). Bilateral disease has been reported to occur in 35% to 85% of patients with these lesions, with an average incidence of approximately 65%. Thus, arteriographic studies should be bilateral. Carotid arteries affected by medial fibrodysplasia are often elongated, and occlusive kinking occurs in approximately 5% of cases.

Coexistent intracranial aneurysms have been documented in 12% to 25% of patients having ECICA fibrodysplasia. Solitary intracranial aneurysms are present in 80% of these patients, with multiple aneurysms occurring in the remaining 20% of patients. Although intracranial arteries are occasionally the site of dysplastic disease, aneurysms seemingly do not develop in the involved vessel. Instead, they appear to evolve as a generalized dysplastic arteriopathy, which increases the likelihood of berry aneurysm formation. The anatomic distribution of aneurysms in patients with medial fibrodysplasia is the same as that in patients not affected with dysplastic ECICA.

Recommendation

The patient was advised to undergo either an open surgical or percutaneous catheter-based dilation of her diseased right internal carotid artery. Conventional surgical dilation was pursued when the patient declined balloon dilation.

■ Surgical Approach

The patient underwent open dilation of her diseased carotid vessel under regional cervical block anesthesia. Rigid dilators were passed through a carotid bulb arteriotomy. She was systematically anticoagulated with heparin (150 U/kg) during the procedure, and this was reversed with protamine (1.5 mg/100 units of heparin) after the arteriotomy was closed. She experienced no intraoperative complications, and a postoperative arteriogram revealed a normal appearing ECICA (Fig. 3-2). She was discharged on her second postoperative day and has remained free of any neurologic signs or symptoms in the intervening 2 years.

Discussion

Operative techniques employed in the management of stenotic ECICA fibrodysplastic lesions have included open graduated intraluminal dilation, percutaneous balloon angioplasty with or without stenting, resection of the diseased vessel with interposition grafting, and angioplasty with patch graft placement. The latter two procedures are uncommon and are usually reserved for treating dissections that have complicated the underlying fibrodysplastic disease.

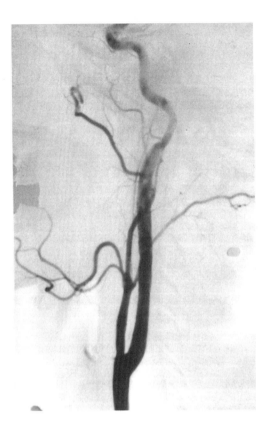

FIGURE 3-2 Postoperative appearance of the dilated ECICA.

Operative exposure of the carotid vessel includes dissection of the entire ECICA to within a few centimeters of the base of the skull. Care must be taken to avoid injury to cranial nerves IX to XII. Extended exposure at the upper cervical levels may be facilitated by subluxation of the mandible. Experience at the University of Michigan supports the use of intermittent traction on the mandible using an external clamp inserted into the angle of the mandible. Others have advocated continuous fixed distraction of the mandible following placement of arch bars.

Since its introduction nearly 35 years ago, graduated intraluminal dilation has been the most common procedure used in the treatment of these lesions. Rigid olive-tip dilators are advanced through an arteriotomy placed in the carotid bulb or distal common carotid artery. Dilators are passed the full length of the ECICA to the base of the skull. Initial dilators are usually 1.5 to 2 mm in diameter, with increasingly larger dilators sequentially advanced until a 5-mm to 6-mm dilator is inserted. Use of instruments with diameters larger than 6 mm should be avoided because they may cause deep dissections or actual disruption of the vessel wall. Balloon dilation through an open arteriotomy during a conventional operative procedure is an alternative to use of a rigid dilator. Back bleeding from the ECICA should allow washout of any dysplastic debris resulting from the dilation. Conclusion arteriography is not routinely performed, but if there are concerns regarding the adequacy of the dilation, it should be done. Conventional shunting usually interferes with the dilation procedure.

Percutaneous balloon angioplasty, with or without stents or stent graft placement, may be useful in treating these lesions. However, to date this approach has not been compared in a clinical trial to the operative use of rigid dilators. Nevertheless, with improved catheter technology and better rescue devices to prevent embolization, this manner of therapy is likely to become much more common.

Therapeutic results in properly selected patients have been generally successful, with approximately 90% of the almost 170 reported cases having had excellent outcomes. However, nearly 5% of these patients have had postoperative neurologic deficits and 1% have died as a consequence of this therapy. Furthermore, follow-up studies, although sporadic in the reported literature, revealed that approximately 2% of patients had late transient ischemic attacks, and late strokes were observed in an additional 2%. Without preoperative randomized studies, conclusive comparisons of open operative procedures, catheter-based interventions, and simple antiplatelet-anticoagulation therapy are inappropriate. Nevertheless, the results of operative dilation for symptomatic ECICA fibrodysplasia justify this therapy in properly selected patients.

Suggested Readings

Chiche L, Bahnini A, Koskas F, et al. Occlusive fibromuscular disease of arteries supplying the brain: results of surgical treatment. *Ann Vasc Surg.* 1997;11:496.

Finsterer J, Strassegger J, Haymerle A, Hagmuller G. Bilateral stenting of symptomatic and asymptomatic internal carotid artery stenosis due to fibromuscular dysplasia. *J Neurol Neurosurg Psychiatry.* 2000;69:683-686.

Manninen HI, Koivisto T, Saari T, et al. Dissecting aneurysms of all four cervicocranial arteries in fibromuscular dysplasia: treatment with self-expanding endovascular stents, coil embolization, and surgical ligation. *Am J Neuroradiol.* 1997;18:1216-1220.

Moreau P, Albat B, Thevent A. Fibromuscular dysplasia of the internal carotid artery: long-term surgical results. *J Cardiovasc Surg.* 1993; 34:465-472.

Stanley JC, Fry WJ, Seeger JF, et al. Extracranial internal carotid and vertebral artery fibrodysplasia. *Arch Surg.* 1974;109:215.

Starr DS, Lawrie GM, Morris GC Jr. Fibromuscular dysplasia of carotid arteries: long-term results of graduated internal dilatation. *Stroke.* 1981;12:196-199.

Stewart MT, Moritz MW, Smith RB III, et al. The natural history of carotid fibromuscular dysplasia. *J Vasc Surg.* 1986;3:305.

case 4

John A. Cowan, Jr., MD, and B. Gregory Thompson, MD

Presentation

A 45-year-old right-handed carpenter with a history of tobacco use is referred to your office because he has recurrent episodes of speech slurring and right arm weakness. The patient states that these episodes began 6 months ago, and that they often occur while he is at work. Each episode lasts approximately 10 to 20 minutes, after which he returns to near full function. No loss of consciousness occurs. On neurological examination, the patient is grossly intact with a mild pronator drift on the right. The patient brings the results of a carotid duplex and arteriogram, which suggests absence of blood flow in the left internal carotid artery (ICA) and no significant ICA disease on the right. He was placed on antiplatelet therapy several months ago with no relief of symptoms.

Recommendation

Urgent computed tomography (CT) scan of the head and cerebral angiogram are recommended. An electrocardiogram and laboratories are obtained.

▪ CT Scan

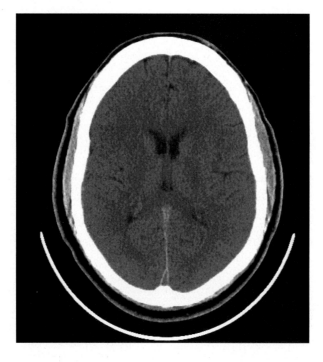

Figure 4-1

CT Scan Report

The noncontrast head CT scan reveals no evidence of stroke or other distinct abnormalities.

Cerebral Angiogram

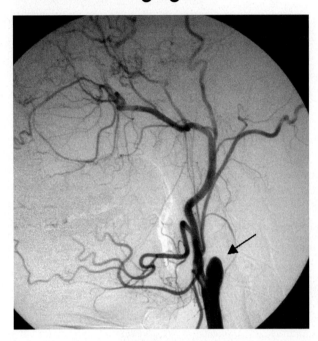

Figure 4-2

Angiogram Report

The cerebral angiogram reveals a 100% occlusion of the left ICA with no significant disease in the right ICA.

Electrocardiogram and Laboratory Results

An electrocardiogram reveals normal sinus rhythm, and blood coagulation studies reveal no abnormalities.

Differential Diagnosis

The constellation of transient aphasia and arm weakness are suggestive of a hemispheric process in the central nervous system. Seizures or cardiac events causing these symptoms would often lead to loss of consciousness, and would be associated with other neurologic or physical symptoms. Thromboembolic (cardiac or other) phenomena, although common, typically result in an isolated neurologic deficit (e.g., arm weakness only, aphasia only, visual complaints only) during a particular episode. In total, the patient may have both arm weakness and speech impairment; however, in this case the patient clearly describes both symptoms simultaneously. In more than 90% of right-handed individuals (more than 70% of left-handers), speech arises from the left hemisphere. Thus transient, stress-related aphasia and right arm weakness are highly suggestive of a low blood flow state in the left ICA distribution. The angiogram solidifies the diagnosis of complete left ICA occlusion and reliance on collateral circulation to the left fontal, temporal, and parietal lobes.

Recommendation

To assess the degree and limits of the patient's collateral circulation, tests that can now be performed include positron emission tomographic (PET) scan, magnetic resonance imaging (MRI) scan with perfusion/diffusion, computed tomographic (CT) scan with perfusion, or xenon CT scanning. In this case, xenon CT scan is ordered.

Xenon CT Scan

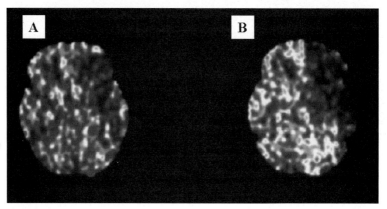

Figure 4-3

Xenon CT Scan Report

Xenon CT scan reveals decreased baseline cerebral blood flow (Fig. 4-3A) and a severe deficit in cerebrovascular reserve (Fig. 4-3B) in the left ICA distribution.

Diagnosis and Recommendations

Complete left internal artery occlusion with symptoms. External carotid artery to internal carotid artery (EC/IC) bypass is recommended.

Surgical Approach

The patient is placed in a Mayfield head-holder to provide 3-point fixation. While the patient is in the supine position, the head is turned to the right. A Doppler probe is then used to demarcate the branches of the superficial temporal artery (STA) in the scalp. After identification of a suitable donor vessel, the head is shaved and prepped in a sterile fashion. A skin incision is made next to the donor vessel so that it can be identified clearly and dissected free from the surrounding connective tissue. The incision is lengthened so that a small craniotomy may be performed beneath the temporalis muscle. A distal branch of the middle cerebral artery is identified on the cortical surface as the recipient vessel. The donor and recipient vessels are joined in an end-to-side anastomosis with an 8-0 monofilament suture. A handheld Doppler probe is used to ensure adequate flow across the anastomosis. When a suitable STA cannot be found, saphenous vein or radial artery can serve as a conduit between the EC and IC circulation.

Postsurgical Angiogram

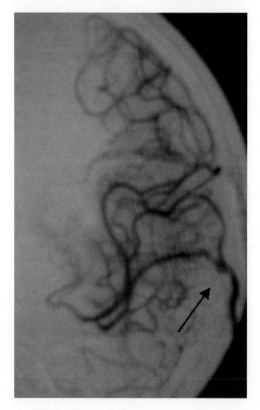

Figure 4-4

Angiogram Report

Anterior-posterior angiogram view reveals restoration of distal middle cerebral artery perfusion via an external carotid artery bypass graft (*arrow*).

Discussion

Complete carotid occlusion is a relatively rare presentation of extracranial carotid artery disease. In many cases, the symptoms due to complete carotid occlusion are hemodynamic in nature rather than thromboembolic. The precise management of these patients remains controversial. In 1985, the EC/IC Bypass Study Group investigators found no statistical difference in stroke prevention between surgery and medical (i.e., antiplatelet therapy) management. This resulted in a dramatic decrease in the number of bypass surgeries performed for stroke prevention. However, several investigators have begun using radiographic tests of cerebral perfusion to select patients at higher risk for hemodynamic stroke. This question is currently being investigated in the multi-institutional Carotid Occlusion Surgery Study (COSS), whose findings should be reported in 2005 or 2006. Until these high-risk populations can be identified,

EC/IC bypass is generally offered to patients failing medical therapy who have symptoms attributable to poor cerebral hemodynamics and who have favorable anatomy for a bypass.

Suggested Readings

EC/IC Bypass Study Group. Failure of extracranial-intracranial arterial bypass to reduce the risk of ischemic stroke. *N Engl J Med.* 1985;313:1191-1200.

Grubb RL, Derdyn CP, Fritsch SM, et al. Importance of hemodynamic factors in the prognosis of symptomatic carotid occlusion. *JAMA.* 1998;280:1055-1060.

Sundt TM. Was the international randomized trial of extracranial-intracranial bypass representative of the population at risk? *N Engl J Med.* 1987;316:814-816.

Yonas H, Smith HA, Durham SR, et al. Increased stroke risk predicted by compromised cerebral blood flow reactivity. *J Neurosurg.* 1993;79:483-489.

Robert Mendes, MD, and Mark Farber, MD

Presentation

A 63-year-old man with a past medical history significant for hypertension and tobacco abuse presents to your office with recent episodes of amaurosis fugax of the right eye and left arm weakness. The episodes last for approximately 3 to 5 minutes, then resolve. He has experienced 3 episodes over the last 2 months. Physical examination reveals a bruit on the right side of the neck, a regular heart rate and rhythm, and no neurologic deficits.

Differential Diagnosis

The most common cause of transient cerebral ischemia is extracranial arterial atherosclerotic disease. The differential diagnosis of these patients also includes cardiac emboli, paroxysmal emboli, fibromuscular dysplasia (FMD), carotid dissection, coils or kinks of the extracranial arteries, aneurysms of the extracranial arteries, and migraine headaches associated with transient neurologic deficits. With this patient's risk factors of age, hypertension, and tobacco abuse, carotid stenosis must be considered the primary diagnosis.

Discussion

Transient cerebral ischemia is a global term encompassing amaurosis fugax, also known as transient monocular blindness (TMB), and lateralizing transient ischemic attacks (TIA). TMB is classically described as having a "curtain over the eye" or "a shade pulled over the eye" that clears in seconds to a few minutes. Lateralizing TIAs commonly manifest as weakness or paresthesia that affect the contralateral body. By definition, the duration of a TIA is less than 24 hours; however, they frequently last only several minutes to an hour before resolving without a residual neurologic deficit. Physicians rarely see patients during attacks, and the history remains the primary factor in establishing a diagnosis.

A patient can experience frequent repetitive neurologic attacks without complete resolution of the deficit between the episodes. If the attacks reproduce the same deficit and there is no progressive deterioration in neurologic function, it is deemed a crescendo TIA. If a progressive deterioration in neurologic function is seen, the patient is described as experiencing a stroke in evolution. In either case, immediate evaluation is necessary and an emergent operation may be required for a surgically correctable lesion.

Flow-related ischemic events are unusual due to an extremely efficient collateral blood supply to the brain, primarily through the circle of Willis. When they do occur, flow-related ischemic events are usually associated with carotid dissections. Most commonly, cerebral ischemic attacks are caused by thromboembolic events from an arterial nidus. The arterial nidus for emboli is usually an atheromatous plaque, but emboli can also originate from lesions caused by

FMD, radiation therapy, or aneurysms of the carotid vessels. A less common source is cardiac emboli, originating from an intracardiac thrombus associated with atrial fibrillation or myocardial infarction. Paroxysmal emboli, which originate from a deep venous thrombus that crosses from the venous to arterial systems via a septal defect in the heart, are a rare cause of cerebral ischemic attacks.

Although angiography has historically been considered the gold standard, the initial diagnostic test is duplex ultrasonography to evaluate the extracranial carotid and vertebral arteries for occlusive lesions. The basic principle of this study is to assess anatomy, using real-time B-mode imaging, and flow dynamics, using quantitative pulsed wave Doppler, to determine the location and severity of disease. The grade of the lesion is characterized by increased velocity spectra recorded proximal to, and at, the point of maximum stenosis. Several studies have compared the accuracy of duplex ultrasound with arteriography, and have determined a close correlation in stenotic estimations. Angiograms should be obtained where duplex cannot accurately determine the severity of the lesion. These situations include proximal common carotid or aortic arch lesions, contralateral carotid occlusion, high bifurcation of the carotid, and discrepancy in symptoms compared to the duplex findings. As technology advances, computed tomographic (CT) angiography and magnetic resonance arteriography (MRA) are becoming more useful diagnostic tools when these issues are encountered.

Recommendation

Obtain duplex ultrasonography of the extracranial vessels.

■ Extracranial Duplex Ultrasound Scan

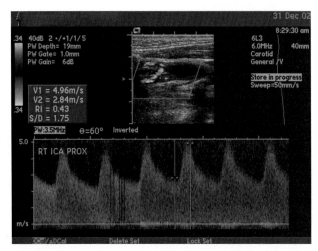

Figure 5-1

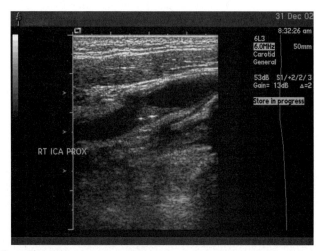

Figure 5-2

Extracranial Duplex Ultrasound Scan Report

Spectral waveform (see Fig. 5-1) and duplex real-time B-mode (see Fig. 5-2) ultrasound scans show a significant (60% to 99%) stenosis of the right internal carotid artery (ICA). Heavy plaque is identified extending from the carotid bulb to the proximal ICA.

Diagnosis and Recommendations

This patient has a symptomatic right ICA stenosis. He is offered a right carotid endarterectomy (CEA) and a life-long aspirin regimen. The expressed benefit of combined surgical intervention and medical management includes an absolute risk reduction of stroke by 17%, and a relative risk reduction of 71% at 18 months. The patient is informed that the operative risks include death, stroke, cranial nerve injury, wound complications, headaches, and restenosis of the carotid artery.

◾ Surgical Approach

The patient is given a regional block to the ipsilateral neck, and provided with mild sedation. A pressure bag is placed in the contralateral hand to provide an intraoperative assessment of the patient's neurologic function. An incision is made anterior to the sternocleidomastoid muscle, and carried through the platysma. The internal jugular vein is identified and retracted laterally. The dissection is carefully continued around the common carotid artery, and control obtained with a vessel loop. The vagus nerve is identified posterior to the carotid artery. The dissection is continued superiorly to the superior thyroid artery and the external carotid artery. Control of these vessels is also established with vessel loops. Care is taken to avoid direct dissection of the carotid bifurcation. The internal carotid artery is further dissected superiorly, well above the distal aspect of the atherosclerotic plaque. The hypoglossal nerve is identified superior to the bifurcation. Further exposure can be obtained superiorly with division of the digastric muscle tendon. However, care must be taken not to injure the glossopharyngeal nerve. The internal carotid is controlled with a vessel loop.

Systemic heparinization is given, a test clamp is performed on the internal carotid artery, and a neurologic assessment is made. Following the assessment, vessels are clamped, and the arteriotomy is made on the anterolateral aspect of the common carotid and extended superiorly beyond the most distal aspect of the internal carotid plaque. If a neurologic deficit was realized during the test clamp, a shunt is placed at this time. The endarterectomy plane is then created, and the plaque is removed (Fig. 5-3). If intimal flaps are present, they are

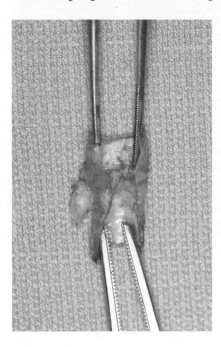

Figure 5-3 Carotid artery plaque after endarterectomy.

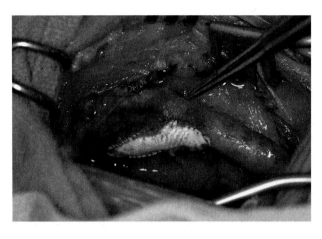

Figure 5-4 Carotid artery patch.

secured with tacking sutures. The arteriotomy is typically closed with a patch; however, an unusually large artery may require primary closure (Fig. 5-4). Back bleeding of the internal carotid is performed to remove any embolic potential (e.g., debris or air) before placing the last few sutures. Arterial flow is restored first to the external carotid and then the internal carotid artery. Duplex ultrasound scan is performed intraoperatively to identify any surgically correctable issues. A drain is placed in the subplatysmal space, and the platysmal layer is approximated, followed by skin closure. The drain is removed on the first postoperative day.

Case Continued

The patient is without neurologic or cranial nerve deficits on postoperative day one. The drain is removed and the patient is discharged from the hospital on aspirin therapy. He is scheduled for a wound check in 2 weeks, and will receive a duplex study in 6 months to initiate routine follow-up of the surgical repair.

Discussion

An understanding of the natural history of the disease process is imperative to the decision-making process aimed at providing therapy to prevent cerebral infarction. The initial mortality of an ischemic stroke approximates 15% to 30%. Survivors have a high risk for recurrent stroke, estimated between 5% and 15% per year, implying that approximately 50% will suffer a second ischemic incident within 5 years.

Patients who experience symptoms (e.g., TIA, TMB) associated with their carotid stenosis are at a higher risk of developing a stroke. The Mayo Clinic study observed 118 patients with TIAs, and discovered the stroke rates at 1, 3, and 5 years were 23%, 37%, and 45%, respectively, if no therapy was administered. This represented a 16-fold increase in the risk of stroke when compared to the age- and sex-adjusted population.

The North American Symptomatic Carotid Endarterectomy Trial (NASCET) is a large prospective study that determined a clear benefit with combined CEA and medical therapy to treat a symptomatic carotid stenosis, when compared to medical therapy alone. This study reported a 30-day operative morbidity and mortality for patients managed with CEA of 5%. At 18 months, a 7% incidence of major stroke occurred in the surgical arm of the trial, compared to a 24% incidence of major stroke in the medical arm of the trial. This difference proved highly significant.

Although the previously stated data provide a general standard, many surgical centers now report lower stroke and fatality rates associated with symptomatic carotid endarterectomies. It is, therefore, important for surgeons to monitor their operative outcomes to appropriately counsel their patients preoperatively.

Suggested Readings

Edwards JM, Moneta GL, Papanicolaou TG, et al. Prospective validation of new duplex ultrasound criteria for 70-99% internal carotid artery stenosis. *JEMU*. 1995;16:3-7.

Hobson RW. Carotid artery occlusive disease. In: Dean RH, Yao JS, Brewster DC, eds. *Current Diagnosis and Treatment in Vascular Surgery*. Norwalk, Conn: Appleton & Lange; 1995:88-104.

Hood DB, Mattos MA, Mansour A, et al. Prospective evaluation of new duplex criteria to identify a 70% internal carotid artery stenosis. *J Vasc Surg*. 1996;23:254-261.

Moneta GL, Edwards JM, Chitwood RW, et al. Correlation of North American Symptomatic Carotid Endarterectomy Trial (NASCET) angiographic definition of 70% to 99% internal carotid artery stenosis with duplex scanning. *J Vasc Surg*. 1993;17:152-159.

Moore WS. Extracranial cerebrovascular disease: the carotid artery. In: Moore WS, ed. *Vascular Surgery: A Comprehensive Review*. 5th ed. Philadelphia: WB Saunders; 1998:555-597.

North American Symptomatic Carotid Endarterectomy Trial Collaborators. Beneficial effect of carotid endarterectomy in symptomatic patients with high-grade carotid stenosis. *N Engl J Med*. 1991;325:445-453.

Sacco RL, Wolf PA, Kannel WB, et al. Survival and recurrence following stroke: the Framingham Study. *Stroke*. 1982;13:290-295.

Schmidt EV, Smirnov VE, Ryabova VS. Results of a seven-year prospective study of stroke patients. *Stroke*. 1988;19:942-949.

Whisnant JP, Matsumoto M, Elveback LR. The effects of anticoagulant therapy on the prognosis of patients with transient cerebral ischemic attacks in a community: Rochester, Minnesota, 1965-1969. *Mayo Clin Proc*. 1973; 48:844-848.

case 6

Gilbert R. Upchurch, Jr., MD, and Gorav Ailawadi, MD

Presentation

A 63-year-old man with a past medical history significant for hypertension and hypercholesterolemia presents to your office after his family physician hears a right-sided neck bruit on routine physical examination. Social history is positive for tobacco use. His medications include a beta-blocker and aspirin. On review of systems, the patient denies evidence of amaurosis fugax, motor or sensory deficits, difficulty with speech, or any previous history of a transient ischemic attack or stroke. On physical examination, the patient has a right-sided carotid bruit. His peripheral upper extremity pulses are all palpable. A duplex ultrasound scan of the carotid arteries is recommended.

▇ Carotid Duplex Ultrasound Scan

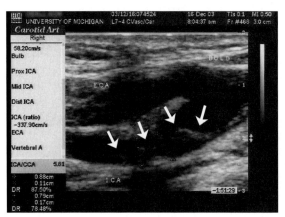

Figure 6-1A

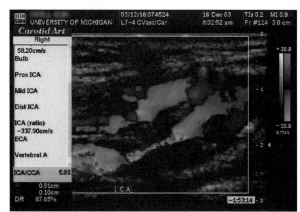

Figure 6-1B

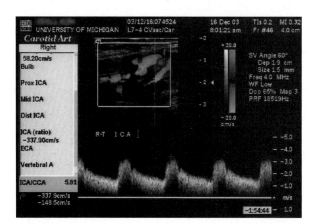

Figure 6-1C

Carotid Duplex Ultrasound Scan Report

Right carotid scan: bulb and internal carotid artery (ICA) show evidence of heterogeneous plaque with 87% diameter stenosis. (*Arrows* denote extent of plaque on Fig. 6-1A.) Figure 6-1B demonstrates plaque with color Doppler. ICA systolic velocity/end diastolic velocity: 338/149 cm/sec; 80% to 99% diameter stenosis (see Fig. 6-1C). External carotid artery (ECA): normal. Vertebral: antegrade.

Right carotid impression: The right carotid study reveals an 80% to 99% diameter stenosis in the bulb/ICA. The distal end of the plaque was seen.

Left carotid impression: The left carotid study reveals no significant disease by image, and velocities are suggestive of a 40% to 60% diameter stenosis in the bulb/ICA. Velocities may be elevated due to contralateral high-grade stenosis.

Differential Diagnosis

This patient has an asymptomatic high-grade right internal carotid artery stenosis. Other pathology may be noted on duplex, including a carotid body tumor, a carotid artery dissection or aneurysm, or reversal of flow in the vertebral artery (secondary to "subclavian steal"). However, given the patient's smoking history, physical examination, and duplex results, the diagnosis is an asymptomatic high-grade right internal carotid artery stenosis.

Discussion

Stroke is the third leading cause of death in the United States, with more than 700,000 strokes and 150,000 deaths annually. Arteriosclerosis of the brachio-cephalic trunk, including the carotid arteries, causes more than 50% of strokes. The events that initiate transformation of a benign carotid bifurcation lesion into a stroke-producing plaque are poorly understood. Initial plaque size, degree of stenosis, and chemical composition of the plaque all are relevant in the evolution of these lesions.

The work-up for a patient who presents with symptomatic or incidental carotid artery stenosis should be systematic. History should be directed at identifying risk factors and prior ischemic events. Physical examination should note signs of cardiac and systemic vascular disease, including assessment of peripheral pulses, examination for bruits, and careful assessment for signs of prior clinical stroke on neurologic examination.

Carotid duplex ultrasonography is the recommended first screening study in patients who are suspected of having carotid artery stenosis. The severity of the ICA lesion can be reliably measured based on the internal carotid to common carotid artery ratio, peak systolic flow, and end diastolic velocities. Magnetic resonance angiography (3D-MRA) with 2D-time-of-flight (2D-TOF) is useful in cases where duplex ultrasonography yields contradictory results or in the elucidation of concomitant intracranial lesions. The traditional "gold standard" diagnostic study for carotid artery stenosis has been angiography, but this study is rarely used now. Carotid angiography, however, was used in most of the randomized studies examining surgery versus medical therapy, justifying the use of carotid endarterectomy (CEA), and therefore serves as the reference standard against which other modalities are compared. It is useful in its ability to identify co-existing lesions of the great vessels and intracerebral arteries. Following a duplex scan, indications for MRA or carotid angiography include cases where symptoms do not correlate with the extent of carotid disease, the top of the plaque is not visualized, the vessel is extremely tortuous, the ipsilateral carotid artery is occluded, or if there is a high carotid bifurcation.

Recommendations

A right carotid endarterectomy (CEA) is recommended, given the patient's age (less than 80 years) and gender (male). A combined 3% risk of ipsilateral stroke and death is quoted. The risk of cranial injury, usually transient, is described as 10% to 15%. Given the patient's age (less than 70 years), lack of diabetes or electrocardiographic abnormalities, and good overall activity status (he is able to walk up a flight of stairs without shortness of breath), no further preoperative cardiac testing is performed. The patient is started on a statin preoperatively.

Case Continued

The patient undergoes appropriate monitoring, including a radial arterial line. A cervical block is placed. After prepping, an incision is made parallel to the anterior sternocleidomastoid muscle. The platysma is divided and the sternocleidomastoid muscle is retracted posteriorly. The carotid sheath is entered, and from this point on in the operation, sharp dissection is utilized. The facial vein is identified, ligated, and divided. Carotid artery dissection is performed with as little manipulation of the artery as possible. The vagus and the hypoglossal nerves are identified and protected. The CCA and the ECA are encircled with vessel loops. The patient is systemically heparinized (100 U/kg), and the ICA is encircled distal to the bulb plaque. After 3 minutes, a test clamp of the ECA and ICA is performed. The patient remains neurologically intact; therefore, the CCA is clamped. An arteriotomy is made in the CCA and extended up the ICA until the top of the plaque is reached. The endarterectomy is begun in the CCA. An eversion endarterectomy of the ECA is performed with good back bleeding. A nicely feathering plaque is removed from the distal ICA. All debris is removed and a synthetic patch is sewn in with fine monofilament suture. Prior to completing the patch, the ECA and ICA are back bled and the CCA is forward bled. The patch is completed. Following patch closure, an intraoperative duplex scan is performed.

▓ Intraoperative Carotid Duplex Ultrasound Scan

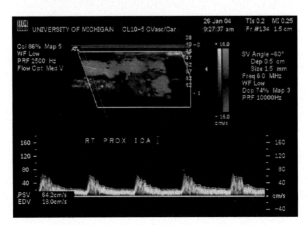

Figure 6-2

Case Continued

The incision is closed and the drapes are removed. The patient is neurologically intact and is transferred to the postanesthesia care unit where he receives an aspirin. The patient is discharged to home the next morning with a follow-up appointment in 2 weeks.

Discussion

Three large clinical studies have been performed that assess the utility of CEA in the setting of asymptomatic carotid artery disease: the Asymptomatic Carotid Atherosclerosis Study (ACAS), the Veterans Affairs Cooperative Asymptomatic Trial (VA Cooperative Study), and the Carotid Artery Stenosis with Asymptomatic Narrowing, Operation versus Aspirin (CASANOVA) studies.

The most widely quoted of these studies is the ACAS, which randomized 1,662 patients with documented carotid artery stenosis of greater than 60% without antecedent ipsilateral cerebrovascular symptoms. Patients were randomized to "best medical therapy" (aspirin) or to aspirin plus CEA. The results demonstrated a significant outcome advantage with aspirin plus CEA when compared to aspirin alone. With a mean follow-up of 2.7 years, the 5-year risk by Kaplan-Meier projection of ipsilateral stroke following CEA was significantly decreased (5.1%) compared to the medical therapy group (11%). In this study, CEA was performed by competent surgeons with a combined 3% or less perioperative morbidity and mortality rate. Men benefited substantially more than women, and experienced a significant reduction in stroke with operative therapy from 12.1% to 4.1%; women had a reduction in stroke risk from 8.7% to 7.3%. This gender difference is often attributed to a higher presurgical stroke rate in women following arteriography. All patients in the surgical arm underwent cerebral angiography, while only 38% of patients in the medical arm underwent angiography. Because evaluation by cerebral angiography is not necessary in many patients with asymptomatic carotid disease, eliminating this risk would have further reduced the stroke rate in the surgical arm from 5.1% to 3.9%. The 30-day perioperative mortality rate in this study was only 1.5%.

It is important to understand that the three aforementioned randomized trials documenting the role of CEA in asymptomatic patients with significant carotid artery stenosis were defined by greater than 60% narrowing by arteriography. These arteriographic measurements relate the size of the lumen within the bulb at the site of disease to the nondiseased distal internal carotid artery. Therefore, arteriographic results should not be confused with duplex ultrasound studies, which measure the actual amount of atherosclerotic material from the outside of the bulb compared to the remaining lumen. The described difference in technique results in an inexact correlation between duplex and angiography. This is important when trying to extrapolate study data from randomized trials to clinical practice today, because duplex ultrasound is often the only preoperative test performed in most patients prior to CEA.

Based on the three randomized clinical trials, CEA is indicated in asymptomatic patients with a carotid artery stenosis of at least 60% by arteriography or approximately 80% by carotid duplex ultrasound scan. The majority of patients with noncomplicated asymptomatic carotid stenosis can be evaluated by duplex alone and do not need to undergo cerebral angiography. Surgeons who perform CEA for asymptomatic carotid disease should perform this operation with a less than 3% perioperative morbidity and mortality.

Recommendations

The patient is seen 2 weeks postoperatively and is doing well. He is encouraged to stop smoking. A follow-up visit is planned at 3 months with a repeat carotid duplex ultrasound scan to assess the rate of ipsilateral carotid artery restenosis. It is imperative to follow the moderate contralateral left ICA stenosis because up to 85% of these patients will progress over time to develop a severe ICA stenosis requiring intervention. After the 3-month follow-up visit, yearly carotid duplex scanning is recommended.

Suggested Readings

Ailawadi G, Stanley JC, Rajagopalan S, Upchurch GR, Jr. Carotid stenosis: medical and surgical aspects. *Cardiol Clin.* 2002;20:599-609.

American Heart Association. *1998 Heart and Stroke Statistical Update.* Dallas: American Heart Association; 1997.

Carotid Artery Stenosis with Asymptomatic Narrowing, Operation Versus Aspirin (CASANOVA) Study Group. Carotid surgery versus medical therapy in asymptomatic carotid stenosis. *Stroke.* 1991;22:1129-1235.

Executive Committee for the Asymptomatic Carotid Atherosclerosis Study. Endarterectomy for asymptomatic carotid artery stenosis. *JAMA.* 1995;273:1421-1428.

Hobson RW, Weiss DG, Fields WS, et al. Efficacy of carotid endarterectomy for asymptomatic carotid stenosis. *N Engl J Med.* 1993;328:221-227.

Huston J III, James EM, Brown RD Jr, et al. Redefined duplex ultrasonographic criteria for diagnosis of carotid artery stenosis. *Mayo Clin Proc.* 2000;75:1133-1140.

Thorvaldsen P, Kuulasmaa K, Rajakangas AM, et al. Stroke trends in the WHO MONICA project. *Stroke.* 1997;28:500-506.

C. Keith Ozaki, MD, FACS

Presentation

A 64-year-old African-American man with a history of essential hypertension and smoking suffers a single 30-minute episode of transient left arm and left leg paralysis. There were no associated speech or visual symptoms, and he describes himself now as back to normal. His current medications are metoprolol and aspirin. Physical examination is remarkable only for a blood pressure of 148/87 mm Hg, and he is completely neurologically intact. Laboratory test results (including lipid panel and hemoglobin A_{1c}), electrocardiogram (ECG), and computed tomographic (CT) scan of the head are normal. Carotid duplex examination reveals a high-grade 80% to 99% proximal right internal carotid artery (ICA) stenosis and no left carotid occlusive disease.

After optimization of his beta-blocker dosage for better blood pressure control, he undergoes an uncomplicated right carotid artery endarterectomy (CEA) under general anesthesia with a shunt. Arterial closure is accomplished with an ePTFE patch. He awakes neurologically intact with a blood pressure of 160/80 mm Hg.

After 2 hours in the postanesthesia care unit, his blood pressure drifts down to 95/60 mm Hg. His pulse is 58 beats per minute (bpm), and he is asymptomatic.

Differential Diagnosis

The differential diagnosis for hypotension after CEA includes hypovolemia (especially if the patient is receiving diuretic therapy for hypertension), cardiac dysfunction, sepsis, anaphylaxis, and neurally mediated mechanisms. This last category includes not only autonomic dysfunction from stimulation of the carotid baroreceptors in the freshly endarterectomized bulb, but also the hypotension may serve as an initial sign of an intracranial event.

■ Approach

Postoperative blood pressure instability after CEA demands thorough bedside evaluation. The accuracy of the blood pressure reading should be verified. The therapeutic strategy depends on the etiology of the hypotension. If non-neural mechanisms (e.g., hypovolemia, cardiac dysfunction) are ruled out, and on examination the patient demonstrates no neurologic deficit suggestive of cerebral ischemia, then alpha agonists (e.g., phenylephrine) may be given via drip infusion to maintain perfusion to vital organs.

Case Continued

Based on this patient's low intraoperative fluid resuscitation record, early post-operative oliguria, unremarkable physical examination results, and normal ECG, intravascular volume depletion is determined to be the cause of his relatively low blood pressure. Exacerbating the hypotension is the patient's persistent bradycardia secondary to his perioperative beta-blockade. He receives one liter of lactated Ringer's solution. Immediately after receiving Ringer's solution, the patient's blood pressure returns to 140/80 mm Hg. Six hours later, his blood pressure is 184/97 mm Hg, and he remains asymptomatic.

Differential Diagnosis

If a patient is in pain or anxious after CEA, then endogenous hormonal responses can drive hypertension postoperatively. Additionally, patients may have missed doses of chronic antihypertensive medications. Other patients after CEA suffer idiopathic postoperative hypertension that stands outside of these known mechanisms.

Approach

Pain therapy is titrated to avoid oversedation, which would impair the ability to perform serial neurologic examinations. For hypertension that is not related to pain, sodium nitroprusside or nitroglycerine hold the advantage of rapid blood pressure reduction and short pharmacologic half-life (permits easy titration).

Discussion

The relatively narrow risk/benefit ratio of CEA and the systemic atherosclerosis in these often high-risk patients demand close perioperative attention to minimize complications. Periprocedural hemodynamic instability is common after CEA. Evolving information would suggest similar alterations in blood pressure and heart rate following percutaneous carotid interventions, such as angioplasty and stenting. Perioperative hypotension and hypertension have been associated with increased incidences of neurologic and cardiovascular events. There are no clearly defined criteria for an acceptable blood pressure range after CEA, and the clinician must consider the patient's baseline pressure. Although based on limited data, many clinicians would consider systolic pressures over 160 or less than 100 to be indications for intervention. Hypotension due to autonomic dysfunction usually resolves within 24 hours of CEA. Idiopathic hypertension after CEA is seen more commonly in patients with preoperative hypertension and high-grade carotid stenosis.

Case Continued

A short course of sodium nitroprusside brings the patient's blood pressure below 140 mm Hg with a pulse rate of 68 bpm. He is restarted on his chronic beta-blocker, and discharged to home on postoperative day one. However, 48 hours postoperatively, he returns to the hospital, complaining of a severe unilateral right orbital and frontal headache, for which he receives acetaminophen without relief. Four hours later he vomits, then suffers a grand mal seizure.

Differential Diagnosis

Neurologic symptoms after a CEA may be driven by extracranial etiologies such as artery-to-artery thromboemboli (platelet-rich emboli from the surface of the endarterectomized artery) or complete thrombosis of the endarterectomized artery. Postoperative neurologic complications may also originate from intracranial causes, such as hemorrhage and cerebral hyperperfusion syndrome.

■ Approach

An emergency duplex ultrasound scan confirms bilateral ICA patency. Head CT scan without contrast serves as an initial screen for intracranial bleeding. Intracranial hypodensities on CT scan may be infarctions or edema. CT scan with perfusion or magnetic resonance imaging (MRI) with diffusion-weighted images (DWI) can help distinguish between infarctions or edema. DWI is a special MRI sequence designed for the detection of cerebral infarction.

■ Head CT and Diffusion Weighted MRI Results

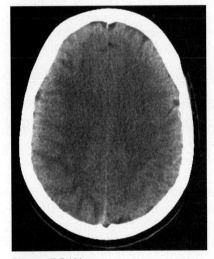
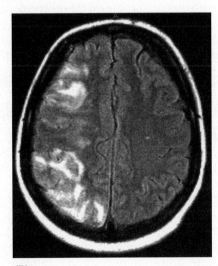
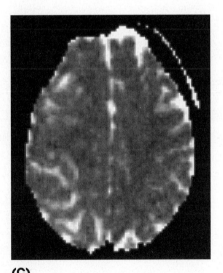

Figure 7-1(A)   (B)   (C)

CT Scan Report

Head CT scan is unremarkable (Fig. 7-1A). Images from a FLAIR (Fluid Attenuation Inversion Recovery) MRI show increased signal intensity in the middle cerebral artery distribution on the right side (see Fig. 7-1B) with no apparent restricted diffusion on the diffusion-weighted images (see Fig. 7-1C). This constellation is not consistent with acute infarction.

Case Continued

The patient partially recovers, but clinically has a dense left hemiplegia. The next day his mental status deteriorates into a coma, and his pupils are bilaterally fixed and dilated. He dies 2 hours later. At autopsy, the endarterectomy site is widely patent and without thrombus. There is a massive right hemispheric hematoma and brainstem herniation through the foramen magnum.

Discussion

After endarterectomy for a high-grade carotid stenosis, the ipsilateral brain vasculature is exposed to perfusion pressures and blood flow substantially higher than it has seen in years. It is theorized that the chronically ischemic intracranial arterioles lose the ability to autoregulate in response to sudden changes in perfusion pressure. When measured by techniques such as brain perfusion CT scan, xenon CT scan, nuclear medicine single-photon emission CT scan, or transcranial Doppler ultrasonography, up to 9% of patients develop early postoperative cerebral blood flow well above that required for metabolic needs, with flows reaching 4 times baseline. Although the majority of these patients suffer no significant clinical consequences from reperfusion, a small portion (estimated 1000 patients in the United States per year) develop severe clinical signs and symptoms from cerebral hyperperfusion syndrome.

The reported incidence of clinically apparent cerebral hyperperfusion syndrome following CEA ranges from 0.04% to 1.2%, and mortality may be as high as 36%. Cerebral hyperperfusion syndrome is not limited to the post-CEA patient. This syndrome may follow stroke, head injuries, and excision of cerebral arteriovenous malformations; it has also been described after carotid angioplasty and stenting. Clinical symptoms and signs include severe ipsilateral headache, seizures, intracranial hemorrhage, and death. Symptoms usually develop within the first 2 weeks postoperatively, with a median of about 3 days. Risk factors that have been described include high-grade carotid stenosis, preoperative and postoperative hypertension, contralateral carotid occlusions, prior cerebral infarcts, use of anticoagulant and antiplatelet agents, and recent contralateral CEA. However, identification of patients who will proceed to complications of cerebral hyperperfusion syndrome remains largely unpredictable.

The pathophysiology of this syndrome probably relates to reactive hyperemia, which leads to cerebral edema and hemorrhage. It shares physiologic features with other reactive hyperemia syndromes, such as ischemia/reperfusion of an ischemic limb, heart, or bowel.

Close monitoring of perioperative blood pressure, and intervention if indicated, is advocated to prevent cerebral hyperperfusion syndrome, even though normotensive patients have developed fatal cerebral bleeding. Intraoperative surgical techniques to reduce blood pressure instability, including minimization of surgical dissection between the origins of the internal and external carotid arteries, may avoid damage to the carotid baroreceptor nerves. Similarly, routine use of lidocaine local anesthetic at the carotid sinus (to blunt autonomic stimulation as the carotid plaque is removed and the bulb re-perfused) may block endogenous pathways that regulate blood pressure and heart rate in the early postoperative period. Because many patients stay in the hospital for only very limited time periods after routine CEA, discharge instructions must emphasize both blood pressure monitoring and control as an outpatient, and immediate medical attention for severe ipsilateral headache. In patients who exhibit early symptoms of cerebral hyperperfusion, the avoidance of antiplatelet and anticoagulant agents has also been advocated, as well as measures to avoid cerebral edema. Rarely, selected patients respond to intracranial decompressive procedures.

Suggested Readings

Ascher E, Markevich N, Schutzer RW, et al. Cerebral hyperperfusion syndrome after carotid endarterectomy: predictive factors and hemodynamic changes. *J Vasc Surg.* 2003;37:769-777.

Bernstein M, Fleming JF, Deck JH. Cerebral hyperperfusion after carotid endarterectomy: a cause of cerebral hemorrhage. *Neurosurgery.* 1984;15:50-56.

McCabe DJ, Brown MM, Clifton A. Fatal cerebral reperfusion hemorrhage after carotid stenting. *Stroke.* 1999;30:2483-2486.

Ouriel K, Shortell CK, Illig KA, et al. Intracerebral hemorrhage after carotid endarterectomy: incidence, contribution to neurologic morbidity, and predictive factors. *J Vasc Surg.* 1999;29:82-87.

Reigel MM, Hollier LH, Sundt TM Jr, et al. Cerebral hyperperfusion syndrome: a cause of neurologic dysfunction after carotid endarterectomy. *J Vasc Surg.* 1987;5:628-634.

Mohammed M. Moursi, MD, FACS

Presentation

A 65-year-old Caucasian man is 45 minutes following a right carotid endarterectomy (CEA), and is now in the recovery room. The patient underwent a CEA for a symptomatic right internal carotid stenosis measuring 86% on preoperative cerebral angiography, with the contralateral side measured as a 35% stenosis. The patient was receiving aspirin preoperatively. The operation was performed under regional anesthesia without the use of a shunt, and the carotid artery was closed with the use of a bovine pericardial patch. Initial intraoperative duplex ultrasound scan at the completion of the endarterectomy showed an intimal flap at the distal extent of the endarterectomy site requiring reopening of the artery and placement of several tacking stitches. Completion duplex ultrasound scan after this repair showed no apparent defects. The patient had no hemodynamic instability during the perioperative period and has demonstrated a normal neurologic exam until this point. Now, 45 minutes after arrival in the recovery room, the patient develops a left-sided hemiparesis involving his upper and lower extremities. In addition, he is now unable to respond to verbal commands.

Differential Diagnosis

The diagnosis with this clinical scenario is clear. This patient has signs and symptoms consistent with an acute stroke after CEA. The diagnostic dilemma involves the etiology for this stroke. The differential for the cause of an ipsilateral acute stroke after CEA includes: (1) intracerebral hemorrhage; (2) watershed infarction; (3) hypoperfusion intraoperatively or postoperatively; (4) hyperperfusion; (5) embolization of atheromatous plaque or thrombus occurring intraoperatively; (6) embolization occurring postoperatively with or without a technical defect at the endarterectomy site (embolic material could be atheromatous plaque, thrombus, or platelet aggregation); (7) thrombosis of the endarterectomy site with or without a technical defect; (8) heparin-induced thrombocytopenia; (9) kink in the artery resulting in low flow; and (10) embolization from a site other than the carotid bifurcation.

Diagnostic Tests

Given that he had a lucent period in the immediate postoperative period and had a completion duplex ultrasound scan that showed no defect, this patient would be best served by simultaneously preparing the operating room for re-exploration and obtaining a duplex scan of the carotid artery to determine patency.

■ Duplex Ultrasound Scan

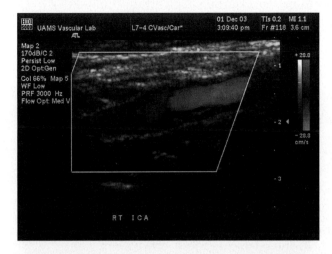

Figure 8-1A

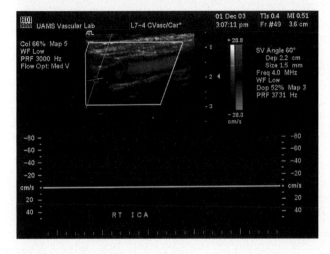

Figure 8-1B

Duplex Ultrasound Scan Report

Duplex ultrasound scan shows an acutely thrombosed internal carotid artery (Fig. 8-1*A*) with Doppler waveform signal indicating no flow (Fig. 8-1*B*).

Diagnosis and Recommendation

The patient has an acute stroke secondary to a thrombosed internal carotid artery endarterectomy site, most likely due to fibrin and platelet adhesion to the endarterectomized surface. Given the thrombosed artery and the short period of time (less than 2 hours) since the CEA, the patient needs emergent re-exploration of the carotid artery. Although the addition of a duplex scan in this situation is somewhat controversial, one of the cornerstones of diagnosis and treatment for an acute stroke after CEA is to determine patency of the artery. With a normal intraoperative duplex scan and a lucent period postoperatively, a duplex scan is recommended. In most hospital settings, this will not delay the required re-exploration, given the portability of the duplex machine and the time required to prepare an operating room. In this situation, the internal carotid artery was thrombosed and re-exploration is indicated. However, had the duplex showed a patent artery with no defects, then exploration could prove to be harmful. In that circumstance, rather than an operation, the patient would require a computed tomographic (CT) scan of the head and possible cerebral arteriography (see Discussion).

Case Continued

By the time the duplex is completed, the operating room is ready and the patient is taken for re-exploration.

Discussion

Once the carotid artery is found to be thrombosed, the patient is given systemic heparin at 100 U/kg IV bolus. In the operating room, the patient can be re-explored under the original regional anesthetic block if the time interval between cervical block and re-exploration is short and if the patient is cooperative. Otherwise, a general anesthetic is administered. The neck incision is opened and the carotid artery is exposed, and the thrombosed artery is confirmed by visual inspection and/or hand-held Doppler. In addition, any kinks or other abnormalities are identified and inspected. The common carotid and external carotid arteries are controlled with vascular clamps, and the arteriotomy is opened; note that no attempt is made to clamp the distal internal carotid artery at this time. Upon opening the artery, the thrombus is removed and the internal carotid is allowed to back bleed into the field; if no back bleeding is observed and there appears to be thrombus extending distally, an embolectomy catheter can be used to gently remove distal clot. Care must be taken to avoid creating a cavernous sinus fistula. Once the thrombus is removed, the endarterectomized surface is inspected for defects. If any defects are identified, they are repaired by either removal of residual plaque or tacking of any intimal flaps. Alternatively, upon opening the artery, platelet aggregation may be identified. Rather than frank thrombus, a defect site may be noted. This should be removed and the defect repaired.

Surgical Approach

The patient undergoes general endotracheal anesthesia, and at exploration the carotid artery is found to be thrombosed. The clot is removed from the distal internal carotid as well as at the endarterectomy site. No obvious defect can be identified. Therefore, an interposition saphenous vein graft is used to replace the proximal internal carotid artery. Low-molecular-weight dextran is started as a continuous drip. Intraoperative duplex ultrasound scan shows a widely patent interposition graft with no defects.

Case Continued

The patient awakes from anesthesia with a mild left upper extremity weakness as his only neurologic defect. The patient is placed on an additional antiplatelet agent along with aspirin. Physical and occupational therapy are initiated, and the patient is eventually sent home to continue his rehabilitation.

▓ Surgical Approach Continued

In this particular case, since no technical defect was observed, the presumed etiology of the thrombosis is fibrin and platelet aggregation and adhesion to the endarterectomized surface. If this is not replaced, the chance of re-thrombosis is high. Therefore, a portion of greater saphenous vein was harvested from the thigh and used as an interposition graft. It is important to initiate pharmacologic antiplatelet therapy both intraoperatively with dextran as well as postoperatively, with another oral antiplatelet agent in addition to aspirin. The neck is then closed; the patient is awakened from the general anesthetic, and is continued on dextran for 24 hours and antiplatelet agents. Care is taken to avoid hypotension in the postoperative period.

Discussion

Carotid endarterectomy has proven to be a beneficial and safe treatment for the prevention of strokes in patients with symptomatic and asymptomatic extracranial carotid artery atherosclerotic occlusive disease. However, acute stroke in the immediate postoperative period remains a recognized complication with centers of excellence reporting a stroke rate in the 1% to 2% range. The management of postoperative stroke after CEA is an area where controversies still exist. Disagreement remains regarding the severity of the deficit that requires re-operation. Areas of disagreement include the role of noninvasive testing and angiography and the window of opportunity when re-operation should be accomplished. To maximize the treatment benefit with this complication, it is imperative to have a clear, well-planned algorithm for a patient who sustains a stroke after CEA, so that action can be undertaken in a timely fashion once the diagnosis is made. This involves a clear understanding of the potential etiological mechanisms of this complication.

Not all strokes after CEA are the same; the timing of the stroke plays a large role in determining etiology and potential treatment options. A patient who undergoes a CEA under general anesthesia and awakens with a neurologic deficit has most likely sustained either an intraoperative hypoperfusion injury or an embolic event secondary to clamping or shunt placement. Upon awakening and identification of the deficit, an interrogation of the carotid artery with duplex to assess patency should be undertaken because the artery will most likely be found to be without thrombus. Re-operation is not recommended due to the potential of extending the ischemic area in the brain with any further clamping of the carotid artery. For the most part, these are locally uncorrectable situations with the likelihood of recovery being poor. Thus, the patient should be considered for a head CT scan and possibly cerebral arteriography with lytic salvage of any thrombosed intracerebral vessels.

In another scenario, a patient may develop a neurologic deficit 1 to 2 days after undergoing a CEA. In this situation, the probable cause is a cerebral hemorrhage and/or edema secondary to hyperperfusion. Hyperperfusion occurs in patients after repair of a high-grade carotid artery stenosis, or in patients who present with severe bilateral stenosis. The symptom complex consists of hypertension, headache, and seizures. Diagnosis is accomplished by CT scan or magnetic resonance imaging (MRI) of the head. Treatment is blood pressure and seizure control.

More commonly, a patient has a lucent period of normal neurologic status after CEA, whether performed under general or regional anesthesia, followed by a stroke in the immediate postoperative period. The most common cause of such a post-CEA stroke is related to a technical error that results in postoperative thromboembolism. In a comprehensive review of 3062 consecutive CEA procedures, Riles et al. found that symptomatic carotid artery thrombosis occurred in 0.8% of patients, but caused 40% of the postoperative strokes. These defects could serve as a point of platelet aggregation and/or initiate thrombus formation. Thromboembolism can occur secondary to errors or defect at the operative site such as an intimal flap, irregularities at the suture lines, a kink caused by elongation after endarterectomy, intramural hematoma, constricting suture line, clamp injury, ledges at the end of the endarterectomy, and/or a rough endarterectomy surface. The cause of the neurologic deficit is usually not due to obstruction of blood flow or ischemia by the thrombus, but rather from embolization of thrombus material as it was forming within the artery, or from embolization originating at the distal extent of the thrombus. In addition, these defects can be the nidus for platelet aggregation, which can also embolize distally. These technical errors can and should be corrected; there is conclusive evidence to recommend decisive surgical management in the treatment of post-CEA thrombosis. If corrected in a timely fashion (1 to 2 hours), there is a high likelihood of significant neurologic recovery. Repair after this time, however, may convert a bland ischemic infarction into a hemorrhagic infarct. Any decision not to perform a re-operation in the presence of a delayed neurologic event should be supported by a study demonstrating a patent internal carotid artery without technical defects. If uncorrected, embolic events could continue to occur, or the artery may progress to complete thrombosis and occlusion. If already thrombosed, restoration of flow to limit ischemia may prove to be beneficial. Rockman et al. showed that in 18 re-explorations performed for an early neurologic deficit, 83.3% clearly showed signs of thrombus or platelet aggregation. Nearly 70% of patients re-explored had either complete resolution of or significant improvement in the deficit that had been present. No patient's condition was worsened by re-exploration.

At exploration, thrombus is removed from the endarterectomy site as well as the distal internal carotid artery, if present; at this stage, some authors suggest an intraoperative cerebral angiogram for identification of intracerebral thromboemboli. If these are identified, catheter-directed intraoperative lytic therapy could be initiated with good results. After these steps, the cause of the thrombosis must be sought. When these defects are identified, a decision must be made regarding the type of repair; if an obvious defect is detected and appears to be the cause of the thromboembolism, or platelet aggregation, local repair with tacking sutures or removal of residual plaque is indicated. If no obvious defect is detected, and platelet fibrin deposition is the presumed etiology, consideration must be given to replacing the proximal internal carotid artery with an interposition saphenous vein graft. In either situation, postoperative antiplatelet therapy with high-molecular-weight dextran and/or another oral antiplatelet agent is recommended.

Suggested Readings

Comerota AJ, Eze AR. Intraoperative high-dose regional urokinase infusion for cerebrovascular occlusion after carotid endarterectomy. *J Vasc Surg*. 1996;24:1008-1016.

Hertzer NR. Postoperative management and complications following carotid endarterectomy. In: Rutherford RB, ed. *Vascular Surgery*. Vol 2. 5th ed. Philadelphia: WB Saunders; 2000:1881-1906.

Paty PS, Darling RC, Cordero JA, et al. Carotid artery bypass in acute postendarterectomy thrombosis. *Am J Surg*. 1996;172:181-183.

Radak D, Popovic AD, Radicevic S, et al. Immediate reoperation for perioperative stroke after 2250 carotid endarterectomies: differences between intraoperative and early postoperative stroke. *J Vasc Surg*. 1999;30:245-251.

Riles TS, Imparato AM, Jacobowitz GR, et al. The cause of perioperative stroke after carotid endarterectomy. *J Vasc Surg*. 1994;19:206-216.

Rockman CB, Jacobowitz GR, Lamparello PJ, et al. Immediate reexploration for the perioperative neurological event after carotid endarterectomy: is it worthwhile? *J Vasc Surg*. 2000;32:1062-1070.

Raul J. Guzman, MD, and Matthew A. Corriere, MD

Presentation

A 61-year-old man with a history of bilateral carotid endarterectomies (CEAs), hypertension, and coronary artery disease presents to your office for follow-up. His most recent CEA was performed on the left side 6 months ago. The right CEA was performed 2 years ago. He remains asymptomatic. Physical examination is notable for a left-sided cervical bruit. You request a carotid duplex study.

Carotid Duplex Ultrasound Scan Report

Right common carotid artery (CCA): occluded.
Right internal carotid artery (ICA): occluded.
Left common carotid artery velocities: 78/29 cm/sec (1% to 15% stenosis).
Left internal carotid artery velocities: 546/278 cm/sec (80% to 99% stenosis).

Differential Diagnosis

Recurrent carotid stenosis (RCS) has an incidence of 4% to 16% in patients evaluated with serial Doppler ultrasound studies following CEA. A stenosis identified within the immediate postoperative period is defined as *residual stenosis* and represents incomplete endarterectomy rather than RCS. Myointimal hyperplasia is usually discovered in patients experiencing recurrence within the first 3 postoperative years, whereas late RCS is more often due to recurrent atherosclerosis.

In symptomatic patients, the differential diagnosis for stroke or transient ischemic attack (TIA) symptoms following carotid endarterectomy includes recurrent carotid stenosis, new-onset atrial fibrillation (or other cardiac sources of embolic disease), vasculitis, and lacunar infarction.

Discussion

A new cervical bruit that develops in an asymptomatic patient after CEA should be evaluated by duplex ultrasound for recurrent carotid stenosis. Patients undergoing CEA should have routine follow-up with duplex ultrasonography. Patients without significant hemodynamic abnormality on initial duplex during the first 6 postoperative months should have the study repeated in 6 months, and thereafter on a yearly basis. Studies demonstrating stenosis greater than 50% should be repeated every 6 months, or sooner if symptoms occur. As many as 50% of patients undergoing reoperation for RCS have an asymptomatic, high-grade lesion that was discovered through duplex ultrasound screening. Patch angioplasty closure of the arteriotomy at the time of primary CEA has been shown to reduce the risk of developing RCS.

Case Continued

The patient is scheduled for arteriography to further evaluate the ICA stenosis noted on duplex.

Arteriogram

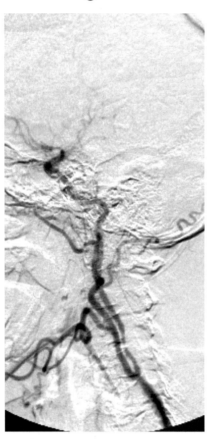

Figure 9-1 Left carotid arteriogram, preoperative.

Arteriogram Report

Left CCA: 30% stenosis located at the origin, which is smooth in appearance.
Left ICA: 80% restenosis 2 cm in length.
Right CCA: occluded.
Right ICA: occluded.

Diagnosis and Recommendation

Recurrent carotid stenosis (RCS), asymptomatic, with contralateral ICA occlusion. This patient is offered a redo left CEA with patch angioplasty. Complications that are discussed with the patient include stroke, myocardial infarction, cranial nerve injury, bleeding, infection, and death.

Discussion

The severity of the stenosis, interval since CEA, medical condition of the patient, status of the contralateral carotid, and presence or absence of symptoms are the key considerations when contemplating operative versus medical management of RCS. Asymptomatic, low-grade, or intermediate-grade lesions may be managed with antiplatelet therapy and followed up with serial duplex studies. The smooth luminal surface associated with myointimal hyperplasia is thought to pose a lower relative risk for embolization than atherosclerotic lesions, and regression of early recurrent lesions has been reported; some authors therefore recommend a higher threshold for operative management of asymptomatic lesions occurring within the first 2 postoperative years. Operative management should be considered for high-grade (greater than 80%) or symptomatic lesions, especially those associated with contralateral carotid occlusion. Preoperative angiography plays an essential role in characterizing the recurrent stenotic lesion, and this anatomic data must be considered in combination with the history and comorbid conditions of the individual patient when selecting the best method of intervention.

Redo CEA with patch angioplasty is the most commonly employed operative intervention for RCS. Small artery size, female sex, continued tobacco abuse, and hyperlipidemia are other identified risk factors for RCS that have been demonstrated less consistently. Although most reported combined stroke-mortality rates for redo CEA approximate those for primary CEA (3% to 5%), it is commonly accepted that redo CEA carries a higher risk for cranial nerve injury (7% to 20%). Repeat dissection frequently necessitates longer operative time, and should therefore be accompanied by routine use of interoperative shunting. Patch angioplasty should be the method of arteriotomy closure whenever possible to reduce the risk for further recurrence.

Carotid angioplasty and stenting has been increasingly employed as a therapeutic modality for early RCS, where myointimal hyperplasia is the most common pathologic finding. Angioplasty and stenting is often performed under local anesthesia with little or no sedation, making it an alternative for patients whose operative risk is thought to be too great for general anesthesia. Bradycardia during balloon inflation and femoral pseudoaneurysm formation are potential complications unique to angioplasty and stenting. However, this procedure carries no risk for cranial nerve injury, and therefore may be a more appropriate option for patients with a history of cranial nerve injury, neck irradiation, radical neck dissection, permanent tracheostomy, limited cervical spine mobility, or other conditions that might predispose to an extraordinarily difficult dissection. Although some centers have suggested short-term death and morbidity rates for carotid angioplasty and stenting that are comparable to redo CEA or carotid reconstruction, the long-term durability of this procedure remains unknown. Traditionally, angioplasty and stenting has not been employed for late RCS, where recurrent atherosclerotic disease is the most common etiology, or for lesions with ulceration, free-floating thrombus, or tortuous arterial anatomy. It remains to be seen whether the emergence of carotid protection devices will expand the application of endovascular management to include these lesions with greater risk for embolic complications. At present, carotid angioplasty and stenting should be considered for patients with early RCS whose risk for redo CEA or other open repair is unacceptably high.

▮ Operative Approach

Redo CEA or carotid reconstruction should be performed through a vertical incision parallel to the anterior sternocleidomastoid, in an approach similar to that employed for primary CEA. Dissection is carried directly through the plane of scar tissue from the previous operation, with lateral reflection of the sternocleidomastoid. Patch angioplasty should be combined with redo endarterectomy whenever possible, and temporary intraoperative shunting should be employed routinely. If redo CEA with patch angioplasty is not possible, several other options exist. Carotid reconstruction with synthetic or saphenous vein graft has been performed in up to 50% of patients undergoing RCS operation in some series, while patch angioplasty alone has been reported with good results in patients with myointimal hyperplasia where endarterectomy is not possible.

Carotid stenting should be performed under local anesthesia; intravenous sedation is infrequently required and should be minimized because it may interfere with intraoperative neurologic assessment. Femoral or direct CCA puncture (in the case of aortoiliac occlusive disease) may be used for access. Balloon inflation during angioplasty is sometimes associated with symptomatic bradycardia, warranting placement or immediate availability of a transvenous pacemaker device during the procedure.

Surgical Approach

The patient is taken to the operating room, where general anesthesia is established and an incision through his existing scar is made and extended cephalad. After lateral reflection of the sternocleidomastoid and internal jugular vein, the common carotid is exposed inferiorly and circumferential control is established. The distal ICA is dissected and redo endarterectomy with polytetrafluoroethylene patch angioplasty is performed. Intraoperative Doppler ultrasound at the conclusion of the procedure is without evidence of residual stenosis. A percutaneous drain is placed at the conclusion of the procedure through a separate stab incision.

Case Continued

The patient is discharged from the hospital on the first postoperative day on aspirin antiplatelet therapy. Postoperative carotid duplex performed one month later shows no evidence of restenosis.

Suggested Readings

Aburahma AF, Bates MC, Stone PA, Wulu JT. Comparative study of operative treatment and percutaneous transluminal angioplasty/stenting for recurrent carotid disease. *J Vasc Surg.* 2001;34:831-838.

Bowser AN, Bandyk DF, Evans A, et al. Outcome of carotid stent-assisted angioplasty versus open surgical repair of recurrent carotid stenosis. *J Vasc Surg.* 2003;38:432-438.

Healy DA, Zierler RE, Nicholls SC, et al. Long-term follow-up and clinical outcome of carotid restenosis. *J Vasc Surg.* 1989;10:662-668; discussion 668-669.

Hertzer NR. Postoperative management and complications following carotid endarterectomy. In: Rutherford R, ed. *Vascular Surgery.* 5th ed. Philadelphia: WB Saunders; 2000:1895-1898.

Hill BB, Olcott CT, Dalman RL, Harris EJ Jr, Zarins CK. Reoperation for carotid stenosis is as safe as primary carotid endarterectomy. *J Vasc Surg.* 1999;30:26-35.

Hobson RW 2nd, Goldstein JE, Jamil Z, et al. Carotid restenosis: operative and endovascular management. *J Vasc Surg.* 1999;29:228-235; discussion 235-238.

Moore WS, Kempczinski RF, Nelson JJ, Toole JF. Recurrent carotid stenosis: results of the asymptomatic carotid atherosclerosis study. *Stroke.* 1998;29:2018-2025.

O'Hara PJ, Hertzer NR, Karafa MT, Mascha EJ, Krajewski LP, Beven EG. Reoperation for recurrent carotid stenosis: early results and late outcome in 199 patients. *J Vasc Surg.* 2001;34:5-12.

Ohki T, Veith FJ, Grenell S, et al. Initial experience with cerebral protection devices to prevent embolization during carotid artery stenting. *J Vasc Surg.* 2002;36:1175-1185.

Ricotta JJ, O'Brien-Irr MS. Conservative management of residual and recurrent lesions after carotid endarterectomy: long-term results. *J Vasc Surg.* 1997;26:963-972.

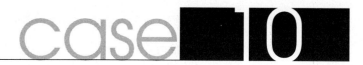

Sean P. Roddy, MD, R. Clement Darling III, MD, and Philip S. K. Paty, MD

Presentation

An 82-year-old right-handed man with hypertension, hypercholesterolemia, history of tobacco use, and coronary artery disease presented with several episodes of amaurosis fugax. He denied other focal symptoms and had no prior stroke. On examination, he had a right carotid bruit. Neurologic examination was unremarkable. A Duplex study from 2 years ago demonstrated an occluded right internal carotid artery (ICA).

Carotid Duplex Report

Normal right common carotid artery (CCA). Occluded right ICA with severe stenosis of the right external carotid artery (ECA). Left carotid system with mild plaque in both the ECA and ICA. Vertebral arteries are patent, with antegrade flow.

Head CT Scan Report

No evidence for intracranial hemorrhage. Global atrophy with no infarct.

Differential Diagnosis

The differential diagnosis for amaurosis fugax focuses on atheroembolism from the heart to the area of brain involved. Although an atherosclerotic plaque may reside in the aortic arch and great vessels, it primarily develops at the carotid bifurcation and usually involves the ICA origin. However, in the setting of an occluded ICA, emboli may be released from the ICA stump or from disease in the ECA. Cardiac thrombus, especially in individuals with atrial fibrillation, valvular heart disease, or ascending aortic disease, has the potential for distal embolization but this is not usually associated with retinal artery events.

Recommendation

Obtain magnetic resonance versus contrast arteriography of the aortic arch and four great vessels. Perform cardiac evaluation, including transesophageal echocardiography.

▨ Arch and Four-Vessel Contrast Arteriogram

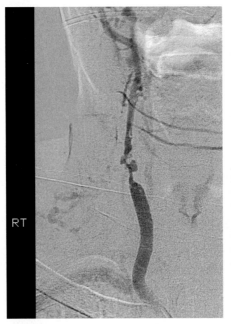 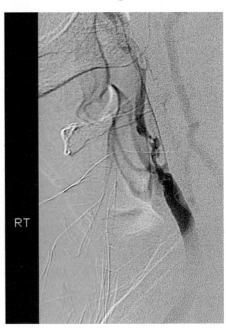

Figure 10-1   **Figure 10-2**

Arteriogram Report

Anteroposterior contrast arteriogram of the right CCA demonstrates ICA occlusion and a stenotic, irregular ECA. Straight lateral contrast arteriogram of the right carotid artery demonstrates ICA occlusion and a stenotic, irregular ECA.

▨ Transesophageal Echocardiogram

Findings: left ventricular ejection fraction of 50%, mild mitral regurgitation, normal ascending aorta, and no atrial or ventricular thrombus.

Diagnosis and Recommendation

From these data, the most likely source of emboli is the stenotic ECA. The ICA stump was occluded on Duplex evaluation 2 years ago, and is therefore less likely the etiology. Recommendation was made for ICA ligation and ECA endarterectomy with patch closure.

▨ Surgical Approach

The carotid artery is exposed through a longitudinal neck incision. The ICA is suture ligated. A CCA and ECA endarterectomy with patch closure is performed.

Case Continued

The patient underwent endarterectomy with polytetrafluoroethylene (PTFE) patch angioplasty. An ulcerated plaque was found at the origin of the ECA.

There were no neurologic sequelae and the patient has remained asymptomatic in 2-year follow-up.

Discussion

A newer alternative recently described by Naylor et al. involves an endovascular approach with a wall graft to exclude the ICA stump and proximal ECA disease. Validation of this technique by others is required.

Suggested Readings

Barnett HJM, Peerless SJ, Kaufman JGE. Stump of internal carotid artery a source for further cerebral embolic ischemia. *Stroke.* 1978;9: 448-456.

Gertler JP, Cambria RP. The role of external carotid endarterectomy in the treatment of ipsilateral internal carotid occlusion: collective review. *J Vasc Surg.* 1987;6:158-167.

Karmody AM, Shah DM, Monaco VJ, Leather RP. On surgical reconstruction of the external carotid artery. *Am J Surg.* August 1978; 136:176-180.

Kumar SM, Wang JCC, Barry MC, et al. Carotid stump syndrome: outcome from surgical management. *Eur J Vasc Endovasc Surg.* March 2001;21:214-219.

Naylor AR, Bell PR, Bolia A. Endovascular treatment of carotid stump syndrome. *J Vasc Surg.* September 2003;38:593-595.

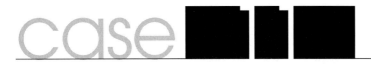

case

Ajay Gupta, MD, and Brian G. Halloran, MD

Presentation

A 65-year-old woman with diabetes mellitus, hypercholesterolemia, active tobacco abuse, and coronary artery bypass graft (CABG) surgery 5 years earlier now presents to the hospital with syncope and chest pain and is admitted for unstable angina pectoralis. Biochemically, she is diagnosed with an acute myocardial infarction. A cardiac catheterization shows occlusion of 2 saphenous vein grafts, diffuse severe stenosis of another saphenous graft, and a widely patent left internal thoracic artery graft. Additionally, 90% stenosis of the proximal left subclavian artery, severe left-ventricular systolic dysfunction with mitral regurgitation, and an ejection fraction of 20% are noted.

Differential Diagnosis

The differential diagnosis for her syncope includes stroke, vertebrobasilar insufficiency, cardiogenic shock or other hypotensive states, epileptic seizure, and metabolic disorders. The predominant cause of her myocardial infarction would be a rupture of an atherosclerotic plaque with subsequent spasm and/or intravascular thrombus formation. Other cardiac causes include ventricular hypertrophy, emboli to coronary arteries, coronary artery vasospasm, arteritis, and low-flow states, such as hypotension.

Case Continued

Upon further questioning, she denies any symptoms consistent with hemispheric stroke, transient ischemic attack (TIA), or amaurosis fugax. She has been physically inactive and denies effort-related pain in the left arm. On physical examination, her right brachial artery blood pressure is 124/80 mm Hg and the left side is 79/58 mm Hg. Heart rate is 66 beats per minute and regular; no murmurs are detected. A bruit is heard in the left side of the neck, and the bilateral carotid pulses are normal. She has easily palpable right brachial and radial pulses; however, the left arm pulses are nonpalpable.

CT Scan Report

A computed tomographic (CT) scan of the head shows mild atrophy with no evidence of ischemic or hemorrhagic stroke.

Duplex Ultrasound Scan

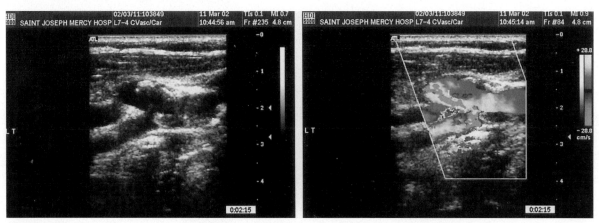

Figure 11-1

Duplex Ultrasound Scan Report

A carotid duplex ultrasound demonstrates 50% to 70% stenosis of the left internal carotid artery. Only mild stenosis less than 30% luminal narrowing is present in the right carotid artery. Vertebral flow is antegrade bilaterally.

Angiogram

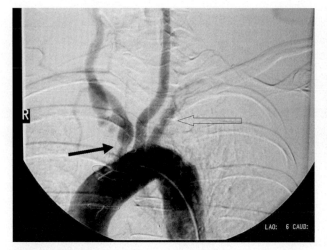

Figure 11-2

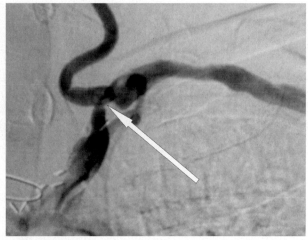

Figure 11-3

Angiogram Report

The arch aortogram (see Fig. 11-2) shows moderate stenosis of both the proximal brachiocephalic artery (*closed arrow*), as well as the proximal left subclavian artery (*open arrow*). Selective catheterization of the left subclavian artery (see Fig. 11-3) shows greater than 95% stenosis of the left subclavian artery just proximal to the takeoff of the left vertebral artery (*white arrow*).

▨ **Angiogram Contiued**

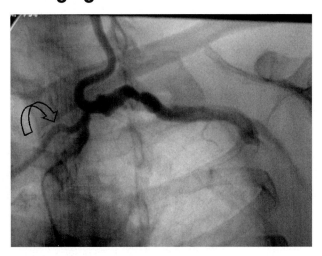

Figure 11-4

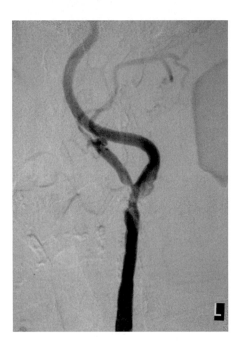

Figure 11-5

Angiogram Report

With delay in the contrast injection, the left internal thoracic artery (see Fig. 11-4) is seen coursing toward the heart (*curved arrow*). Selective injection into the left common carotid artery (see Fig. 11-5) also shows significant plaque at the carotid bifurcation compromising both the internal and external carotid arteries.

Diagnosis and Recommendation

Probable coronary subclavian steal syndrome with possible vertebrobasilar insufficiency. Although this patient's symptoms are not related to exertion of the left arm to produce a "classic" steal syndrome, she has critical stenosis of the proximal left subclavian artery, placing her myocardium at ischemic risk via the internal thoracic artery graft.

Because of her recent myocardial infarction and weakened heart, as well as moderate stenosis of the left carotid bifurcation, she is offered a left carotid-subclavian artery bypass with concomitant carotid endarterectomy under regional anesthesia.

Surgical Approach

The operation is performed through 2 incisions. A transverse incision is made superior and parallel to the clavicle. The scalene fat pad is elevated and care taken to preserve the phrenic nerve, as well as to avoid injuring the thoracic duct. After dividing the scalenus anticus from the first rib, the subclavian artery is dissected just distal to the vertebral and internal thoracic arteries.

The second incision is longitudinal along the anterior border of the sternocleidomastoid muscle for standard exposure of the carotid bifurcation. A tunnel is then bluntly developed between the two incisions underneath the sternocleidomastoid muscle, but anterior to the internal jugular vein.

Following systemic heparinization, proximal and distal control of the subclavian artery is obtained and a 6-mm expanded polytetrafluoroethylene (ePTFE) graft is anastomosed in an end-to-side fashion. After restoring flow to the subclavian artery, the carotid vessels are clamped and a standard endarterectomy is performed. The graft is then sewn to the carotid arteriotomy, also in an end-to-side manner, thus acting as a patch angioplasty for the closure.

Prior to completion of the carotid anastomosis, the vessels and graft are flushed of debris and air. Intraoperative continuous wave Doppler ultrasonography confirms adequacy of the revascularization.

Case Continued

The patient is neurologically intact, and is discharged home the next day. She is seen for an office follow-up 3 weeks later. Blood pressure in each arm is 150/82 mm Hg, and she has palpable pulses in the left brachial and radial arteries. A duplex ultrasound at that time and then 6 months later finds no restenosis of the carotid artery and a widely patent carotid-subclavian bypass. Although she has no further cardiac problems, she continues to smoke.

Discussion

Compared to the lower extremities, atherosclerotic occlusive disease of the upper extremities is relatively rare. The left subclavian artery is the most common aortic arch branch affected by atherosclerosis, which is possibly due to a more acute angle of origin of this vessel producing turbulence. Other occasional causes of stenosis or occlusion include Takayasu's arteritis, acute or chronic aortic dissection, external compression by tumor of the thoracic outlet, and embolism.

Most patients with significant arterial occlusive disease in the proximal subclavian artery are asymptomatic. This may only be recognized by a discrepancy of more than 25 mm Hg in the bilateral brachial artery systolic pressures. Because the vertebral and internal thoracic arteries are major branches of the proximal subclavian artery, they may serve as collateral vessels to provide more distal flow to the arm. Reversed flow through these arteries can be seen on duplex ultrasound or angiographically. More often than not, patients still remain asymptomatic even in the setting of this reversed flow.

Classic subclavian steal syndrome refers to neurologic symptoms of cerebral ischemia that are initiated by ipsilateral arm exercise. This may clinically manifest as posterior cerebral symptoms such as episodic syncope, diplopia, vertigo, and ataxia from a hemodynamic reduction in vertebrobasilar flow. However, even anterior and middle cerebral hemispheric symptoms can occur if concomitant carotid disease or inadequate collaterals from the circle of Willis are present.

Coronary subclavian steal syndrome (CSSS) refers to reversed flow from an *in situ* internal thoracic-coronary bypass, thereby producing symptoms of cardiac ischemia. Even more rare than vertebral subclavian steal syndrome, CSSS has only been reported on the left side of the body. Early onset of symptoms within 4 months of CABG is usually due to a preexisting hemodynamically significant lesion of the subclavian artery. Late onset disease, such as reported here, is often due to atherosclerotic disease of the proximal subclavian artery. The approach to therapy for subclavian steal syndromes varies with the clinical setting. Risk factor modification (smoking cessation and control of hypertension, diabetes, and hyperlipidemia) is essential. Patients are also educated about preventing injury and reducing exercise of the affected arm. Invasive treatment of subclavian steal syndromes is necessary for patients with symptoms such as stroke or TIA, vertebrobasilar insufficiency, myocardial ischemia, incapacitating arm claudication, or limb ischemia at rest.

When indicated, the treatment of choice is percutaneous transluminal angioplasty (PTA) and/or stent placement of the subclavian lesion. Although PTA/stent can be effective in restoring stenotic vessels to normal diameter or even re-establishing a lumen to occluded segments, this intervention is contraindicated when the subclavian lesion is too close to the origin of the vertebral (or internal thoracic) artery, as was the case in our patient. The long-term efficacy of percutaneous treatment in the subclavian vessel has not been fully established. Extra-anatomic revascularization is the most frequent form of surgical correction. Direct endarterectomy of the subclavian artery should be abandoned due to the fragility of the vessel. A carotid-subclavian bypass is generally performed with ePTFE conduit, because this prosthetic material has a reported better patency rate than saphenous vein graft (likely due to fewer problems with kinking). A carotid endarterectomy should be done simultaneously for hemodynamically significant stenosis of the carotid bifurcation. Overall patency of 95% at one year and 73% at 5 years has been reported for carotid-subclavian bypass. Alternative revascularization options include axillary-axillary artery bypass, and transposition of the subclavian artery onto the side of the carotid artery.

Suggested Readings

Gray WA, et al. Head or heart? *N Engl J Med.* 1999; 341:1458-1462.

Lee SR, et al. Simultaneous coronary-subclavian and vertebral-subclavian steal syndrome. *Circ J.* 2003;67:464-466.

McIntyre KE, et al. Subclavian steal syndrome. Available at: http://www.emedicine.com. Accessed October 24, 2003.

Ouriel K, et al. *Atlas of Vascular Surgery: Operative Procedures.* Philadelphia: WB Saunders; 1998: 214-217.

Paty PSK, et al. Surgical treatment of coronary subclavian steal syndrome with carotid subclavian bypass. *Ann Vasc Surg.* 2003;17: 22-26.

Michael J. Naylor, MD, and Mark Iafrati, MD

Presentation

A 59-year-old man complains of bilateral arm pain, numbness, tingling, and difficulty using both arms. He has numerous medical problems, including peripheral vascular disease. His recent medical history is significant for implantation of an iliac artery stent. Past medical history includes coronary artery disease, chronic obstructive pulmonary disease, and resection of a bladder tumor. He has been a heavy smoker for much of his life. Interestingly, he denies any history of stroke, transient ischemic attack, or amaurosis fugax. On physical examination, blood pressure in the right arm is 70/42 mm Hg, and in the left arm is 72/45 mm Hg. He has no palpable arm pulses. The brachial, ulnar, and radial pulses are obtained using a handheld Doppler probe.

Differential Diagnosis

The differential diagnosis of bilateral arm pain, numbness, and tingling includes neurologic-stroke (TIA), degenerative joint or musculoskeletal disease, atypical chest pain from a cardiac origin, and vascular-ischemic claudication from supra-aortic occlusive disease.

CT Scan Report

A CT scan of the head revealed no evidence of a stroke.

▓ Coronary Angiogram With Arch Arteriogram

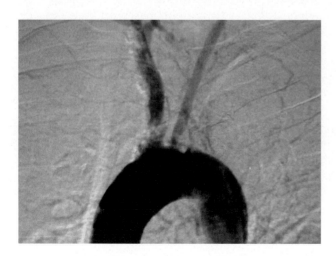

Figure 12-1

Angiogram Results

Severe aortic arch atherosclerosis with 80% stenosis of the innominate artery is noted. The right subclavian artery is occluded distal to the vertebral artery. There is moderate stenosis of the origin of the right vertebral artery. Bilateral carotid bifurcation disease is identified, as well as stenosis of the right internal carotid artery. The left subclavian artery is occluded. Also seen is critical stenosis of multiple coronary arteries, including the left anterior descending, the diagonal, and the right coronary artery.

Diagnosis and Recommendation

Significant brachiocephalic occlusion/stenosis of the innominate artery, the right and left subclavian artery, and right internal carotid artery. In addition, there is 3-vessel coronary disease. You plan a 3-vessel coronary artery bypass grafting and brachiocephalic reconstruction through a median sternotomy.

Discussion

Reconstruction of the innominate artery was first described in the early 1950s. Wylie and DeBakey then described large series in the subsequent two decades. Most of these series included atherosclerotic disease of the brachiocephalic, subclavian, and carotid arteries grouped together. Several recent reports detail surgical techniques specifically pertaining to the innominate artery.

The 3 general categories of surgical treatment for innominate artery atherosclerosis include endarterectomy, extra-anatomical bypass (cervical repair), and transthoracic bypass. The goal of innominate artery reconstruction is primarily to provide increased perfusion to the brain.

The majority of patients in the most series have undergone a transthoracic approach via a median sternotomy. In a large series by Kieffer, 135 (91%) of the 148 patients had a median sternotomy, and the majority (78%) had a bypass graft originating from the ascending aorta. Endarterectomy was performed in 22%, often using Wylie's technique, which involves clamping the transverse aortic arch. Others had an open endarterectomy of the arch and supra-aortic vessels on cardiopulmonary bypass. The remainder had endarterectomy using the cervical approach. The authors noted that a significant number of patients had innominate artery reconstruction combined with carotid endarterectomy and coronary artery bypass grafting.

Another series by Berguer advocates treating patients based on their individual cardiopulmonary risk and the anatomic location of the atherosclerotic lesion. Patients with significant cardiopulmonary risk or a history of mediastinal operation are preferentially treated with cervical operations. Cervical or extra-anatomic procedures include axillo-axillary bypass, carotid-carotid bypass, and a crossover graft such as left subclavian to right carotid bypass. Also in this category is carotid or subclavian transposition. In contrast, the transthoracic technique is preferred for complex arch reconstructions.

With regard to cervical repairs, prosthetic grafts have been shown to be superior to vein grafts. This is perhaps because of a near perfect size match, and the fact that the vein graft can be compressed during neck motion. An interesting technical note is that a crossover bypass graft can be placed in the retroesophageal space, which shortens the graft length significantly and is less apparent to the patient in the subcutaneous tissues of the neck.

Transthoracic repair of innominate artery atherosclerotic lesions can be performed with an endarterectomy or bypass procedure. The technique of endarterectomy includes clamping the aortic arch near the origin of the innominate while avoiding the left common carotid artery. It is often difficult to terminate the endarterectomy at the aortic wall, and tacking sutures often are needed. This technique is most appropriate for focal, isolated innominate lesions, which are uncommon. Transthoracic repair begins with a sternotomy and can include neck incision or clavicular incisions, depending on the lesion complex. Some have advocated a mini or partial upper sternotomy. The proximal end of a Teflon or Dacron graft is anastomosed to the aorta using a side-biting clamp on the transverse arch. The distal component of the bypass graft can then be anastomosed end to end to the innominate artery with oversewing of the proximal stump. Alternatively, an end-to-side anastomosis can be performed above the area of narrowing or occlusion. Most often, multiple distal vessels need inflow. The important technical note is that one should generally not utilize bifurcated grafts. Instead, additional side arms should be attached to the primary graft. This eliminates the problem of the complex bifurcated grafts taking up too much space within the closed mediastinal space, leading to possible graft compression. However, in selected cases where space permits, bifurcated grafts can occasionally be used with excellent outcome.

Operative mortality following surgical repair of the innominate artery for occlusive disease ranges from 3% to 20%, depending on the series. However, recent reports have mortality less than 5% for a large group of patients. The most frequent complication after either type of repair is myocardial infarction, followed by stroke. Other morbidity includes major postoperative bleeding, infection, and graft thrombosis. Ten-year overall survival of these patients approximates 50%, which is similar to the 10-year survival after many other vascular procedures; most patients succumb to their underlying coronary artery disease. Overall primary patency reported by Berguer et al. is 82% for cervical repairs and 88% for transthoracic repairs.

▌ Surgical Approach

A standard right neck incision is made and the right carotid artery is exposed. Attention is then turned to the sternotomy and the coronary bypass grafting. After coronary revascularization, a large side-biting clamp is applied to the ascending aorta, so as not to interfere with the saphenous vein bypasses (Fig. 12-2). An end-to-side anastomosis is performed with a 14 × 7-mm Dacron bifurcated graft using 3-0 monofilament suture in a running fashion. The short common graft trunk improves graft lie. The graft is then tunneled to the right neck. The endarterectomy is performed and the distal limb of the graft is anastomosed

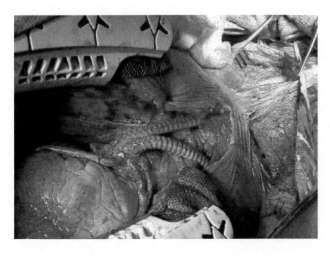

Figure 12-2 Surgical exposure via a median sternotomy with a bifurcated ascending aorta to bilateral carotid artery bypass.

circumferentially to the arteriotomy, through which the endarterectomy is performed using 6-0 monofilament suture.

Next, the left common carotid artery is exposed through a transverse cervical incision 2 cm above the clavicle. The area of the left common carotid artery, which was by palpation disease free, is then prepared. After proximal and distal control is obtained, a longitudinal arteriotomy is performed, and the anastomosis is created between the left limb of the graft and the left common carotid, using 5-0 monofilament suture in a running manner. After completion of the brachiocephalic reconstruction, the graft is covered with bovine pericardium, as well as the native pericardium, and the chest is closed.

Case Continued

The patient recovers promptly and is discharged in excellent condition on the fourth postoperative day.

Recommendation

Future plans for this patient include extra-anatomic bypass of his carotid to subclavian on both sides in a sequential manner. This will address his bilateral subclavian stenoses, which are symptomatic.

Discussion

Percutaneous transluminal angioplasty (PTA) with stenting is an important alternative to surgical reconstruction of the aortic arch. Endovascular techniques have numerous perceived advantages over open surgical methods. These include the minimal invasive nature, lack of general anesthetic, easier patient acceptance, shorter intensive care unit and inpatient stay, and perhaps lower overall cost. The primary disadvantage is reduced patency rates.

Upon review of the literature, no direct comparisons between open surgical and endovascular therapies have been performed. However, several moderate-sized case series are available. Sullivan et al. from the Cleveland Clinic reported on endovascular treatment of supra-aortic lesions using PTA and stenting in 83 patients, including 7 innominate artery lesions. In this report, all innominate lesion stents were initially successful. A list of complications in the overall series includes access related (brachial hematoma, arteriovenous fistula, brachial pseudoaneurysm, femoral pseudoaneurysm); embolic (brachial artery, left internal mammary); technical (covering the origin of the left vertebral, common carotid artery dissection, stroke); and other (acute renal failure, congestive heart failure, myocardial infarction). The authors state that it is technically easier to access the innominate from the right brachial; however, brachial interventions carry a higher risk of complication at the access site. The authors suggest "the results, both initial and late, of various treatment options for atherosclerotic lesions of the supra-aortic trunks seem to favor surgical therapy, especially when complete occlusions are included. The addition of intravascular stents seems to have improved the results of balloon angioplasty alone, but prospective, randomized comparisons are not available." In addition, they suggest that short stenoses of the innominate and subclavian arteries may be the most suitable for endovascular repair, especially in patients at high risk for open repair.

In 2002, Huttl et al. published the most extensive experience with innominate artery disease treated endovascularly using primary angioplasty without stenting. This study included 89 patients with 84 stenoses and 5 short occlusions of the innominate artery, with surgery reserved for unsuccessful PTA or long-segment innominate occlusion. The authors accessed the arterial system through the femoral artery in most cases. Notably, until 1996, stents were unavailable in Hungary, where Huttl et al. performed their study. Therefore, between 1996 and 1999, only one PTA with a stent was performed in a patient who had residual stenosis following PTA. Cumulative primary patency following primary PTA of the innominate artery in this series was 98% at 6 months and 93% between 16 and 117 months. Secondary patency was 100% at 6 months and 98% between 16 and 117 months. Of the patients in this study, 61% became symptomless, 32% improved, and 7% showed no improvement. Only one stroke occurred in 89 patients.

Despite these outstanding results, fear of cerebral embolization with the development of a major stroke seems a logical concern. During angioplasty, embolic particles can arise at virtually any step of the procedure. The balloon/stent dilation appears to produce the greatest risk for embolization. Several authors have described techniques to decrease the risk of cerebral embolization. The list includes antiplatelet medications (aspirin, ticlopidine, or clopedigrel), careful atraumatic technique, patient selection, stent implantation, and cerebral protection devices. As mentioned previously, only one stent was used in the Hungarian experience without the use of cerebral protection devices. Overall, Huttl's report (as well as several earlier studies) shows a very low risk of embolization during an innominate PTA, even without cerebral protection devices. Although stenting has been shown to improve patency in most vascular beds, Huttl's long-term patency of 93% with PTA alone will be difficult to improve upon with stenting.

In contradistinction to the Cleveland Clinic experience, Huttl et al. sumarized their experience with PTA of the innominate with stronger recommendations. "In this study we have confirmed in a large series (n = 89) of innominate artery PTAs that it is a safe and effective procedure with an excellent initial success rate, without any lethal complication, with a lower complication rate than the surgical option and with similar long-term patency rate as for surgery. PTA should be the treatment of choice in cases of symptomatic innominate artery stenosis and a short occlusion (less than 1 cm in length); surgery is indicated if PTA (and/or stent insertion) is unsuccessful or in the case of long occlusion."

Endovascular therapies for lesions clearly have a role in the treatment of focal lesions and high-risk patients. As surgeons become more facile with these techniques and instrumentation is improved, endovascular therapy will likely take on a more central role in the treatment of innominate artery occlusive disease.

Suggested Readings

Berguer R, Morasch M, Kline R. Transthoracic repair of innominate and common carotid artery disease: immediate and long-term outcome for 100 consecutive surgical reconstructions. *J Vasc Surg.* 1998;27:34-42.

Brewster D, Moncure A, Darling C, Ambrosino J, Abbott W. Innominate artery lesions: problems encountered and lessons learned. *J Vasc Surg.* 1985; 2:99-112.

Cormier F, Ward A, Cormier J, Laurian C. Long-term results of aortoinnominate and aorto-carotid polytetrafluoroethylene bypass grafting for atherosclerotic lesions. *J Vasc Surg.* 1989;10:135-142.

Huttl K, Nemes B, Simonffy A, Entz L, Viktor B. Angioplasty of the innominate artery in 89

patients: experience over 19 years. *Cardiovasc Intervent Radiol.* 2002;25:109-114.

Kieffer E, Sabatier J, Koskas F, Bahnini A. Atherosclerotic innominate artery occlusive disease: early and long-term results of surgical reconstruction. *J Vasc Surg.* 1995;21:326-337.

Queral L, Criado F. The treatment of focal aortic arch branch lesions with Palmaz stents. *J Vasc Surg.* 1996;23:368-375.

Sullivan T, Gray B, Bacharach J, et al. Angioplasty and primary stenting of the subclavian, innominate, and common carotid arteries in 83 patients. *J Vasc Surg.* 1998; 28:1059-1065.

case ■ 13

Susan L. Hickenbottom, MD, and Douglas J. Quint, MD

Presentation

A 33-year-old right-handed man presents to the emergency department with a 30-minute episode of difficulty finding his words, numbness and tingling on the right side of his face and in his right arm, and mild weakness of his right hand. These symptoms came on suddenly, then gradually resolved over the next 10 to 15 minutes; he was completely back to normal within a half hour. He has no medical problems and takes no medications. He has never had an episode like this previously. He was involved in a minor motor vehicle accident (MVA) about 2 weeks earlier, in which he was a restrained passenger in a car that was rear-ended. Other than some mild neck pain and headache since the accident, he has had no other complaints and did not seek medical attention until today. On physical examination, blood pressure in the right arm is 120/64 mm Hg. Cardiac examination is normal, and no carotid bruits are auscultated. He has some mild paraspinal muscle tenderness in the neck, especially on the left. Neurologic exam is entirely normal. Blood chemistries are normal, as is a noncontrast computed tomography (CT) scan of the head (not shown).

Differential Diagnosis

The most serious cause of transient, focal neurologic symptoms is a transient ischemic attack (TIA), although the differential diagnosis for these symptoms is extensive and includes partial complex seizure, complicated migraine, demyelinating processes, and psychiatric conditions, such as panic attacks or conversion disorder. Patient history, neurologic examination, and diagnostic work-up can often help differentiate between these possibilities.

Discussion

As compared to elderly patients, in whom the etiology of stroke is most often atherosclerotic, patients under the age of 40 with suspected TIA or stroke have a much broader differential diagnosis. In addition to atherosclerosis, potential etiologies for "stroke in the young" include nonatherosclerotic large artery disease (arterial dissection, fibromuscular dysplasia, moyamoya disease, vasculitis, and other vasculopathies); cardioembolism (bacterial endocarditis, intracardiac shunt, rheumatic heart disease); hypercoaguable states (antiphospholipid antibody syndrome; sickle cell disease; disseminated intravascular coagulation; thrombotic thrombocytopenic purpura; deficiencies of protein C, protein S, or antithrombin III; factor V Leiden mutation and other gene mutations); substance abuse; migraine headache; pregnancy and puerperium-related causes; and genetic syndromes. The specific etiology of stroke in the young remains unclear (cryptogenic) in up to 40% of patients, even after extensive evaluation.

Case Continued

In this young patient with symptoms suggestive of a TIA, no traditional vascular risk factors, and history of recent MVA, suspicion for an arterial dissection as the cause of his symptoms should be high. A head and neck magnetic resonance imaging (MRI) scan and magnetic resonance arteriography (MRA) to assess the patient for possible carotid dissection is ordered.

■ Head and Neck MRI and MRA

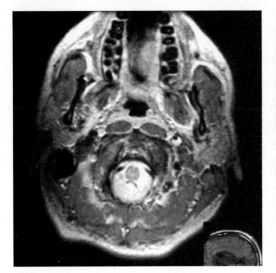

Figure 13-1

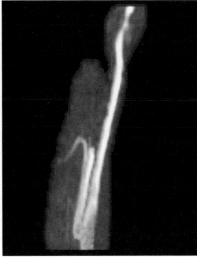

Figure 13-2

MRI and MRA Reports

An axial T1 MRI image of the neck demonstrates a left carotid artery dissection with intramural hematoma ("crescent sign"), a pathognomonic finding for dissection. An MRA for the same patient again demonstrates the left internal carotid artery (ICA) dissection with probable dissecting aneurysm ("pseudoaneurysm").

■ Conventional Angiography

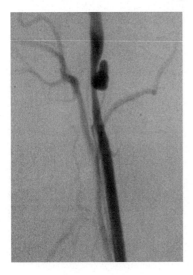

Figure 13-3

Conventional Angiography Report

Conventional angiography done a few days later in the same patient demonstrates the left ICA and clearly shows the dissecting aneurysm.

Diagnosis and Recommendations

Left extracranial internal carotid artery dissection. The patient is started on intravenous heparin and warfarin with plans to continue systemic anticoagulation (goal International Normalized Ratio [INR] 2.0 to 3.0) for 3 months; at that time, imaging studies will be repeated to evaluate the need for continued anticoagulation.

Discussion

Prior to the introduction of noninvasive neuroimaging, carotid artery dissection was thought to be a relatively rare occurrence. However, with the advent of MRI and other noninvasive modalities, dissection is being diagnosed in many patients who present with very mild or no neurologic symptoms, and is now recognized as the most common cause of stroke in those under the age of 40.

Dissections usually arise from an intimal tear, which allows blood under arterial pressure to enter the wall of the artery and form an intramural hematoma. The blood dissects through the arterial media, sometimes emerging again in the distal lumen and sometimes tracking outward into the adventitia to form a dissecting aneurysm, or pseudoaneurysm.

Most dissections are involved with some type of trauma, although it may be mild, such as turning the head while backing up a car. Even with careful history taking, a provoking traumatic incident may not be identified in up to 50% of cases, and these dissections are referred to as "spontaneous." Dissections may also be associated with various connective tissue disorders, such as Marfan's syndrome, Ehlers-Danlos type IV, fibromuscular dysplasia, and cystic medial fibrosis. However, testing for a connective tissue disorder is not indicated in typical spontaneous dissection, and is typically pursued only in patients with multiple dissections or phenotypic suggestion of an underlying disorder.

Pain in the head, neck, or face occurs at the moment of dissection in up to 80% of patients with dissection, and can be a major clue to the etiology of stroke. An ipsilateral Horner's syndrome (oculosympathetic palsy) is seen in 50% of cases, although it may be subtle and identified only if looked for carefully. Rarely, carotid artery dissection may also be accompanied by other cranial nerve palsies (IX, X, XI, and XII, with facial palsy and even ischemic optic neuropathy very rarely reported). Stroke or TIA symptoms may appear at the time of dissection, but typically occur days to weeks after dissection, and are thought to result from thromboembolic events rather than hemodynamic compromise.

Conventional angiography (CA) had long been the gold standard in the diagnosis of arterial dissections because it shows the arterial lumen and often demonstrates the irregular, tapering appearance of the luminal stenosis seen in dissection. However, pathognomonic features, such as a double lumen or intimal flap, are seen in fewer than 10% of cases. Magnetic resonance angiography (MRA) techniques are now rapidly replacing CA as the standard imaging modality to identify dissection. The resolution of MRA approaches that of CA; moreover, MRA is noninvasive, decreasing the risk of complications for the patients.

In addition, fat-suppressed MR axial images of the neck demonstrate intramural hematoma, and MRI is superior in cases where luminal stenosis or occlusion is nonspecific in appearance. CT angiography is also emerging as another noninvasive imaging modality for dissection, but may be susceptible to the same imaging pitfalls as CA and MRA when stenosis or occlusion has nonspecific appearance. Carotid ultrasound will often not show the site of dissection, but in 90% of cases an abnormal flow pattern will be seen.

Systemic anticoagulation initially with intravenous heparin and then warfarin (goal INR 2.0 to 3.0) for 3 to 6 months is usually advocated, presuming that most neurologic complications arise from distal embolization from arterial thrombosis sealing intimal tears. However, no randomized clinical trials have ever been performed in patients with carotid dissection, and thus no evidence-based data are available to support this practice. Therefore, antiplatelet therapy with aspirin or similar agents may be an acceptable alternate treatment option, especially in patients with contraindications to systemic anticoagulation and those at high risk from systemic anticoagulation. Of note, several case series have reported good results for patients with dissection treated with thrombolytic therapy within 3 hours of stroke onset, and therefore dissection in and of itself should not be considered a contraindication for thrombolytic treatment for acute ischemic stroke.

Given the current lack of data, a reasonable strategy would be to manage dissection patients with warfarin for 3 months and then repeat MRA imaging studies. If recanalization has occurred or if the vessel remains completely occluded, anticoagulation can be discontinued and the patient started on antiplatelet therapy. If luminal irregularities are seen, anticoagulation can be continued for another 3 months with re-imaging at that time. Recanalization occurs within the first weeks to months after dissection in approximately two thirds of patients.

Prognosis of stroke secondary to dissection is related to the severity of the initial ischemic event, but overall is more favorable than for other stroke syndromes. In general, prognosis for those with mildly symptomatic or asymptomatic carotid artery dissection is very good, and several studies have shown excellent or complete recovery in more than 80% of patients with angiographic signs of dissection.

Surgical Approach

Most arterial dissections heal spontaneously. Surgical or endovascular treatment should be reserved for patients who have persistent ischemic symptoms despite maximal medical therapy, or who have complications associated with enlarging pseudoaneurysms. Surgical treatment can include ligation of the artery, with or without accompanying extracranial-intracranial arterial bypass surgery. Successful endovascular stenting has been described in several case series and is likely associated with less morbidity than surgery, but long-term results of stenting are not known.

Case Continued

Your patient has been treated with warfarin for 3 months and returns for re-imaging with MRI.

▨ MRA

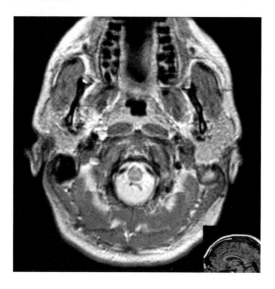

Figure 13-4

MRI Report

MRI demonstrates resolution of the dissection.

Case Continued

You discontinue the warfarin, and recommend the patient take an 81-mg aspirin daily for the next 6 months.

Suggested Readings

Derex L, Nighoghossian N, Turjman F, et al. Intravenous tPA use in acute ischemic stroke related to internal carotid artery dissection. *Neurology*. 2000;54:2159-2161.

Kasner SE, Hankins LL, Bratina P, et al. Magnetic resonance angiography demonstrates vascular healing of carotid and vertebral artery dissections. *Stroke*. 1997;28:1993-1997.

Kremer C, Mosso M, Georgiadis D, et al. Carotid dissection with permanent and transient occlusion or severe stenosis: long-term outcome. *Neurology*. 2003;60:271-275.

Saver JL, Easton JD. Dissection and trauma of cervicocerebral arteries. In: Barnett HJM, Mohr JP, Stein BM, Yatsu FM, eds. *Stroke Pathophysiology, Diagnosis, and Management*. New York: Churchill Livingstone; 1998:769-786.

Schievink WI. Spontaneous dissection of the carotid and vertebral arteries. *N Engl J Med*. 2001;344:898-906.

Zetterling M, Carlstrom C, Konrad P. Internal carotid artery dissection. *Acta Neurol Scand*. 2000;101:1-7.

case 14

Candace Y. Williams, BS, and Gilbert R. Upchurch, Jr., MD

Presentation

A 50-year-old man with a history of chronic obstructive pulmonary disease (COPD) and hypertension presents to your office after he was seen by his primary care physician for evaluation of a slowly enlarging right anterior neck mass. The patient has no other symptoms. Social history is positive for a 35 pack-year smoking history and occasional alcohol use. Family history is non-contributory. On physical examination, a soft compressible 3-cm mass is felt in the right anterior triangle of the neck. The mass can be moved laterally, but not vertically (Fontaine sign). No bruits or thrills are present. Neurologic examination is within normal limits.

Differential Diagnosis

The differential diagnosis for an anterior neck mass in an adult male includes thyroid neoplasms; multinodular goiter; metastatic head and neck cancer to cervical lymph nodes, tumors of the salivary gland, parotid gland, larynx, or parathyroid. Other considerations include lymphoma, carotid body tumor, carotid aneurysm, or lymphadenitis. Less likely diagnoses include a branchial cleft cyst, thyroglossal duct cyst, or ectopic thymus, parathyroid, or thyroid tissue. Given the patient's smoking history, cancers of the head and neck and carotid body tumors are the most likely diagnoses.

Recommendations

Based on clinical assessment and subsequent differential diagnosis, a complete blood count with differential (CBC), thyroid-stimulating hormone (TSH) level, and anterior neck ultrasound (US) scan with Doppler flow are ordered to evaluate the etiology of the mass.

Case Continued

The patient was found to have a normal CBC and TSH. The results of his US scan follow.

▨ Ultrasound Scan

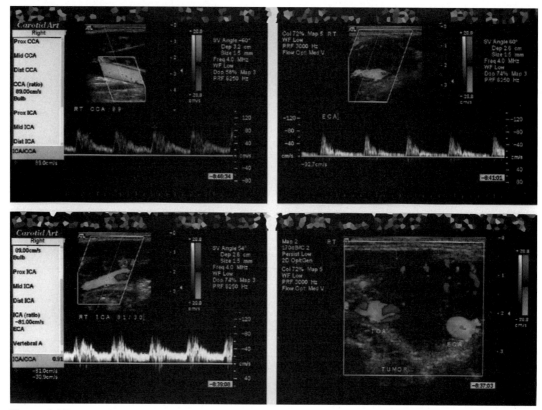

Figure 14-1

Ultrasound Scan Report

Color-flow duplex sonography reveals a 3.7 × 4.2-cm solid hypoechoic, hyper-vascular mass nestled in the right carotid bifurcation (see Fig. 14-1, *lower right panel*). Note splaying of the internal and external carotid artery. The right common carotid artery (CCA), internal carotid artery (ICA), and external carotid artery (ECA) all were found to have normal velocities, suggestive of no significant atherosclerotic disease.

Diagnosis

Carotid body tumor (CBT).

Discussion

Carotid body tumors (CBTs) are rare neoplasms constituting less than 0.5% of all tumors. They occur equally in men and women primarily in their fourth and fifth decades and are more likely to occur in the Caucasian population. Arising from the paraganglion cells of the carotid body, these tumors are adherent to the adventitia of the internal and external carotid arteries posterior to the bifurcation. CBTs are highly vascular, being supplied by the external carotid artery

(ECA) and ascending cervical artery branches. Most CBTs occur sporadically, but about 10% are familial in nature. These differ from sporadic cases by earlier occurrence, multiple tumor growths, and autosomal dominant transmission. Familial cases have been linked to germline mutations in the mitochondrial complex II succinyl dehydrogenase B, C, and D subunit genes, which have potential to induce tumorigenesis. Although the exact etiology of the sporadic tumor is unknown, examining the normal function of the carotid body may provide clues. The carotid body functions as a chemoreceptor stimulated by hypoxia, hypercapnia, and acidosis to regulate ventilation. During conditions of chronic hypoxia, such as patients living in high altitudes or those with COPD, the carotid body enlarges and histologically develops cellular hyperplasia that is similar in appearance to the benign-appearing CBTs. Because CBTs have been associated with high altitudes and COPD, chronic hypoxia is possibly an etiologic factor.

Clinically, CBTs usually present as a slowly enlarging asymptomatic anterior neck mass that typically causes no pain. Eventually, as the tumor grows larger, compression of the airway or invasion of adjacent cranial nerves leads to chronic cough, local discomfort, pain, fullness, numbness, dysphagia, and hoarseness. Other rare associated symptoms include headaches, dizziness, palpitations, tachycardia, hypertension, photophobia, and diaphoresis, which may suggest a functional, catecholamine-producing CBT. On examination, CBTs can feel soft and compressible or can be firm, smooth, and lobulated. They are mobile in the lateral direction, but cannot be moved longitudinally, a characteristic described as the Fontaine sign. Many CBTs are pulsatile, like aneurysms, but unlike aneurysms, are not expansile. In addition, in about 40% of cases, a bruit can be heard over the mass.

Laboratory studies to be performed include urine and serum catecholamine levels if patient has symptoms of a functional tumor. Helpful radiographic studies for the diagnosis and preoperative evaluation of a CBT include US, computed tomography (CT), magnetic resonance imaging (MRI), and selective carotid angiography. It is important that imaging modalities give an accurate diagnosis of CBT, because biopsy of the vascular lesion could result in disastrous hemorrhage. Traditionally, selective carotid angiography has been the gold standard for confirmation of a carotid body tumor. Angiography evaluates the entire brachiocephalic and cerebrovascular tree for occult tumors, atherosclerosis, aneurysms, and other anatomic variations as well as tumor size, extent, blood supply, and aberrant vasculature for the CBT. However, angiography is limited by potential complications including hematomas, arterial dissection, false aneurysm, distal embolization, contrast reactions, and rarely stroke. Color flow carotid artery duplex US is a noninvasive method used to visualize CBTs in the carotid bifurcation, estimate lesion size and vascularity, and screen vessels for tumor encasement or atherosclerotic disease.

Two other helpful modalities are CT and MRI. Both CT and MRI can be useful to evaluate large lesions; multiple tumors; proximal, distal, and intracranial extension of tumors; and encasement of vessels. Computed tomography has been utilized to classify CBT in terms of associated morbidity risks with resection. Known as the Shamblin classification system, it divides CBT into well-localized and easily resectable tumors (group 1); the larger tumors densely adhered to vessels and partially surrounding vessels (group 2); and the largest of tumors that encase the carotid arteries and adjacent nerves (group 3). In addition, MR angiography (MRA) may be utilized to reconstruct the vasculature and evaluate for aberrant vessels. Finally, due to the slow but relentless growth of CBTs, as well as a rare potential for metastasis, all CBTs should be resected. Observation or radiation should be considered only in the severely debilitated or very elderly patient because the natural history of the CBT is to continue to grow, invade, and compress adjacent structures, causing neurovascular injury. Once patients with CBTs have been treated, additional therapy includes screening US scans for relatives and genetic counseling.

Recommendations

Given that the patient most likely has a CBT and also has hypertension, he should be evaluated for elevated catecholamines. In addition, an MRI study is recommended to establish the Shamblin classification of resection difficulty, as well as to assess for additional lesions. An angiogram is recommended to evaluate the vasculature. Following completion of these studies, the patient should be scheduled for resection of the CBT.

Case Continued

The patient's serum and urine catecholamine levels were within normal limits. The results of the MRI and angiogram are shown below.

MRI

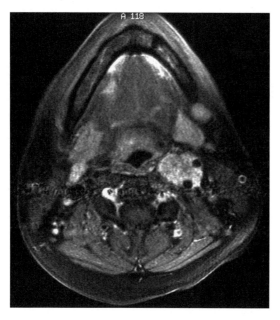

Figure 14-2

MRI Report

A 3-cm enhancing mass is noted between the ICA and ECA. The tumor appears densely adhered to the vasculature and partially surrounds the vessels. No other lesions are noted.

Selective Carotid Angiogram

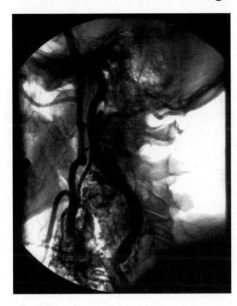

Figure 14-3

Angiogram Report

A 3-cm hypervascular mass is noted splaying the carotid bifurcation. Vascular supply appears to come from the ECA. Coil embolization was performed.

Surgical Approach

A well-planned operative approach is necessary to ensure complete tumor resection and reduce perioperative morbidity. Preoperative planning should involve a complete neurologic examination to assess tumor involvement of cranial nerves, as well as to establish a preoperative neurologic baseline for postoperative monitoring. Next, the need for preoperative embolization must be assessed. With the use of percutaneous catheters to selectively embolize the ECA with thrombogenic particles, large hypervascular tumors may be more easily resected with reduced risk of intraoperative hemorrhage in tumors greater than 5 cm. However, this procedure is associated with a risk of embolization of the occluding particles to the brain, causing stroke or transient ischemic attacks. Therefore, the benefits of this technique must be weighed against risks.

General anesthesia is preferred over local technique to allow for better airway control and less movement of the operative field. Nasotracheal intubation is also better than oral intubation because it allows for optimal exposure with greater upward displacement of the floor of the mouth during paramandibular dissection. If the CBT is known to extend high along the ICA, subluxation of the ipsilateral mandible should also be performed for better exposure. Next, cerebral monitoring should be established with the use of continuous recorded electroencephalographic (EEG) monitoring of the scalp. Preparation of a saphenous donor vein site for possible arterial reconstruction is wise. Following a standard carotid exposure, a systematic dissection should be performed to avoid injury. Bipolar electrocautery should be used for bloodless dissection along the tumor surface to avoid injury to adjacent arteries and nerves. Dissection should occur in the periadventitial plane to avoid intraoperative hemorrhage and weakening of the carotid vessels. The dissection begins with identification of the common carotid artery at the level of the omohyoid muscle and careful dissection of the vagus nerve. Next, separation of the ECA-associated hypoglossal, superior laryngeal, and marginal mandibular branch of facial nerves from the tumor should be achieved. Finally, in the last and most difficult portion of the tumor dissection, the ICA, proximal hypoglossal nerve, upper vagus nerve, pharyngeal branch of vagus nerve, spinal accessory nerve, and glossopharyngeal nerves may be associated with the tumor. In addition, if the tumor is densely adhered to the vasculature at any point, temporary (5 to 10 minutes) clamping of the common carotid artery after systemic heparinization may be performed to reduce pulsatile movement of the field. Once the tumor has been resected, but prior to closure, any enlarged ipsilateral lymph nodes should be removed. A closed suction drain may be placed.

Case Continued

The patient underwent complete resection of a CBT. He was monitored overnight in the surgical intensive care unit and was then transferred to the general care floor. The patient experienced no difficulty breathing or swallowing; the neck drain produced minimal serous fluid and was removed after 24 hours. Prior to discharge from the hospital on postoperative day 3, on neurologic examination, the patient demonstrated tongue deviation to the right side.

Discussion

The patient is most likely experiencing postoperative deficit in the hypoglossal nerve. This is often temporary and occurs in 20% of patients, along with deficits in the marginal mandibular nerves. Permanent deficits occur in 4% of patients and are related to tumors that arise in the vagus nerve. The risk of cranial nerve deficits increases dramatically with tumor volumes greater than 7 cm^3. Other complications associated with CBT resection include postoperative stroke in 2% to 4% of patients, but perioperative mortality is less than 2%. In addition, in patients who undergo bilateral CBT excision, carotid body dysfunction after operation can lead to severe hypertension, labile blood pressure, palpitations, headaches, and hypoventilation during the first 24 to 72 hours after operation.

Case Continued

The patient was observed for 5 years following the procedure with interval CT studies and both neurologic and neck examinations. Family members were also screened with US and neck examination, and did not have CBT or other paraganglion tumors. The patient's hypoglossal cranial nerve deficit resolved within 6 months. The patient has remained disease free with no recurrence or metastasis of the CBT.

Discussion

Resection can be complete and curative in 95% of patients with CBT. Metastases occur in less than 5% of cases, and usually in the setting of incomplete resection. When present, metastases may be present in the local lymph nodes, liver, lung, and bone, and occasionally the brain. Recurrences occur in 5% to 10% of patients and are often associated with familial cases.

Suggested Readings

Basal BE, Myers EN. Etiopathogenesis and clinical presentation of carotid body tumors. *Microsc Res Tech*. 2002;59:256-261.

Hallett JW, Nora JD, Hollier LH, et al. Trends in neurovascular complications of surgical management for carotid body and cervical paragangliomas: a fifty-year experience with 153 tumors. *J Vasc Surg*. 1988;7:284-291.

La Muraglia GM, Fabian RL, Brewster DC, et al. The current surgical management of carotid body paragangliomas. *J Vasc Surg*. 1992;15:1035-1045.

Moore WS, Colburn MD. Carotid body tumors. In: Fischer JE, Baker RJ, eds. *Mastery of Surgery*. 4th ed. Philadelphia: Lippincott Williams & Wilkins; 2001:397-408.

Nora JD, Hallett JW, O'Brien PC, et al. Surgical resection of carotid body tumors: long-term survival, recurrence, and metastasis. *Mayo Clin Proc*. 1998;63:348-352.

Wang SJ, Wang MB, Barauskas TM, Calcaterra TC. Surgical management of carotid body tumors. *Otolaryngol Head Neck Surg*. 2000;123:202-206.

Westerband A, Hunter GC, Cintora I, et al. Current trends in the detection and management of carotid body tumors. *J Vasc Surg*. 1998;28:84-93.

case 15

Jonathan D. Gates, MD

Presentation

A 51-year-old man presents to the emergency department with a stab wound sustained 12 hours ago to the right side of the neck. He describes a tender mass around the area. He admits to mild clumsiness and numbness in his left hand and left leg, but denies stridor, vocal changes, or other neurologic symptoms. Examination reveals that he has a 2-cm stab wound to zone II of the right neck just anterior to the sternocleidomastoid muscle with a moderate-sized firm hematoma without crepitus (Fig. 15-1). He is not in respiratory distress and has no stridor on auscultation of the neck. There is no active bleeding from the neck wound. The patient is hemodynamically stable and has no other wounds. Neurologic examination reveals a mild left pronator drift and mild decrease to light touch sensation in the left arm and left leg. A computed tomography (CT) scan of the neck is recommended.

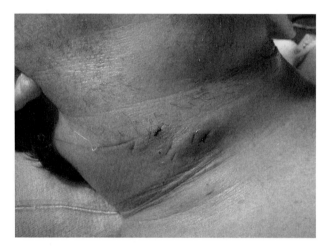

Figure 15-1 Stab wound to neck.

■ CT Scan of Neck With IV Contrast

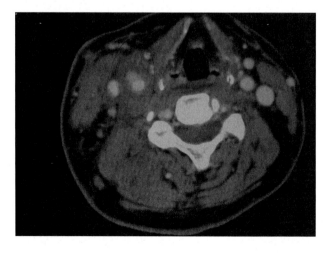

Figure 15-2

CT Scan Report

An extraluminal collection of intravenous contrast at the distal common carotid artery is apparent.

Differential Diagnosis and Recommendations

This man has suffered a single stab wound to the neck with a moderate hematoma. It is essential to determine the depth of this wound through local exploration. If the wound is small, it must be explored with the use of local anesthesia to enlarge the wound to determine whether or not it has penetrated the platysma. If the wound is large and gaping, often elevation of the tissue is sufficient to determine that the platysma has been violated.

There is no evidence for airway compromise. Airway control is paramount with penetrating wounds to the neck. If there is any question as to the adequacy of the airway, he should be intubated. Clinically, he has evidence for a mild right hemispheric stroke. At the top of the differential, one must consider penetrating injury to the carotid artery with an acute mild stroke. Given that the patient is hemodynamically stable and the wound has penetrated deep to the platysma, further work-up is essential and appropriate. If this patient was actively bleeding from the stab wound, he should be moved to the operating room emergently without further work-up.

Preoperative CT scan of the head is essential in this stable patient to delineate the absence or presence of the suspected stroke and determine whether there is a hemorrhagic component. CT scan with intravenous contrast has become an excellent screening test for arterial injuries in some locations, the neck being one of them. Magnetic resonance angiography (MRA) may aid in the diagnosis of arterial injury, but requires the patient be moved to the MR suite, rendering the patient less available for ongoing care. Angiography supplies additional information and is perhaps more sensitive with respect to minor intimal injury. Angiography also introduces the option for a percutaneous solution to the problem. At this time, angiography remains the gold standard for evaluation of carotid artery injury. In addition, given the depth of the injury, one must consider injury to the digestive tract.

■ CT Scan of Head

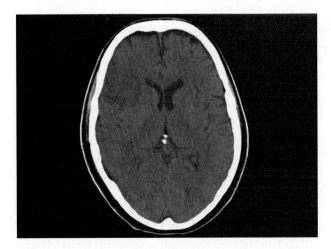

Figure 15-3

CT Scan Report

CT scan of the head without intravenous contrast shows a 3-cm nonhemorrhagic stroke in the right frontal lobe anterior to the motor strip.

Arteriogram

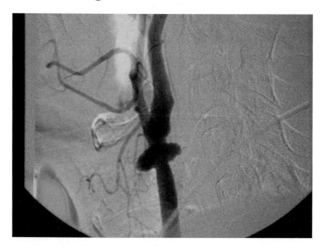

Figure 15-4

Arteriogram Report

Arteriogram of the right carotid artery demonstrates a pseudoaneurysm of the common carotid artery with patent internal and external carotid arteries.

Three-Dimensional CT Scan

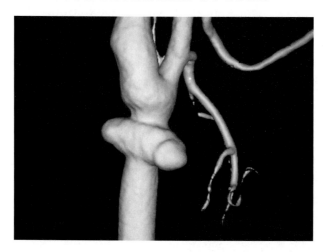

Figure 15-5

CT Scan Report

Computerized 3-dimensional reconstruction of the right common carotid artery injury shows a pseudoaneurysm of the common carotid artery.

Diagnosis

This patient has a contained pseudoaneurysm of the right common carotid artery with a moderate-sized bland infarct of the right frontal lobe. This is a symptomatic lesion in that a platelet plug must have formed at the site of the injury or from turbulence within the pseudoaneurysm and embolized to the brain. The carotid lesion also may rupture, given the tenuous nature of the wall of the pseudoaneurysm. Clinically, the stroke is relatively small. Radiographically, it is of moderate size and hemorrhagic transformation is of concern.

Recommendation

Percutaneous solutions to arterial pathology have evolved from the early embolization of end vessels, to stent placement, and currently covered stents for larger defects in the wall of arteries. A covered stent could be placed across the lesion with occlusion of the external carotid artery to maintain flow through the internal carotid artery. The risk of doing so includes the need for anticoagulation during and after the procedure.

Continuous intravenous heparin anticoagulation for the duration of the procedure is less of a concern than the need for Integrilin after the procedure to ensure stent patency. This may represent a risk of transformation of the bland infarct into a hemorrhagic infarct. In addition, CT scan of the neck raises the issue of a foreign body. If the wound were to become infected, the presence of the covered stent may complicate the situation. One must continue with the evaluation of the aerodigestive tract using bronchoscopy and either endoscopy or barium swallow.

Surgical options include exploration and repair of the arterial injury with intravenous heparin intraoperatively and aspirin perioperatively. The risk of intracranial bleeding would be less, and this would allow definitive evaluation of the airway and digestive tract as well with possible removal of the foreign body.

Surgical Approach

Electroencephalography (EEG) monitors are placed on the head, and the patient undergoes general anesthesia. The right side of the neck is carefully positioned for maximal exposure and the neck, chest, and lower leg are prepped and draped so as to provide exposure for a potential median sternotomy for proximal control, if needed. In addition, leg preparation allows harvesting of the saphenous vein for patch angioplasty. In vascular trauma, one must anticipate the unexpected, and be prepared for proximal and distal control of the common carotid and internal/external carotid arteries, respectively, so as to minimize hemorrhage prior to addressing the pseudoaneurysm. If the common carotid injury is lower in the neck, then proximal control may indeed require a median sternotomy to control the innominate artery. Once the arteries are exposed and controlled, heparin is given and the skin and overlying tissues superficial to the pseudoaneurysm are opened (Fig. 15-6). The pertinent arteries are clamped and the pseudoaneurysm exposed to define the injury. The majority of the anterior wall of the common carotid artery is disrupted. The artery is opened longitudinally from the common carotid artery into the internal carotid artery. If EEG were not available, one could measure the stump pressure of the internal carotid artery or place an indwelling shunt. Once the back wall is repaired with 6-0 Prolene, a saphenous vein patch is secured to the arteriotomy in usual fashion and the shunt, if used, is removed prior to completion of the anastomosis (Fig. 15-7). A Jackson-Pratt drain is placed through a separate incision, and the platysma and skin are closed separately. The patient's neurologic exam is evaluated upon emergence from anesthesia. Follow-up CT scan of the head demonstrated no further exacerbation of the previously noted frontal stroke.

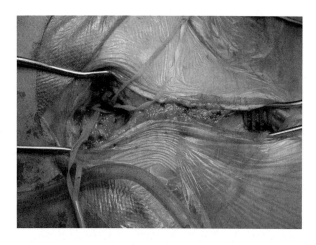

Figure 15-6 Intraoperative photograph demonstrates proximal and distal control of the common carotid and the internal/external carotid arteries.

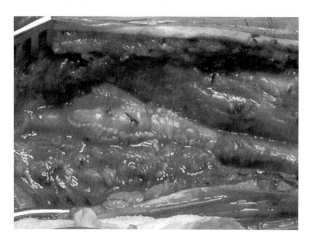

Figure 15-7 Intraoperative photograph demonstrates the carotid artery after repair of the posterior common carotid artery and patch angioplasty of the anterior portion with restoration of flow.

Discussion

Penetrating wounds deep to the platysma require further investigation. This may take the form of mandatory exploration or a more selective approach. When choosing the selective approach, it is understood that an aggressive work-up should ensue, looking for injury to the aerodigestive tract or vascular system. Once the diagnosis of the arterial injury is made, it should be addressed through a surgical or endovascular approach.

Suggested Readings

Kuehne JP, Weaver FA, Papaicolaou G, et al. Penetrating trauma of the internal carotid artery. *Arch Surg.* 1996;131:942-948.

Liekweg WG, Greenfield LJ. Management of penetrating carotid injury. *Ann Surgery.* 1978; 188:587-592.

Parodi JC, Schonholtz C, Ferreira LM, Bergen J. Endovascular stent graft for treatment of arterial injuries. *Ann Vasc Surg.* 1999;13: 121-129.

Ramadan F, Rutledge R, Oller D, et al. Carotid artery trauma: a review of contemporary trauma center experiences. *J Vasc Surg.* 1995; 21:46-56.

Thal ER, Snyder WH, Hays RJ, Perry MO. Management of carotid artery injuries. *Surgery.* 1974;76:955-962.

Vladimir Grigoryants, MD, Narasimham L. Dasika, MD,
and Gilbert R. Upchurch, Jr., MD

Presentation

A 30-year-old woman is referred for evaluation of dysphagia. Her past medical history is unremarkable. Physical examination reveals no abnormalities. Her upper extremity blood pressures are equal in the right and left arms. Endoscopy reveals a posterior extraluminal mass, which appears pulsatile. Esophageal manometry reveals no significant peristaltic abnormalities. Previous diagnostic testing includes an upper gastrointestinal barium swallow, which was ordered by her primary care physician.

■ Barium Swallow

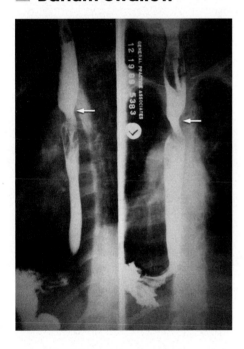

Figure 16-1

Barium Swallow Report

Barium swallow shows a posterior proximal filling defect in the proximal esophagus (*arrow*), suggestive of extrinsic compression.

Differential Diagnosis

The differential diagnosis of dysphagia is broad and includes malignant and benign tumors of the esophagus, esophageal strictures and webs, diverticula, peristaltic disorders of the esophagus, and extrinsic compression of the esophagus by adjacent masses or vascular structures. Given the finding suggestive of extrinsic compression and its pulsatile nature, an aberrant right subclavian artery should be suspected in this patient.

Discussion

An aberrant right subclavian artery is present in up to 1% of the population. This condition results from an embryologic defect involving the right fourth aortic arch and right dorsal aorta. In this condition, the right subclavian artery comes off the aorta distal to the left subclavian artery. The aberrant artery crosses the midline posterior to the esophagus in 80% of patients, anterior to the esophagus in 15%, and anterior to the trachea in 5%. Symptoms occur in a minority of patients and include dysphagia (dysphagia lusoria), cough, shortness of breath, right arm claudication when stenosis of the artery is present, embolism to the right upper extremity or the brain when the artery is aneurysmal, and severe upper gastrointestinal hemorrhage resulting from arterial erosion into the esophagus. Compressive symptoms may or may not be associated with the presence of an aneurysm.

Angiography is the gold standard for diagnosing this rare vascular anomaly. A chest x-ray may demonstrate a mediastinal mass when an aneurysm of the aberrant right subclavian artery is present. A contrast study of the esophagus frequently shows a posterior filling defect. Endoscopy allows exclusion of mucosal abnormalities and may detect pulsatility of the compressed area of the esophagus. Computed tomographic (CT) imaging shows the relationship of the artery relative to the surrounding mediastinal structures, provides information about the diameter of the artery, and shows whether an aneurysm is present. A combination of CT scanning and angiography is necessary for adequate preoperative planning.

Recommendation

CT scan of the chest and angiography.

■ Chest CT and Chest Angiography

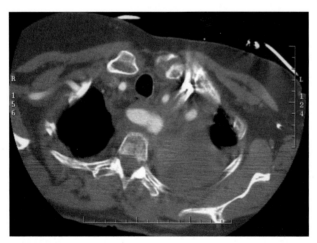

Figure 16-2

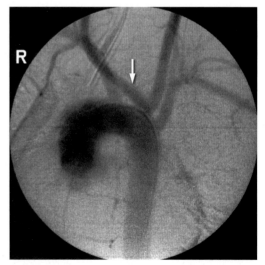

Figure 16-3

Chest CT and Chest Angiography Reports

Chest CT scan illustrates the retroesophageal course of an aberrant right subclavian artery. (This CT scan was obtained from a patient who also had a ruptured aortic arch aneurysm.) Aortic arch angiography demonstrates the aberrant right subclavian artery arising from the proximal descending thoracic aorta (*arrow*).

Diagnosis and Recommendation

Aberrant right subclavian artery compressing the esophagus. Transposition of the aberrant right subclavian artery to the right common carotid artery is planned. The patient is informed that resolution of dysphagia is expected after this procedure. Risks of the operation are discussed with the patient. Risks include stroke, bleeding, infection, thrombosis, embolism, and death, as well as injury to the esophagus, trachea, recurrent laryngeal nerves, right brachial plexus, and phrenic nerve.

Surgical Approach

Transposition of the right subclavian artery to the right common carotid artery, with transection of the right subclavian artery to the left of the esophagus, is a good option when no aneurysm is present. This procedure is performed through a right supraclavicular incision. The aberrant subclavian artery is identified and mobilized behind the esophagus to allow transection to the left of the esophagus. The distal end of the artery is anastomosed to the right common carotid artery in an end-to-side fashion. The proximal stump is oversewn. The surgeon should be aware that the ipsilateral vertebral artery may arise from the common carotid artery and the thoracic duct may enter the right jugulosubclavian junction in these patients. Injury to the thoracic duct may result in a persistent chylothorax. Other described techniques include use of a prosthetic interposition graft for a carotid to subclavian bypass or an aortosubclavian bypass.

Case Continued

The aberrant right subclavian artery is approached and mobilized through the right supraclavicular incision. The patient undergoes transposition of the right subclavian artery to the right common carotid artery. The proximal stump appears broad based. No anomalies of the vertebral artery or the thoracic duct are found.

Discussion

The origin of the artery frequently appears broad based, known as Kommerell's diverticulum. Resection of the stump of the artery, or the Kommerell's diverticulum, is not necessary.

Case Continued

The procedure is concluded uneventfully. An intraoperative duplex scan shows a patent anastomosis. The patient is extubated and is transferred to the recovery room. Neurovascular examination in the operating room and recovery room reveals a strong right radial pulse and no evidence of distal embolism or neurologic deficits. The patient reports resolution of dysphagia at 4 weeks postoperatively.

Discussion

Aneurysms of the aberrant right subclavian artery are usually found at or near the origin of the artery and are believed to result from degeneration of the Kommerell's diverticulum. Even if asymptomatic, these aneurysms should be treated because they present a high risk of rupture (up to 50%), thrombosis, or embolism. The aneurysms are best approached and excised through a left posterolateral thoracotomy. Stent graft repair of an aneurysm of the aberrant right subclavian artery has been described. Patients with aneurysms of the aberrant right subclavian artery should be screened for abdominal aortic aneurysms because their concomitant presence is common.

Suggested Readings

Austin EH, Wolf WG. Aneurysm of aberrant subclavian artery with a review of the literature. *J Vasc Surg.* 1985;2:571-577.

Davidian M, Kee ST, Kato N, et al. Aneurysm of an aberrant right subclavian artery: treatment with PTFE covered stengraft. *J Vasc Surg.* 1998;28:335-339.

Gomez MR, Bernatz PE, Forth RJ. Arteriosclerotic aneurysm of an aberrant right subclavian artery. *Dis Chest.* 1968;54:63-66.

Kieffer E, Bahnini A, Fabien K. Aberrant subclavian artery: surgical treatment in thirty-three adult patients. *J Vasc Surg.* 1994;19:100-111.

Rosa P, Gillespie DL, Goff JM, et al. Aberrant right subclavian artery syndrome: a case of chronic cough. *J Vasc Surg.* 2003;37:1318-1321.

Stone WM, Brewster DC, Moncure AC. Aberrant right subclavian artery: varied presentation and management option. *J Vasc Surg.* 1990;11:812-817.

James M. Estes, MD

Presentation

A 65-year-old woman presents with a 3-week history of intermittent right-hand numbness, dizziness, and flashing colored lights in both eyes. The episodes last a few minutes and then completely subside. Her past medical history includes type 2 diabetes mellitus, hypertension, hyperlipidemia, and hypothyroidism. Physical examination reveals bilateral cervical bruits and a markedly diminished brachial pulse in the left arm.

Differential Diagnosis

This patient's neurologic symptoms are consistent with both vertebrobasilar and hemispheric ischemia. The flashing colored lights suggest involvement of the visual cortex in the posterior cerebrum, and the dizziness may be related to ischemia of other hindbrain structures. These symptoms are indicative of symptomatic subclavian steal.

The hand and arm numbness suggest ischemia in the distribution of the middle cerebral artery, implicating a critical carotid lesion as a cause, most likely from a hemodynamic and not embolic etiology in this case. An angiogram is ordered.

▪ Aortogram

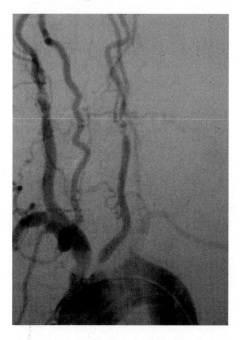

Figure 17-1

Arch Aortogram Report

Arch aortogram demonstrates severe proximal left subclavian artery disease, a moderately severe lesion in the proximal left common carotid artery, and severe left carotid bifurcation disease.

▨ Arteriography

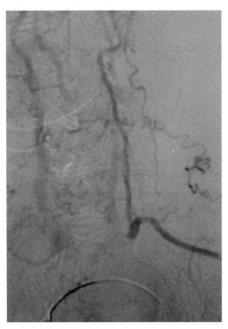

Figure 17-2

Arteriography Report

Delayed arteriographic sequence demonstrates retrograde left vertebral flow and filling of the subclavian artery distal to the occlusive lesion.

Discussion

Evidence of subclavian artery disease is occasionally discovered on routine physical examination in older patients with atherosclerotic risk factors. However, surgical reconstruction for this condition is unusual and represents less than 5% of arterial cases in busy academic centers, according to Evans and Shepard. The Joint Study of Extracranial Arterial Occlusion found associated subclavian or innominate disease in 17% of patients undergoing arteriography for suspected carotid disease, according to Fields and Lemak.

The true incidence of severe subclavian artery disease is largely unknown, because most patients are asymptomatic and are discovered incidentally after finding either decreased pulses or a lower blood pressure in one arm. Symptoms generally reflect vertebrobasilar insufficiency and typically include dizziness, visual symptoms, and syncope. The classic symptoms of vertebrobasilar insufficiency induced by arm exercise are uncommon, and in most cases the symptoms are provoked by orthostatic maneuvers or excessive dosages of antihypertensives. Arm claudication may be present as well, but overt arm or hand ischemia is uncommon and usually indicates multilevel occlusive disease. The presence of hemispheric or ocular symptoms suggests coexisting carotid bifurcation disease.

A subset of patients who have had coronary bypass using the left internal mammary artery (LIMA) may present with recurrent angina due to hemodynamically limiting subclavian disease proximal to the LIMA origin. This condition is referred to as *coronary steal syndrome.*

The initial diagnostic test of choice is duplex ultrasound imaging. Often the subclavian lesion can be identified, and the presence of retrograde vertebral flow confirms the diagnosis of subclavian steal. It is also crucial to assess the carotid bifurcations, because significant coexisting disease is common and should be considered for treatment. Arteriography is the definitive test because it provides a more detailed view of overall anatomy, particularly the origins of the great vessels, which are difficult to identify with ultrasonography.

Treatment is indicated when symptoms of cerebral or arm ischemia are present. The most common surgical procedures performed are the carotid-subclavian bypass and subclavian-carotid transposition. Our preference is bypass using a short 8-mm polytetrafluoroethylene (PTFE) graft, because the transposition requires much more proximal dissection of the subclavian artery, putting the thoracic duct, phrenic nerve, and vertebral artery at greater risk of injury.

If the ipsilateral carotid artery is not suitable for inflow, extra-anatomic configurations such as axillo-axillary, subclavian-subclavian, and even femoro-subclavian bypasses can be constructed. However, direct great vessel reconstruction is preferred in these circumstances, using a graft off the ascending aorta in patients medically fit enough to tolerate median sternotomy.

Endovascular treatment of subclavian disease has emerged as an important therapeutic option. In general, long-term patency is reduced compared with surgical reconstruction. Yet, this approach may be more desirable for patients with severe comorbidities or active myocardial ischemia from coronary steal. Results are better for focal lesions, and the available data are mixed regarding outcome following angioplasty with stenting compared with angioplasty alone.

Diagnosis and Recommendation

Symptomatic left subclavian steal and carotid atherosclerosis.

Left carotid endarterectomy, intraoperative retrograde angioplasty/stenting of the proximal left common carotid artery, carotid-to-subclavian bypass using 8-mm PTFE.

Case Continued

This patient has both a symptomatic subclavian steal and ipsilateral carotid bifurcation disease. Surgical management is complicated by the moderate focal stenosis of the left common carotid origin, which precludes its use as inflow for a carotid subclavian bypass. You elect to perform a carotid-to-subclavian bypass and carotid endarterectomy with endovascular treatment of the common carotid artery disease, because the lesion is focal and the remainder of the artery is normal. The alternatives of aorto-carotid/subclavian bypass or extra-anatomic reconstruction are less desirable for this patient because of her age.

Surgical Approach

The patient is positioned similar to carotid endarterectomy, with the neck extended and rotated to the right. Electroencephalographic (EEG) monitoring is employed. The steps in the procedure are planned so as to minimize cerebral ischemia and allow for shunting as needed.

The subclavian artery is dissected out through a medial supraclavicular incision. The clavicular head and a portion of the sternal head of the sternocleidomastoid muscle are divided. The phrenic nerve is gently retracted medially and the anterior scalene muscle divided, exposing the subclavian artery.

A second incision is made along the anterior border of the sternocleidomastoid muscle. The carotid artery is fully dissected out, as for carotid endarterectomy. A tunnel is made posterior to the jugular vein for the bypass, and the distal subclavian anastomosis is performed to an 8-mm externally supported PTFE graft.

Test clamping of the common carotid artery is performed, and no EEG changes are noted. An arteriotomy is made in the proximal common carotid artery and a short 9-Fr sheath is passed proximally. An 8-mm self-expanding stent is placed across the lesion, followed by an 8-mm angioplasty balloon. The stent is positioned to flare slightly into the aortic lumen. Angiography is performed.

■ Angiography

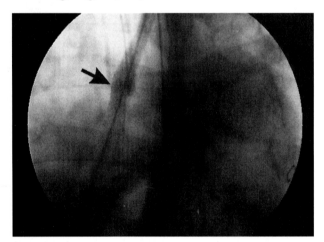

Figure 17-3

Angiography Report

Intraoperative completion arteriogram following primary stenting and touch-up angioplasty of the proximal common carotid artery reveals no residual stenosis. (*Arrow* indicates treated area of vessel.)

■ Surgical Approach Continued

The proximal anastomosis of the subclavian bypass is then constructed to the common carotid arteriotomy used for sheath access. The clamp is positioned above the anastomosis, and carotid endarterectomy is performed using a Dacron patch closure. The carotid endarterectomy is performed last to prevent stasis thrombus from forming in the endarterectomized artery during carotid stenting. The wounds are closed over a closed suction drain.

Case Continued

Postoperatively, the patient is neurologically intact and has a normal blood pressure in the left arm.

Discussion

This case illustrates the utility of combined surgical and endovascular treatment options for complex great vessel disease. Although the carotid stent could have been placed preoperatively, a retrograde intraoperative approach is chosen to protect the cerebral circulation from potential atheroembolization, because exposure of the artery is required for the endarterectomy and bypass.

The precise role of surgical versus endovascular treatment for subclavian artery occlusive disease has yet to be defined. At experienced centers, according to Cina et al., carotid-subclavian bypass can be done with a very low complication rate and 5-year patency rates of 90%, and is the procedure of choice in patients who are acceptable operative risks. Endovascular treatment is a good option for patients with severe comorbidity and high operative risk, but confers inferior long-term patency, ranging from 59% to 68% (4-year follow-up) in Schillinger's experience with 113 patients. Their data also suggests that long-term patency is better with angioplasty alone, as in-stent restenosis occurred frequently, though Henry et al. found no difference in long-term patency for stenting versus angioplasty alone.

In summary, intervention for subclavian artery occlusive disease is uncommon, but is indicated in those with symptoms of cerebral or arm ischemia, as well as cardiac ischemia in patients with LIMA bypass and proximal subclavian disease. Several therapeutic options are available, ranging from endovascular techniques to direct arch reconstruction. Appropriate therapy should be individualized based on anatomy and comorbidity to maximize long-term durability and minimize periprocedural risk.

Suggested Readings

Cina CS, Safar HA, Lagana A, et al. Subclavian carotid transposition and bypass grafting: consecutive cohort study and systematic review. *J Vasc Surg.* 2002;35:422-429.

Evans JR, Shepard AD. Upper extremity occlusive disease. In: Ernst CB, Stanley JC, eds. *Current Therapy in Vascular Surgery.* 2nd ed. Philadelphia: BC Decker; 1991:178-181.

Fields W, Lemak N. Joint study of extracranial arterial occlusion. *JAMA.* 1972;222:1139-1143.

Henry M, Amor M, Henry I, et al. Percutaneous transluminal angioplasty of the subclavian arteries. *J Endovasc Surg.* 1999;6:33-41.

Schillinger M, Haumer M, Schillinger S, et al. Risk stratification for subclavian artery angioplasty: is there an increased rate of restenosis after stent implantation? *J Endovasc Therapy.* 2001;8:550-557.

case 18

Randall Harada, MD, and Sanjay Rajagopalan, MD

Presentation

A 43-year-old man who is an assembly line worker presents with pain and discoloration in all 4 extremities. He previously noted a discolored area in the tip of his right fourth and fifth fingers approximately a month ago. He also previously noted pain in his feet bilaterally with exertion that seems to have gotten worse, with constant pain when he goes to bed at night. The pain is relieved by elevation of his feet or with the use of narcotics. He also notes redness in his feet that seems to be worse with dependency. He has not been able to work the last 2 weeks owing to these symptoms. On further questioning, he notes increasing cold intolerance in his upper and lower extremities over the last 2 years, which he attributes to his age. Past medical history is unremarkable for prior medical illness or rheumatologic disease. He smoked 2 to 3 packs of cigarettes a day for the past 25 years and cannot quit. His medications currently include Tylenol with codeine. There is no history of migraine medication or ergot-type derivative use. Although he has worked as an assembly line worker, his job does not include exposure to vibratory tools. There is no family history of premature atherosclerotic vascular disease or death. On physical examination, the patient is afebrile with normal blood pressures in the upper extremities. Examination of the right upper extremities reveals a healed ulcer measuring 2 mm on the tip of the right fourth digit. Radial pulses are normal. Allen's test reveals severe blanching of the right hand on occlusion of the radial artery, suggesting occlusion of the radial artery at the wrist. No Osler nodes or Janeway lesions are noted. Examination of the lower extremities reveals normal femoral, popliteal, and dorsalis pedis pulses, but an absent posterior tibial artery pulse on the left lower extremity. Cardiac examination is normal, with no murmurs or rubs on auscultation. No bruits are appreciated.

Differential Diagnosis

The presentation is one of an individual with advanced signs of ischemia in his lower and upper extremities, and Raynaud's symptoms. These symptoms are concerning for small vessel disease involvement in both upper and lower extremities, and are therefore suggestive of a systemic process. The presence of a healing ulcer in the upper extremity (evidence of tissue loss) rules out primary Raynaud's syndrome. The differential diagnosis includes diseases that involve small and medium vessels of both the upper and lower extremities. Consideration should also be given to infectious etiologies (eg, infective endocarditis) or intracardiac sources of embolism. Table 18-1 lists potential considerations.

Table 18-1. Etiologic considerations

Large Vessel Obstructive Disease	Small Vessel Obstructive Disease	Vasospasm

Atherosclerotic
Aneurysmal
• TOS
• Traumatic
• Kawasaki's
• FMD
Vasculitis
• Giant cell (Takayasu's)
• Radiation
	Blood dyscrasias
	• Cryoglobulins
	• Myeloproliferative disease
	• Multiple myeloma (especially
	  Waldenström's macroglobulinemia)
	Buerger's disease
	Embolic
	  • Atheromatous plaque
	  • Heart, innominate, subclavian
	  • Aneurysms
	    Innominate, subclavian,
	    axillary, brachial, ulnar
	Henoch-Schönlein purpura
	Hypercoagulable states
	  • Antiphospholipid syndrome
	  • AT-III, protein C, S deficiency
	  • Lupus anticoagulant
	  • Heparin induced thrombocytopenia
	Vasculitis
	  • Scleroderma
	  • CREST
	  • Rheumatoid arthritis
	  • Systemic lupus erythematosus
	  • Polymyositis/dermatomyositis
	  • MCTD
	Miscellaneous
	  • Frostbite
		Large vessel vasospasm
		• Cocaine
		• Ergotamine
		• Methamphetamine
		• Cannabis
		Small vessel vasospasm
		  • Primary Raynaud's
		  • Secondary Raynaud's

AT-III = anti-thrombin III; CREST = calcinosis, Raynaud's phenomenon, esophageal involvement, sclerodactyly, telangiectasia (syndrome); FMD = fibromuscular dysplasia; MCTD = mixed connective tissue disease; TOS = thoracic outlet syndrome.

Recommendation

A complete evaluation is ordered, including laboratory studies as outlined in Table 18-2 and Figure 18-1.

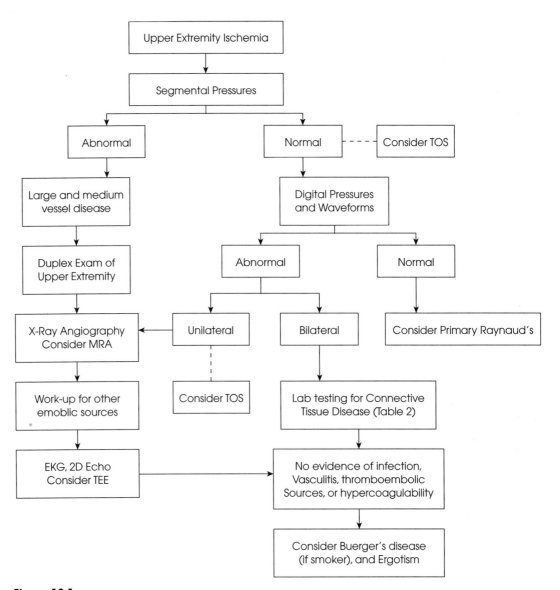

Figure 18-1

Table 18-2. Laboratory testing in patients with suspected small vessel disease

General Laboratory Testing	Laboratory Tests for Secondary Raynaud's and Obstructive Disease
Complete blood count Chemistry profile	Mini hypercoagulability screen*
Erythrocyte sedimentation rate	Antinuclear antibody and rheumatoid factor, extractable nuclear antigens
Hepatitis screen	Serum protein electrophoresis Complement levels, cryoglobulins Anticentromere antibody

*Mini hypercoagulability screen includes antiphospholipid antibodies, lupus anticoagulant, antithrombin III, protein C (activity) and protein S levels, factor V Leiden, and prothrombin gene mutation.
For large artery obstruction, one may consider performing this work-up in addition, when appropriate.

Evaluation Report

Complete blood counts, total cholesterol, lipid profile, and homocysteine levels are normal. A work-up for collagen vascular disease, hypercoagulability (including antiphospholipid antibodies, antithrombin III, protein C, and protein S activities) are normal. Erythrocyte sedimentation rate (ESR) is 15 mm/h and the level of C-reactive protein (CRP) is low.

A transthoracic echocardiogram followed by a transesophageal echocardiogram does not reveal a cardiac or aortic (ascending arch and portion of descending) source.

Segmental pressures in the upper extremity reveal symmetric diminution in pressures at the level of the fingers with a decrease in pressures in most fingers of both upper extremities (40 mm > in the right fourth and fifth digits, with damped waveforms in these digits, normal finger pressures should be > 80 mm Hg).

Upper extremity duplex testing reveals patent brachial and axillary arteries without evidence of aneurysm or occlusion.

An ankle brachial index (ABI) and segmental pressures of the lower extremity revealed an index of 0.9 in the right and 0.9 in the left. Toe brachial indices were 0.3 bilaterally with monophasic waveforms in all digits of the feet.

Recommendation

A 3-dimensional contrast-enhanced magnetic resonance arteriography (MRA) is ordered of the abdomen and lower extremities, using floating table or bolus chase technique, to rule out concomitant large-vessel disease in the pelvis and thighs.

▓ Contrast-Enhanced MRA

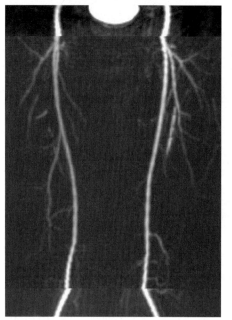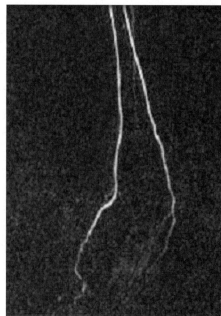

Figure 18-2   **Figure 18-3**

MRA Report

MRA of the lower extremities (Fig. 18-2) does not reveal large-vessel occlusive disease (iliac and femoral arteries were patent bilaterally). However, it does reveal an occlusion of the left posterior tibial artery at its origin with reconstitution at the ankle by collaterals. Disease of the tibioperoneal system was noted with incomplete visualization of the pedal vessels bilaterally.

Two-dimensional MRA (Fig. 18-3; digital subtraction images) of the right foot shows nonopacification of the pedal vessels.

Diagnosis

This man has systemic disease that selectively affects small and medium vessels of the upper and lower extremities. The patient also has symptoms suggestive of Raynaud's syndrome. The major etiologies to consider in this case are related to infectious, embolic, and vasculitic causes, and Buerger's disease. Specific aspects of this case that are of interest and enable one to arrive at the diagnosis are as follows. **Unilateral versus bilateral symptoms:** Bilaterality of symptoms and signs (asymptomatic involvement of digits) suggests a systemic process. **Tissue necrosis in the upper extremity** excludes primary Raynaud's, which is intermittent and shows complete resolution in between attacks. Moreover, the lower extremity symptoms in this case are suggestive of a systemic diagnosis. Digital ulcerations are most commonly caused by vasculitis (50% to 75% of all cases); half of the vasculitis cases are caused by primary Sjögren syndrome (PSS), the syndrome of calcinosis, Raynaud's phenomenon, esophageal involvement, sclerodactyly, and telangiectasia (CREST), Buerger's, and complications of atherosclerosis (eg, embolism). The presence of foot claudication suggests small-vessel involvement often seen in Buerger's disease. However, foot claudication is by no means specific for Buerger's disease (it may also be seen with thromboembolization). Smoking history is almost invariably present, and the absence of smoking should render the diagnosis of Buerger's disease suspect.

Case Continued

Based on the preponderance of evidence, diagnosis by exclusion, and the strong history of smoking, Buerger's disease is the most likely diagnosis. Atherosclerosis is unlikely in view of the distal nature of involvement and the concomitant involvement of the upper extremities.

Discussion

Buerger's disease (thromboangiitis obliterans) is a nonatherosclerotic segmental peripheral arterial disease primarily affecting small- and medium-sized vessels of the arms and legs. It is strongly associated with current or recent tobacco use and appears to be more common in countries with heavier tobacco use. The disease has a male predominance with an onset before age 45 to 50 years. Affected patients often first notice dysesthesias, Raynaud's phenomenon, and pedal claudication. Ischemic rest pain, ulceration, superficial migratory thrombophlebitis, and digital gangrene are characteristics of disease progression. Multiple limbs are nearly always involved, even in cases where clinical signs and symptoms exist in a single limb. Hence, an Allen test may be positive even in the setting of only lower extremity pain and ulceration.

Diagnosis is by exclusion, as detailed above. Commonly measured markers for inflammatory disease (ESR, CRP) and autoantibodies (antinuclear antibody, rheumatoid factor) are usually normal or negative. Proximal sources of emboli should be considered as part of the differential diagnosis and may be evaluated by transthoracic or transesophageal echocardiogram, depending on clinical suspicion. Arteriography typically shows segmental occlusive lesions of distal vessels surrounded by "corkscrew" or "tree-root" collateral vessels in the absence of atherosclerosis. These findings are suggestive, but not pathognomonic. An excisional biopsy is rarely needed, but can be obtained from amputations or acute superficial phlebitis for confirmation of the diagnosis. Histopathologic analysis of an acute phase lesion may demonstrate the classic findings of inflammatory cellular thrombi, with relative sparing of the vessel wall and preservation of the internal elastic lamina. Chronic lesions are characterized by organized thrombus and fibrosis.

The following clinical criteria are used most commonly for the diagnosis: (1) age younger than 45 years and current (or recent past) history of tobacco use; (2) presence of distal extremity ischemia (claudication, rest pain, ischemic ulcers, or gangrene) documented with noninvasive vascular testing; (3) laboratory tests to exclude autoimmune diseases, hypercoagulable states, and diabetes mellitus; (4) exclusion of a proximal source of emboli by means of echocardiography and arteriography; (5) consistent arteriographic findings in the involved and clinically noninvolved limbs.

Recommendations

Treatment approaches in Buerger's disease are outlined in Table 18-3. The initial approach in this patient should be the complete cessation of tobacco use, including smoking, chewing, or using nicotine-replacement products. A large

Table 18-3. Treatment approaches in Buerger's Disease

General Recommendations
Smoking cessation
Exercise
Avoid trauma
Treat infection with antibiotics

Local Wound Care
Lubricate skin with lanolin-based cream
Lamb's wool between toes in case of ulcers or gangrene

Medical Treatment
Control pain (narcotics may be needed)
Calcium channel blockers (amlodipine or nifedipine) if severe Raynaud's
Aspirin and/or clopidogrel
Iloprost
Spinal cord stimulator
Endoscopic sympathectomy

Surgical
Infrainguinal bypass with vein
Surgical sympathectomy

majority of patients who quit smoking will avoid disease progression and amputations. If he continues to have active disease, despite reports of tobacco cessation, testing for urinary nicotine or cotinine should be considered prior to evaluation for other less definitive medical or surgical therapies.

Pain control: In patients with intractable pain due to lower or upper extremity involvement, sympathectomy (thoracic or lumbar) using endoscopic means may be considered. Spinal cord stimulator treatment may also be of benefit in patients with recalcitrant pain.

Concomitant medical therapy: Although no prospective evidence exists regarding the benefit of therapies such as antiplatelet agents, statins, or anticoagulation in patients with Buerger's disease, antiplatelet therapy with aspirin and/or Clopidogrel is probably reasonable. In this patient, who has a severe vasospastic component, a calcium channel antagonist was initiated (Amlodipine 5 to 10 mg/day). If ongoing tissue loss occurs, treatment with prostaglandin analogues, such as Iloprost, may be beneficial. There is also anecdotal data about the use of angiogenic growth factors, such as vascular endothelial growth factor (VEGF), in these patients. Surgical revascularization is rarely performed because of poor target vessels and the diffuse distal predilection of the disease, as seen in this patient, and because of the usually good response following tobacco cessation. Vascular reconstruction may be considered in patients with bypassable disease and severe nonhealing ulcers or ischemic rest pain who have quit smoking. Infrainguinal bypass using autogenous vein grafts from a series in Japan revealed 5-year patency rates of less than 50% in patients with Buerger's disease, with patency rates directly related to smoking continuation.

Suggested Readings

Dilege S, Aksoy M, Kayabali M, Genc F, Senturk M, Baktiroglu S. Vascular reconstruction in Buerger's disease: is it feasible? *Surg Today.* 2002;32:1032-1047.

Joyce JW. Buerger's disease (thromboangiitis obliterans). *Rheum Dis Clin North Am.* 1990; 16:463-470.

Mills JL, Porter JM. Buerger's disease (thromboangiitis obliterans). *Ann Vasc Surg.* 1991;5: 570-572.

Olin JW, Young JR, Graor RA, Ruschhaupt WF, Bartholomew JR. The changing clinical spectrum of thromboangiitis obliterans (Buerger's disease). *Circulation.* 1990;82 (suppl IV):3-8.

Olin JW. Thromboangiitis obliterans (Buerger's disease). *N Engl J Med.* 2000;343:864-869.

case 19

Robert W. Thompson, MD, and Michel A. Bartoli, MD

Presentation

A 28-year-old female postal clerk presents to your office with a 3-year history of left hand, arm, and neck pain. She also experiences left upper extremity numbness and tingling that are aggravated by use, especially with the arm elevated, as well as occipital headaches. All of these complaints began several months after an automobile collision in which the patient suffered a hyperextension strain to the neck, but had no definitive cervical spine injury. Her symptoms did not improve with several courses of physical therapy, and she was advised to continue working despite the discomfort. Over the past year, she eventually found it too painful to work; her symptoms progressed to the extent that she often has difficulty sleeping at night. The patient has seen 7 different physician specialists over the past 2 years without insight into the cause of her symptoms, and she has not experienced any symptomatic improvement with a variety of different treatment modalities. Previous evaluations have included cervical spine and shoulder radiographs, computed tomography (CT) and magnetic resonance imaging (MRI) of the head and neck, and nerve conduction and electromyography studies. The results from all of these tests have been described to be normal.

Differential Diagnosis

A large number of conditions have to be considered in the initial differential diagnosis of this patient's symptoms. This list includes cervical spine arthritis, degenerative disc disease or spinal stenosis, post-traumatic cervical spine strain, and fibromyalgia of the trapezius muscles. Shoulder tendinitis or other degenerative joint conditions should also be considered, along with acromioclavicular impingement syndrome, epicondylitis, ulnar nerve (cubital tunnel) entrapment syndrome, and median nerve (carpal tunnel) compression syndrome. The diffuse and nonspecific nature of her complaints might also make it necessary to consider a peripheral neuropathy or multiple sclerosis. Given the frequent lack of objective findings on previous evaluations, it is also important to include even psychogenic causes of her symptoms and the possibility of secondary gain.

Diagnostic Testing

Most of the entities in this differential diagnosis can be evaluated either by specific elements of the physical examination or by diagnostic tests that yield positive findings in the presence of the condition. For example, the presence of degenerative cervical spine disease or disc herniation on CT scan could provide definitive evidence of these conditions. Alternatively, negative test results can also definitively exclude some of the diagnoses in question; thus, the absence of focal slowing of nerve conduction over the wrist excludes carpal tunnel syndrome. In this case, the results of previous evaluations have effectively eliminated a problem restricted to the cervical spine, the shoulder joint, or a single peripheral nerve distribution. In this situation, a diagnosis of neurogenic thoracic outlet syndrome (TOS) begins to emerge as a distinct possibility.

Neurogenic TOS is an uncommon condition often not considered until other entities have been excluded and there is ongoing symptomatic deterioration. Unfortunately, there are no single aspects of the physical examination or specific diagnostic tests that can confirm or exclude a diagnosis of neurogenic TOS. Establishing a diagnosis of neurogenic TOS thereby depends on a constellation of subjective symptoms and corroborative findings on physical examination that fit into a typical clinical pattern, combined with the exclusion of other, more common conditions.

Case Continued

Physical examination reveals a cool left hand without signs of ischemia, thromboembolism, or venous congestion. The left arm has a full range of motion with pain, numbness, and tingling induced by abduction to 180 degrees. There is tenderness upon palpation of the left supraclavicular space with reproduction of left hand symptoms. Muscle spasm is detectable along the border of the left trapezius and sternocleidomastoid muscles. There is pain and tenderness along the medial border of the scapula.

In performing the Adson test, the left radial artery pulse is not easily palpable with the arm at rest, but is present. The pulse seems to dampen with the arm positioned at 90 degrees abduction or higher. The right radial pulse is also diminished at rest, but is palpable in all arm positions. The patient is unable to complete an elevated arm stress test (EAST), due to the development of severe left arm and hand pain within 10 seconds of arm elevation. Examination of the right upper extremity is completely normal.

Diagnosis

The most probable diagnosis is neurogenic TOS. The factors supporting the diagnosis are the history of previous neck trauma and progressive symptoms affecting the entire arm and hand. The absence of a previous diagnosis despite multiple tests and evaluations is also supportive of neurogenic TOS. Although numbness and tingling in the hand are often considered worrisome symptoms, pain is the most disabling and predominant symptom for which treatment is directed. The findings on examination that support neurogenic TOS include localized muscle spasm and tenderness over the left scalene triangle, with reproduction of hand symptoms on palpation. Although positional ablation of the radial pulse suggests compression of the subclavian artery within the scalene triangle, this is a common finding even in asymptomatic individuals; the pulse examination therefore offers little insight into the nature of the symptoms. The most important finding is difficulty completing the EAST: a positive test is highly suggestive of neurogenic TOS, whereas a negative result calls the diagnosis into question.

Neurogenic TOS is thought to arise as a result of individual anatomy that predisposes to neurovascular compression, combined with some form of trauma to the scalene muscles. One of the anatomical factors associated with TOS is the presence of a congenital cervical rib. Radiographs should be inspected to evaluate whether such an anomaly is present, because it may help to solidify the diagnosis and influence management decisions.

Radiographs

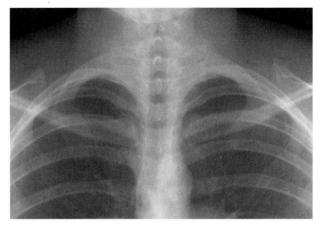

Figure 19-1

Radiology Report

Normal radiographs of the upper chest and cervical spine, with no evidence of cervical rib.

Discussion

In some cases where TOS is suspected, one must consider the possibility of subclavian artery compression resulting in formation of a post-stenotic subclavian aneurysm. These lesions are usually clinically silent until they produce thromboembolism with occlusion of distal vessels within the upper extremity. Because the clinical presentation of this complication may be subtle, the examiner must be sure that any changes in perfusion of the hand do not represent ischemia. When physical examination is equivocal or in cases where a cervical rib is present, it is useful to consider magnetic resonance (MR) arteriography as a noninvasive test by which to rule out the presence of a subclavian aneurysm.

Magnetic Resonance Arteriography

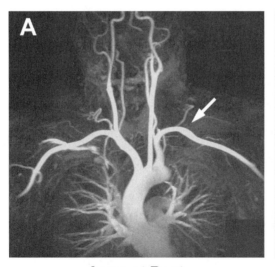
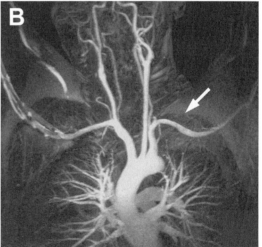

Arms at Rest
Arms Elevated

Figure 19-2

MRA Report

A contrast-enhanced MR angiogram was performed to evaluate the left subclavian artery (*arrows*) at the level of the thoracic outlet. With the arms at rest, the subclavian arteries exhibit a normal contour and luminal caliber, without signs of occlusive disease or aneurysmal dilatation (Fig. 19-2, panel *A*). With the arms elevated above the head, the subclavian arteries remain patent without signs of positional occlusion (Fig. 19-2, panel *B*). The results of this study are normal.

Recommendation

A trial of physical therapy specifically targeted toward relief of neurogenic TOS is recommended. Although the patient has not improved with previous courses of therapy, it is unlikely that these efforts were undertaken with the specific diagnosis of TOS. Because therapy for TOS differs from that given for other related conditions, this treatment should be conducted by a therapist with expertise, interest, and experience in management of TOS. Adjunctive measures should be recommended, including use of anti-inflammatory medications and muscle relaxants. Use of narcotic pain medications is not recommended.

Case Continued

After 8 weeks of physical therapy, the patient has had no change in symptoms. The therapist reports that the patient has made minimal improvement in pain-free range of motion and that her progress is limited by ongoing pain with activity.

Diagnosis and Recommendation

This patient may be considered to have neurogenic TOS refractory to conservative treatment, and surgical decompression is recommended. The patient is informed that a substantial improvement in symptoms can be expected in approximately 70% of patients following appropriate surgical treatment, but that complete long-term relief of all symptoms (ie, "cure") is unlikely. It is emphasized that ongoing physical therapy and rehabilitation will remain an essential part of her overall treatment. Potential complications of surgery are discussed, including nerve or vascular injuries and temporary dysfunction of the phrenic and/or long thoracic nerves, with an incidence in experienced hands of less than 2%.

Surgical Approach

The recommended approach to this problem is supraclavicular exploration with complete resection of the anterior and middle scalene muscles. Any associated fibrous bands and muscle anomalies within the scalene triangle are also resected. Complete brachial plexus neurolysis is added to remove any associated fibroinflammatory tissue that may be contributing to nerve irritation. It is recommended that first rib resection be included in the decompression procedure, although some specialists advocate preservation of the first rib when it appears that adequate decompression has been accomplished by scalenectomy alone. Following decompression, the brachial plexus nerve roots are surrounded with Seprafilm in an effort to reduce postoperative adhesions. A closed-suction drain is placed within the operative field, and is removed several days later. Use of the affected extremity is not restricted following operation, and physical therapy is resumed within the first 2 weeks. Liberal use of antiinflammatory agents, muscle relaxants, and narcotic pain medications is recommended during the first 4 to 6 weeks after surgery.

Discussion

The central goal of thoracic outlet decompression is to remove the structural elements of the scalene triangle that contribute to nerve root compression and irritation. This has traditionally been focused on resection of the first rib at the base of the scalene space. However, greater appreciation for the role of the anterior and middle scalene muscles has led to renewed emphasis over the past decade on the need for scalenectomy, with or without rib resection. It has also become appreciated that scar tissue surrounding the brachial plexus nerve roots may play an important role in nerve irritation.

Several different operative approaches for thoracic outlet decompression have been described, including (1) transaxillary first rib resection; (2) supraclavicular scalenectomy with or without first rib resection; and (3) posterior thoracotomy with first rib resection. Although the transaxillary approach allows removal of the first rib, it is usually not feasible to perform complete scalenectomy, brachial plexus neurolysis, or vascular reconstructions, if necessary, without repositioning the patient and using an alternate incision. In contrast, all of these procedures can be performed through the supraclavicular approach. Although there is no evidence that outcomes are different with any of these approaches, the risk of injury appears to be lowest with supraclavicular exploration. Supraclavicular exploration also has the advantage that any associated procedures involving the subclavian artery or vein can be readily performed through the same exposure.

Suggested Readings

Cheng SW, Reilly LM, Nelken NA, Ellis WV, Stoney RJ. Neurogenic thoracic outlet decompression: rationale for sparing the first rib. *Cardiovasc Surg*. 1995;3:617-624.

Hempel GK, Shutze WP, Anderson JF, Bukhari HI. 770 Consecutive supraclavicular first rib resections for thoracic outlet syndrome. *Ann Vasc Surg*. 1996;10:456-463.

Juvonen T, Satta J, Laitala P, Luukkonen K, Nissinen J. Anomalies at the thoracic outlet are frequent in the general population. *Am J Surg*. 1995;170:33-37.

Lindgren KA, Oksala I. Long-term outcome of surgery for thoracic outlet syndrome. *Am J Surg*. 1995;169:358-360.

Novak CB. Conservative management of thoracic outlet syndrome. *Semin Thorac Cardiovasc Surg*. 1996;8:201-207.

Reilly LM, Stoney RJ. Supraclavicular approach for thoracic outlet decompression. *J Vasc Surg*. 1988;8:329-334.

Sanders RJ, Jackson CG, Banchero N, Pearce WH. Scalene muscle abnormalities in traumatic thoracic outlet syndrome. *Am J Surg*. 1990;159:231-236.

Sanders RJ, Raymer S. The supraclavicular approach to scalenectomy and first rib resection: description of technique. *J Vasc Surg*. 1985;2:751-756.

Sanders RJ. *Thoracic Outlet Syndrome: A Common Sequelae of Neck Injuries*. Philadelphia: JB Lippincott; 1991.

Thompson RW, Petrinec D, Toursarkissian B. Surgical treatment of thoracic outlet compression syndromes. II. Supraclavicular exploration and vascular reconstruction. *Ann Vasc Surg*. 1997;11:442-451.

Thompson RW, Petrinec D. Surgical treatment of thoracic outlet compression syndromes. I. Diagnostic considerations and transaxillary first rib resection. *Ann Vasc Surg*. 1997;11:315-323.

Urschel HC Jr. The transaxillary approach for treatment of thoracic outlet syndromes. *Semin Thorac Cardiovasc Surg*. 1996;8:214-220.

Matthew J. Eagleton, MD

Presentation

A 27-year-old male construction worker, with a past medical history significant for a right clavicle fracture following a motor vehicle accident several years ago, presents to the emergency department with the complaint of new onset of numbness and tingling in his right arm. The paresthesias involved the forearm and hand. Associated with the paresthesias, he complains of a cold sensation in the hand, but denies any pain or weakness. The patient reports one episode similar to this in the past that resolved spontaneously. The patient works with a jackhammer and used it for the 3 days prior to presentation. He smokes one pack of cigarettes per day and has done so for 2 years. On physical examination, the right hand is cool with sluggish capillary refill. There is no palpable radial or ulnar pulse on the right, and Doppler signals over these arteries are absent. There is a palpable brachial pulse. The right clavicle has a mild bony prominence at the site of previous fracture, but there are no other masses in this region. The remainder of his physical examination is normal.

Differential Diagnosis

The differential diagnosis for upper extremity ischemia includes diseases that can be attributable to the small or large arteries of the arm. Diseases affecting the small arteries include Raynaud's syndrome, connective tissue diseases, Buerger's disease, and occupational-related disease (eg, continued work with vibratory machinery). Diseases of the large arteries of the arm include atherosclerosis, arteritis, and thromboembolism. The main sources of thromboembolism include the heart and aneurysms in the more proximal arterial tree. In this young, otherwise healthy patient who smokes, works with a jackhammer, has a history of a right clavicle fracture, and has unilateral upper extremity ischemia, the etiologies to consider most significantly are Buerger disease, an occupational-related disease due to the use of vibratory machinery, or an embolic event from a more proximal aneurysm that has formed secondary to thoracic outlet compression on the subclavian artery.

Recommendation

Based on clinical assessment and the subsequent differential diagnosis, an arch and right upper extremity arteriogram are ordered.

▨ Arteriogram

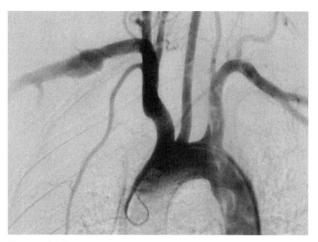

Figure 20-1

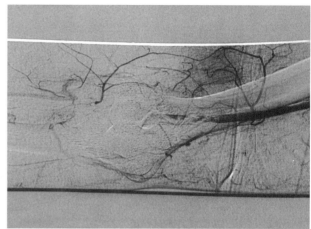

Figure 20-2

Arteriogram Report

A fusiform focal aneurysm of the right subclavian artery at the level of an old clavicular fracture is present. The remainder of the right brachiocephalic and subclavian arteries is unremarkable. There is an occluded right brachial artery just below the level of the elbow consistent with thromboembolic disease. There is reconstitution of right radial and right ulnar arteries via recurrent radial and recurrent ulnar collaterals.

Diagnosis

Acute limb ischemia due to a thromboembolism that originated in a subclavian artery aneurysm.

Discussion

Aneurysms of the subclavian and axillary arteries are rare, accounting for less than 1% of peripheral artery aneurysms. Of the brachiocephalic aneurysms, the subclavian artery aneurysm is the most common, with the right subclavian artery involved more frequently than the left. There are a variety of causes of subclavian artery aneurysms, and the most frequent etiology is variable from series to series. Thoracic outlet compression and atherosclerosis are the 2 main culprits. Thoracic outlet compression with post-stenotic dilation usually affects the distal subclavian artery and proximal axillary artery, whereas more proximal aneurysms are due to atherosclerotic degeneration. Intrathoracic aneurysms occur more frequently in men, whereas more distal lesions associated with thoracic outlet compression are seen more commonly in women. Up to 50% of patients presenting with subclavian artery aneurysms will have concomitant aneurysms in other locations, most commonly the aorta or contralateral subclavian artery.

Axillary artery aneurysms are usually caused by blunt or penetrating trauma, the most common form of which is chronic crutch use. Other traumatic events include attempts at venous cannulation in this region, fracture dislocation of the arm and shoulder, and radiation injury. A variety of other diseases are known to be associated with the development of axillary artery aneurysms including connective tissue disorders, tuberous sclerosis, sarcoidosis, and several of the arteritides.

In both subclavian and axillary artery aneurysms, patients present with symptoms in more than two thirds of the cases. Symptoms are generally related to compression of the aneurysm on adjacent structures, ischemic complications from thromboembolism, or rupture. Subclavian artery aneurysms often present with symptoms of compression that manifest as chest wall or shoulder pain, or facial swelling secondary to compression of the superior vena cava. Horner's syndrome has been described as a manifestation of a large subclavian artery aneurysm. In addition, both subclavian and axillary artery aneurysms can present with symptoms of upper extremity paresthesias secondary to the aneurysmal compression on the brachial plexus. Thromboembolism is the second most common cause of symptoms in subclavian artery aneurysms. Distal thromboembolism can occur, resulting in upper extremity ischemia. In addition, retrograde propagation of the thrombus can occur, with subsequent embolization into the cerebrovascular circulation resulting in transient ischemic attacks or stroke. Many patients experience repetitive small emboli that result in a more chronically diseased outflow bed in the arm. Following thromboembolism, patients can present with mild symptoms of ischemia due to the multiple collateral channels supplying the arm. In addition, they may present with digit ischemia that may mimic Raynaud's syndrome. Subclavian artery aneurysm and axillary artery aneurysm rupture is rare. Rupture is most often seen in patients with large aneurysms, infected aneurysms, or traumatic pseudoaneurysms.

The history and physical examination are important in distinguishing the symptoms of an axillary or subclavian artery aneurysm from other etiologies. The upper extremity ischemia, caused by distal embolization in patients with axillary and subclavian arterial aneurysms, can mimic several pathologies including Raynaud syndrome, collagen vascular disease, immunologic disorders, and hypercoaguable states. An axillary or subclavian artery aneurysm should be suspected in patients presenting with evidence of upper extremity ischemia and any symptoms suggestive of aneurysmal compression on adjacent structures. In addition, any history of clavicular, shoulder, upper extremity, or neck trauma should raise suspicion of an axillary or subclavian artery aneurysm. On physical examination, evidence of decreased perfusion in the upper extremity may exist, although given the excellent collateral blood flow to the arm, patients may not have an immediately threatened limb. A pulsatile mass may be palpable in the supraclavicular or infraclavicular regions. The most common pulsatile mass in this region, however, is often due to a tortuous common carotid artery or subclavian artery and not an aneurysm.

Depending on the patient's presentation, noninvasive studies should be performed on the upper extremity, including segmental blood pressure measurements and digital duplex waveform analysis. Laboratory testing, including complete blood counts, serum chemistries, erythrocyte sedimentation rates, antinuclear antibody, and a hypercoaguable work-up, may be helpful in discerning the etiology. Bony abnormalities, if found on physical examination, should be further evaluated with plain radiographs. A useful tool to look for the presence of a subclavian artery or axillary artery aneurysm is duplex ultrasonography. Arteriography is generally necessary, particularly when patients present with symptoms of ischemia. Arch and upper extremity arteriography are useful for preoperative planning, as it can define the location and extent of the aneurysm and its location relative to other structures, such as the common carotid artery and vertebral artery. An angiogram will also help determine the degree of disease present in the outflow vessels of the arm, which may have multiple sites of occlusion or stenosis from repeated episodes of thromboembolism.

Recommendations

Because the patient presented with acute limb ischemia, but without an immediately threatened limb, thrombolysis can be initiated in an attempt to clear the distal arterial bed of thrombus burden. Thromboemboli, however, can be resistant to thrombolysis due to the chronic nature of the clot that has embolized. In patients presenting with immediately threatened limbs, operative thromboembolectomy is indicated.

Case Continued

Thrombolytic therapy of the brachial artery restores patency of the brachial, radial, and ulnar arteries within 24 hours. At this point the patient has a warm, pink hand with palpable radial and ulnar pulses. The paresthesias resolved.

Recommendations

The diagnosis is an embolic event from the fusiform subclavian artery aneurysm. Although emboli often do not respond to thrombolytic therapy, this patient has complete resolution. The patient at this point is offered repair of the subclavian artery aneurysm and thoracic outlet decompression. The complications mentioned to him include bleeding, infection, risk of phrenic nerve and brachial plexus palsy, recurrent embolization, thrombosis of the bypass graft, and pneumothorax.

▌ Surgical Approach

The patient undergoes repair of the subclavian artery aneurysm with placement of an interposition polytetrafluorethylene (PTFE) graft. The operation is performed through a supraclavicular incision. The anterior scalene muscle is divided, taking care to avoid injury to the phrenic nerve, and the underlying artery is exposed. Proximal and distal control of the subclavian artery is obtained, and after the patient is given systemic heparin, the vessel is occluded. An endoaneurysmorrhaphy is performed to decrease the risk of brachial plexus injury, and an interposition PTFE graft is placed. The anastomoses are sewn with running monofilament suture in an end-to-end fashion. Due to the callus formed at the site of the prior clavicle fracture, the first rib is resected to decompress the thoracic outlet. The wound is closed in layers. The patient is placed on aspirin therapy in the postoperative period.

Discussion

The treatment for subclavian and axillary artery aneurysms is endoaneurysmorrhaphy with arterial replacement using either a prosthetic graft or an autogenous graft. All symptomatic aneurysms should be repaired, as well as asymptomatic aneurysms that are larger than 2 cm in diameter.

Proximal left subclavian artery aneurysms are approached through a left posterolateral thoracotomy entering the thorax through the fourth rib space. Intrathoracic right subclavian artery aneurysms are best approached through a median sternotomy. Aneurysms in these regions are generally reconstructed using prosthetic grafts. More distal subclavian artery aneurysms are approached through a supraclavicular and/or infraclavicular incision, while axillary artery aneurysms are approached through an infraclavicular incision with an extension, or separate incision, on the arm. The operative team must be ready to obtain more medial control of these vessels, through a sternotomy or thoracotomy, if the situation requires. In some cases, when there is redundant artery and a short aneurysm, resection of the aneurysm is possible with a primary end-to-end anastomosis of the remaining artery. Generally, however, an interposition graft is used. It is recommended that most aneurysms be repaired via endoaneurysmorrhaphy, as opposed to complete aneurysm resection, as this decreases the risk of injury to the adjacent brachial plexus. This is particularly true of large aneurysms. Depending on the size match and length required, the conduit used to perform the repair can vary from prosthetic graft material, to hypogastric artery, to a vein graft. Obviously, in situations such as a trauma where local wound contamination may be significant, preference is given to autogenous conduits. In patients with poststenotic dilation of the subclavian artery, a first rib resection is performed at the time of aneurysm repair. Outcomes from repair of subclavian and axillary artery aneurysms have been excellent with minimal morbidity and mortality.

Experience with endovascular repair of subclavian and axillary artery aneurysms is limited, but growing. This approach has most commonly been applied to patients who have suffered a traumatic injury to these vessels. The feasibility of placing covered stents in these regions has proven successful, but the long-term outcomes are not known.

Suggested Readings

Bower TC, Pairolero PC, Hallet JW, et al. Brachiocephalic aneurysms: the case for early recognition and repair. *Ann Vasc Surg*. 1991; 5:125-132.

Bower TC. Subclavian and axillary artery aneurysms. In: Ernst CB, Stanley JC, eds. *Current Therapy in Vascular Surgery*. 4th ed. St. Louis: Mosby; 2001:190-195.

Clagett GP. Upper extremity aneurysms. In: Rutherford RB, ed. *Vascular Surgery*. 5th ed. WB Saunders Philadelphia; 2000:1356-1369.

Nehler MR, Taylor LM, Moneta GL, et al. Upper extremity ischemia from subclavian artery aneurysm caused by bony abnormalities of the thoracic outlet. *Arch Surg*. 1997;132:527-532.

Pairolero PC, Walls JT, Paine W, et al. Subclavian axillary artery aneurysms. *Surgery*. 1981;90:757-763.

Schoder M, Cejna M, Holzenbein T, et al. Elective and emergent endovascular treatment of subclavian artery aneurysms and injuries. *J Endovasc Ther*. 2003;10:58-65.

Xenos ES, Freeman M, Stevens S, et al. Covered stents for injuries of subclavian and axillary arteries. *J Vasc Surg* 2003;38:451-454.

case 21

Raymond M. Shaheen, MD, and Jon S. Matsumura, MD

Presentation

A 42-year-old right-handed mechanic with no significant past medical history presents to your office with a 4-month history of pain and cyanosis of the right second, third, fourth, and fifth fingers. He complains of small ulcers on his third and fifth fingertips for over 2 months. His occupation involves repetitive striking of tools using the palmar surface of an open hand. He denies using tobacco or illicit drugs.

Differential Diagnosis

Pain, ulceration, and color changes are common symptoms and signs of extremity ischemia; others include gangrene, cold intolerance, paresthesias, weakness or fatigue, and exertional cramping or weakness. The differential diagnosis for extremity ischemia can be categorized into diagnoses that commonly affect the lower extremities and those that are usually isolated to the upper extremities. The former include atherosclerosis, cardiac embolization, hypercoagulable states, and thromboangiitis obliterans. The latter include Raynaud's syndrome, vasculitis (eg, systemic lupus, rheumatoid arthritis), radiation arteriopathy, arterial thoracic outlet syndrome, iatrogenic arterial injury, injections from drug abuse, vibrational injury, and hypothenar hammer syndrome.

Case Continued

The patient has normal upper extremity pulses and equal arm blood pressures. Allen's test is performed, and results are normal with patent radial, ulnar, and palmar arch arteries. Superficial ulcerations of the tips of the right third and fifth digits are noted.

Thrombophilia Studies Report

Negative for deficiencies of protein C and S, and antithrombin III. Homocysteine level is normal, and there is no lupus anticoagulant, anticardiolipin antibody, factor V Leiden mutation, or prothrombin gene 20210 mutation.

Collagen Vascular Disease Studies Report

Negative for elevations in erythrocyte sedimentation rate (ESR), C-reactive protein (CRP), and autoantibodies, such as antinuclear antibodies (ANA), rheumatoid factor (RF), and complement levels.

Arteriogram

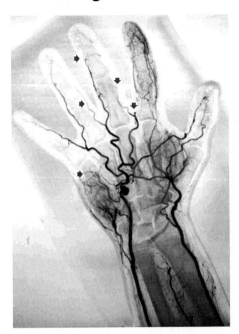

Figure 21-1

Arteriogram Report

Selective arteriography showed aneurysmal degeneration of the palmar ulnar artery with embolic occlusion of multiple digital arteries (*solid black arrows*).

Diagnosis

The patient's history of occupational repetitive striking of his hands, with no other significant past medical history, and arteriography demonstrating abrupt embolic occlusion of digital vessels in the runoff pattern of the more proximal palmar ulnar artery lesion are most consistent with a diagnosis of *hypothenar hammer syndrome*.

Thromboangiitis obliterans (Buerger's disease) is a nonatherosclerotic segmental inflammatory disease of small and medium vessels in the extremities, which is strongly associated with smoking. These patients differ from other candidate inflammatory diagnoses (eg, systemic lupus erythematosus, rheumatoid arthritis) in that the usual inflammatory or immunologic markers (ie, acute phase reactants such as ESR, CRP, and autoantibodies, such as ANA, RH, and complement levels) are normal. Raynaud's syndrome is characterized by *episodic* attacks of vasospasm of arterioles of the distal extremities, usually in female patients and usually with a bilateral pattern. This patient has no history of cardiac arrhythmia and a negative hypercoagulable evaluation, making cardiac embolization or thrombophilia unlikely. Although iatrogenic arterial injury or injection drug abuse with digital embolization could be consistent with the radiographic findings, he has no physical examination findings or social history to support these diagnoses.

Recommendation

This patient is offered excision and reconstruction of the ulnar artery aneurysm, which is the most likely embolic source of his digital vessel occlusions.

Surgical Approach

Axillary block is obtained and a longitudinal palmar incision is performed. Identification and resection of an ectatic palmar ulnar artery segment correlating with the arteriographic findings is performed. The greater saphenous vein at the ankle (better size match than in the thigh) is used as an interposition graft. Saline solutions containing heparin and papaverine are used to prepare the vein and irrigate the arterial targets to minimize vasospasm and thrombus formation. A spatulated end-to-end anastomosis is performed with 7-0 polypropylene sutures in interrupted fashion.

Discussion

The predisposing factor in the development of hypothenar hammer syndrome is repetitive use of the palm of the hand by striking or pushing hand tools. This mechanism of injury involves the hook of the hamate bone striking the unprotected superficial palmar branch of the ulnar artery, which may lead to aneurysmal degeneration and/or thrombosis. Recent studies have also suggested that the pathophysiology may involve focal fibromuscular dysplasia as a predisposing risk factor for the development of hypothenar hammer syndrome in patients with occupational repetitive striking of the hands. Subsequent embolization may occlude digital arteries, with resultant severe vascular insufficiency and ulceration. Arteriography remains the gold-standard diagnostic test, and can help direct surgical management. Ultrasonography may be useful in assessing patients noninvasively, and digital pressures can determine the patency of digital arteries. Ultrasound can also identify some ulnar artery aneurysms that may be missed by arteriography due to the presence of mural thrombus.

All patients with hypothenar hammer syndrome should be counseled about minimizing further trauma to the hands. Treatment of asymptomatic ulnar artery occlusions is primarily nonoperative. Patients with mild symptoms also are treated nonoperatively. Padding and refraining from repetitive trauma to the hands can be associated with significant clinical improvement and avoid surgical intervention.

Reconstruction is the preferred approach for patients with significant ischemic changes, particularly when there is ulnar artery occlusion or a patent embolizing source. Thrombolysis may be a beneficial adjunct by reestablishing flow to recently embolized digital vessels in the acute setting. Occasionally, thrombolysis may uncover an unsuspected ulnar artery aneurysm. Patent and embolizing palmar ulnar arteries require either ligation (in the setting of a patent palmar arch without skin ulceration), or interposition vein reconstruction.

Vascular reconstruction with a short graft and normal inflow is often successful. Most patients with hypothenar hammer syndrome can obtain a high degree of functional restoration and remain gainfully employed with avoidance of the inciting repetitive traumatic injury.

Suggested Readings

Birrer M, Baumgartner I. Images in clinical medicine. Work-related vascular injuries of the hand—hypothenar hammer syndrome. *N Engl J Med.* 2002;347:339.

Conn J Jr, Bergan JJ, Bell JL. Hypothenar hammer syndrome: posttraumatic digital ischemia. *Surgery.* 1970;68:1122-1128.

Ferris BL, Taylor LM Jr, Oyama K, et al. Hypothenar hammer syndrome: proposed etiology. *J Vasc Surg.* 2000;31:104-113.

Taylor LM Jr. Hypothenar hammer syndrome. *J Vasc Surg.* 2003;37:697.

Vayssairat M, Debure C, Cormier JM, Bruneval P, Laurian C, Juillet Y. Hypothenar hammer syndrome: seventeen cases with long-term follow-up. *J Vasc Surg.* 1987;5:838-843.

case 22

Derek T. Woodrum, MD, and Gilbert R. Upchurch, Jr., MD

Presentation

A 62-year-old man is referred to your office by his primary care physician after a recent diagnosis of an abdominal aortic aneurysm (AAA). The AAA was incidentally found when the patient underwent a computed tomography (CT) scan for chronic low back pain. His back pain has been unchanged over the past several years. On initial questioning, he denies abdominal or groin pain. His medical history includes tobacco use, hypertension, and degenerative joint disease. His medications include hydrochlorothiazide for hypertension and ibuprofen for osteoarthritis.

He has been relatively sedentary since retiring. However, he can walk up a flight of stairs without becoming short of breath. He denies symptoms of angina or lower extremity claudication. On physical examination, blood pressure is 140/80 mm Hg, and heart rate is 82 beats per minute. His abdominal examination reveals a well-healed right lower quadrant appendectomy scar, and a nontender pulsatile mass just above the umbilicus. His femoral pulses are 2+, and he has 1+ dorsalis pedis and posterior tibialis pulses bilaterally. The remainder of his examination is normal.

◻ Outside CT Scan of the Abdomen and Pelvis With Intravenous Contrast

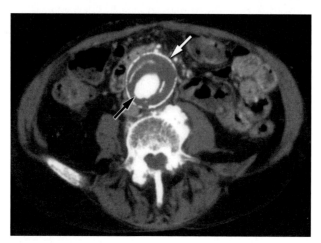

Figure 22-1

CT Scan Report

A 5.7-cm infrarenal AAA is present. (Figure 22-1 shows the typical appearance of an AAA.) No evidence of contrast extravasation is seen. The aneurysm begins 2 cm below the renal arteries and ends at the aortic bifurcation (not seen in this image). Note the difference in diameter between the blood flow channel (*black arrow*) and the aortic wall (*white arrow*).

Imaging Features

An abdominal aorta is defined as aneurysmal when its diameter is greater than 50% over baseline. A normal aorta is approximately 2 to 2.5 cm in diameter, so an AAA is present when the diameter reaches 3 to 3.5 cm. Aneurysms have many anatomic variations, and may be saccular or fusiform. The shape is an important consideration, because the aortic diameter can be overestimated if a cross-sectional image (CT scan) is taken orthogonal to the aneurysm's long axis. The relationship of the renal arteries to the proximal extent of the aneurysm should be noted. An infrarenal aneurysm has a proximal "neck" of uninvolved aorta below the renal arteries. The distal extent of the aneurysm is also important. Although some AAAs end at the bifurcation, many extend into one or both of the common iliac arteries, sometimes necessitating concomitant repair.

Discussion

AAA is a common condition that carries a high mortality. More than 30,000 open AAA repairs were performed in the year 2000, with AAAs responsible for more than 16,000 deaths. The prevalence of unruptured AAAs is certainly much higher than reflected in the operative numbers, given the frequently undiagnosed nature of this mostly silent condition. Patients with insurance and good access to health care are more likely to have their AAA diagnosed—not necessarily by physical examination, but usually by other diagnostic studies.

The pathogenesis of AAA is multifactorial. Its causes fall into at least 4 categories: proteolytic degradation of the aortic wall connective tissue; inflammation and subsequent immune response; biomechanical wall stress; and molecular genetic factors. It is hypothesized that an initial insult to the aortic wall (possibly atherosclerosis, infection, microdissection, or localized biomechanical wall stress) stimulates an immune response through an unknown mechanism that turns on a pathway wherein proteolytic enzymes degrade the medial wall proteins, causing an aneurysm. All of these processes are undoubtedly affected by the patient's genetic predisposition. A single cause for AAA formation is unlikely to be revealed.

AAAs should be repaired electively to prevent the tragedy of rupture. Ruptured AAAs carry a mortality of at least 70%, but frequently this is much higher. Even if the patient survives long enough to make it to the operating room, there is still only a 50% chance of survival to hospital discharge. The decision to electively repair an AAA depends mainly on its maximal diameter. The risk of rupture for an AAA is typically expressed as the likelihood of rupture in the following year. An aortic diameter of less than 4 cm carries almost no risk of rupture in the following year; these aneurysms should be observed with serial diameter measurements by duplex ultrasound. However, the 1-year rupture rate begins to rise quickly: 0.5% to 5%/year for AAA 4 to 5 cm, 3% to 15%/year for AAA 5 to 6 cm, 10% to 20%/year for AAA 6 to 7 cm, and as high as 50%/year when an AAA reaches 8 cm in size. Other factors that may increase the likelihood of AAA rupture at a given diameter are chronic obstructive pulmonary disease, female gender, rapid expansion rate, hypertension, and smoking. The current general consensus for the average patient (especially male) is that an AAA less than 5.5 cm in size may be followed, unless rapid expansion is noted.

Recommendation

Prior to the widespread utilization of CT scans, abdominal radiographs would occasionally reveal AAAs by visualizing calcification of the aneurysm sac. More recently, 3-dimensional reconstructions from CT scans have proved useful in preoperative planning. Traditional angiography may show an aneurysm, but frequently its diameter measurements are not accurate, because the luminal plaque within an aneurysm sac may still have a blood flow channel of relatively normal diameter (see Fig. 22-1). A 3-dimensional CT scan is recommended.

◼ CT Scan With 3-Dimensional Reconstructions

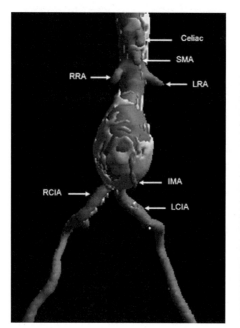 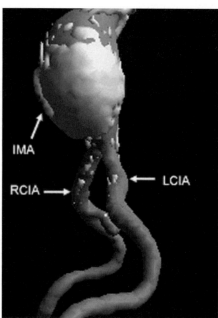

Figure 22-2   **Figure 22-3**

CT Scan Report

Anterior-posterior and left lateral 3-dimensional reconstructions of an infrarenal AAA ending at the aortic bifurcation show a moderate amount of atherosclerotic plaque (*colored yellow*). The blood flow channel is also dilated. The proximal aortic neck is conical (increases by greater than 10% over 1.5 cm; *celiac* = celiac artery; *SMA* = superior mesenteric artery; *RRA/LRA* = right/left renal artery; *RCIA/LCIA* = right/left common iliac artery).

Diagnosis and Recommendation

Infrarenal AAA without extension into the iliac arteries. The patient is offered an open repair of his AAA, given his young age and conical proximal aortic neck. The patient and his family are quoted an approximately 2% to 5% perioperative mortality. Many studies have investigated the relationship between hospital volume and outcome following AAA repair. When other variables are controlled, high-volume hospitals (more than 30 open AAA repairs per year) have an overall lower mortality after AAA repair (there is a 1.7 times greater risk of death at a low-volume hospital).

Surgical Approach

The abdomen is widely prepped and draped. Adequate exposure is very important in this operation; a midline incision is made. Alternatively, some surgeons utilize a transverse incision or a retroperitoneal approach. After dissecting the duodenum off the aorta, proximal control is obtained below the renal arteries, and distal control is obtained of the common iliac arteries. Brisk diuresis is established with mannitol and furosemide. Following heparin administration, the iliac arteries are clamped distally, then the proximal intrarenal aorta is clamped. The aneurysm sac is then opened longitudinally, and the aortic thrombus removed. All lumbar arteries are oversewn. The inferior mesenteric artery (IMA) is briskly back bleeding and is oversewn. A prosthetic tube graft is sewn in place with monofilament suture. Once the graft is in place and the patient is hemodynamically stable, the aneurysm sac is closed over the graft. The retroperitoneum is closed to prevent subsequent aortoduodenal fistula. The abdomen is closed in the standard fashion. The patient is admitted to the intensive care unit for routine postoperative care.

Case Continued

The patient does well the first night after the operation, but the next afternoon you are called by the nurse to the bedside. The patient's blood pressure has been trending down over the past 2 hours, and he has increasingly required intravenous fluids to keep his blood pressure in the normal range. Also, the nurse tells you that he passed a bloody bowel movement. On physical examination, he appears unwell, and has diffuse abdominal tenderness and guarding. His peripheral pulses remain palpable. Emergency laboratory studies reveal a metabolic acidosis and a stable hematocrit.

Differential Diagnosis

This patient's change in clinical course is concerning. The decrease in blood pressure could be due to intravascular hypovolemia, cardiac shock, sepsis, or bleeding. With decreasing blood pressure and abdominal pain after aortic surgery, bleeding is always the first concern. This is less likely in this patient with a stable hematocrit. It is unusual for a patient to have any bowel movement in the first couple days after an AAA repair, and a bloody stool suggests colonic ischemia. Generally, postoperative mesenteric ischemia occurs in the colon supplied by the IMA. The blood flow through the IMA is variable in the setting of an AAA. Many times, the IMA has thrombosed prior to the operation with its ostia occluded by plaque and thrombus. Otherwise, it is often oversewn during the operation. Collateral blood flow from the superior mesenteric artery and superior hemorrhoidal arteries are usually sufficient to supply blood flow to the lower colon. If not, the colon may become ischemic and ultimately progress to frank necrosis.

Diagnosis and Recommendation

Probable colon ischemia. The patient should undergo an emergent endoscopy for definitive diagnosis.

Case Continued

The patient undergoes flexible sigmoidoscopy, which reveals frank, circumferential necrosis of the sigmoid and descending colon. Broad-spectrum antibiotics are administered, and he is returned to the operating room for a partial colon resection, during which the left colon is removed, and a transverse colostomy is created. The rectum is stapled off (Hartman's procedure). His postoperative course is protracted, but relatively uneventful. He eventually recovers and does well.

Discussion

Severe colon ischemia is rare after AAA repair, occurring less than 1% of the time. However, it carries a high degree of morbidity and a significant mortality rate. IMA reimplantation may not affect the incidence of colon ischemia. The key to successful treatment of postoperative colon ischemia is early detection and removal. A high index of suspicion should lead to early endoscopy if any symptoms or signs of colonic ischemia occur.

Additional Considerations

Preoperative preparation for patients scheduled to undergo major vascular surgery is very important. Excellent assessment tools and algorithms are available to aid in decisions regarding the need for preoperative cardiac testing. The patient is less than 70 years of age, has no cardiac history or symptoms, has a normal EKG, and has reasonable exercise tolerance. He should be started on a beta-blocker preoperatively and continued at least 3 months postoperatively, but does not need additional cardiac testing. He should also be counseled on the benefits of smoking cessation and strongly encouraged to do so.

Suggested Readings

Ailawadi G, Eliason J, Upchurch Jr. GR Current concepts in the pathogenesis of abdominal aortic aneurysm. *J Vasc Surg.* 2003;38:584-588.

Axelrod DA, Henke PK, Wakefield TW, et al. Impact of chronic obstructive pulmonary disease on elective and emergency abdominal aortic aneurysm repair. *J Vasc Surg.* 2001;33:72-76.

Boxer LK, Dimick JD, Wainess RM, et al. Payer status is related to differences in access and outcomes of abdominal aortic aneurysm repair in the United States. *Surgery.* 2003;134:142-145.

Brewster D, Cronenwett J, Hallet J, et al. Guidelines for the treatment of abdominal aortic aneurysm. *J Vasc Surg.* 2003;37:1106-1117.

Dimick JD, Stanley JC, Axelrod DA, et al. Variation in death rate after abdominal aortic aneurysmectomy in the United States: impact of hospital volume, gender, and age. *Ann Surg.* Apr 2002;235:579-585.

Fleisher L, Eagle K. Lowering cardiac risk in noncardiac surgery. *N Engl J Med.* 2001;345:1677-1682.

Upchurch Jr GR, Proctor MC, Henke PK, et al. Predictors of severe morbidity and death after elective abdominal aortic aneurysmectomy in patients with chronic obstructive pulmonary disease. *J Vasc Surg.* 2003;37:594-599.

Peter L. Faries, MD, Rajeev Dayal, MD, Scott Hollenbeck, MD,
Albeir Mousa, MD, and K. Craig Kent, MD

Presentation

The patient is a 77-year-old man who was discovered to have an abdominal aortic aneurysm (AAA) by ultrasound performed for evaluation of intermittent right upper quadrant discomfort. The ultrasound demonstrated no cholelithiasis, thickening of the gallbladder wall, or dilatation of the common bile duct and was not remarkable for findings other than an AAA. A subsequent CT scan is ordered.

■ CT Scan

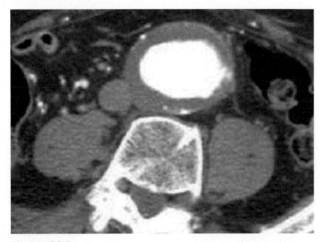

Figure 23-1

CT Scan Report

CT scan confirms the presence of a 7.9-cm AAA.

Differential Diagnosis/Treatment Options

The diagnosis of an asymptomatic AAA has been established using radiographic studies. There is no evidence of rupture or acute expansion. Further decisions regarding treatment must now incorporate evaluation of the patient's overall condition, ability to tolerate surgery, life expectancy, and likelihood of aneurysm rupture. Given the large size of the aneurysm, rupture within 12 months is likely. Intervention is therefore indicated for the prevention of rupture, if the patient does not have a terminal illness and if he is able to tolerate surgical repair.

Case Continued

The patient's ability to tolerate conventional open aneurysm repair should be evaluated. Upon obtaining additional history, it is determined that the patient requires elevation of his head on 2 pillows to sleep at night, he cannot ascend a flight of stairs due to the onset of significant dyspnea, and he awakens 2 to 3 times a night to urinate. He has a 45 pack-year history of smoking, but discontinued smoking 10 years ago. Physical examination demonstrates an 8-cm pulsatile abdominal mass that is nontender. He has excellent femoral pulses bilaterally. His colostomy site from his prior abdominal-perineal resection is intact and functioning well, and the loss of abdominal domain from his prior abdominal surgery does not significantly limit his ambulation. He has 2+ pedal edema without ulceration or evidence of venous insufficiency.

Further cardiac and pulmonary evaluation is ordered.

Report of Diagnostic Tests

An echocardiogram and adenosine thallium stress test are performed. The patient is demonstrated to have global ventricular hypokinesis with a markedly reduced ejection fraction of 20%. There are fixed myocardial perfusion defects in the left anterior and lateral wall regions, but no reversible perfusion defects.

Pulmonary function tests indicate significantly reduced pulmonary capacity and functional reserve with forced expiratory volume in 1 second (FEV_1) of 0.9 L.

Recommendation

Several factors suggest that this patient will be at significantly increased risk for morbidity and mortality if conventional AAA repair is performed. His cardiac and pulmonary capacity is considerably reduced. In addition, the presence of a stoma and the loss of abdominal domain make his a "hostile" abdomen and increase the difficulty of conventional repair. Therefore, this patient should be considered for endovascular repair of his AAA using a stent graft.

Discussion

Anatomic evaluation is performed to determine if a stent graft will be successful in excluding the aneurysm from the arterial circulation, thereby preventing aneurysm rupture. To achieve aneurysm exclusion, undilated arterial areas must be present proximal and distal to the aneurysm. These fixation zones in the immediate infrarenal aorta proximally and common iliac arteries distally allow for sealing of the aneurysm and prevent arterial flow into the aneurysm sac. An undilated aortic segment at least 10 mm in length must be present distal to the renal arteries. Excessive angulation of the pararenal aorta may also prevent adequate stent graft fixation and sealing. Normal common iliac arteries must also be present to achieve fixation and sealing in those regions. Alternatively, the stent graft may be extended to the external iliac arteries; however, this requires occlusion of the internal iliac arteries that may be associated with ischemic complications of the pelvis and gluteal region. The vessels used to access the aorta must also be of an adequate caliber to allow passage of the endovascular stent graft. Typically, this is carried out from the femoral arteries through the external iliac arteries.

The current patient undergoes a contrast-enhanced spiral CT scan with images obtained at 2.5-mm intervals to allow measurement of the proximal aortic and common iliac artery diameters. Three-dimensional reconstruction of the CT scan can be used to determine the length of the arterial segment that is to be excluded by the stent graft. That is the distance from the distal-most renal artery to the bifurcation of the common iliac arteries bilaterally. Alternatively, length may be determined using contrast angiography performed with a calibrated catheter with radiopaque marks at 1-cm intervals. These measurements are used to determine the length of the stent graft.

CT Scan and Angiogram

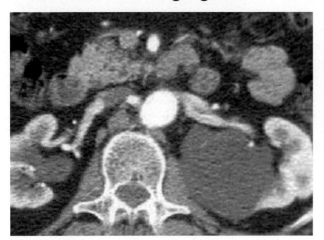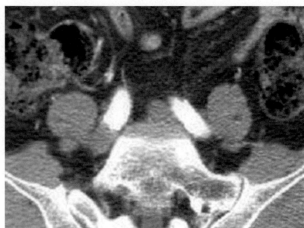

Figure 23-2

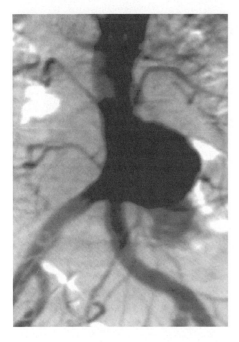

Figure 23-3

CT Scan and Angiogram Report

The proximal aortic fixation zone is determined to be 25 mm in diameter and 18 mm long. The common iliac arteries are 14 mm in diameter, and the distance from the renal ostia to the iliac bifurcations is 147 mm on the right and 152 mm on the left.

The most appropriate course of management for the treatment of this patient is endovascular AAA repair. He possesses arterial anatomy that will allow successful exclusion of the aneurysm by placement of a stent graft. He exhibits multiple factors that would place him at increased risk for conventional repair. He has a large AAA and no terminal conditions, so he is likely to die from aneurysm rupture if repair is not performed.

Surgical Approach

Repair is performed in the operating room on a radiolucent table. The patient may receive local, epidural, or general anesthesia. Because he exhibits significant pulmonary disease, regional anesthesia without the requirement for intubation is preferable. The abdomen and legs are prepared in a sterile manner in the event that conversion to open repair becomes necessary. It is likely to be of value to exclude the stoma site from the sterile field. Exposure of the common femoral arteries is performed bilaterally, and an angiographic guide wire is introduced into the abdominal aorta. A flush catheter is placed in the aorta over the wire to allow the performance of angiography. A stiff guide wire is placed through a selective angiographic catheter from the contralateral femoral artery. After administration of systemic anticoagulation, an arteriotomy is created at the site where the stiff guide wire is introduced. The main body of the stent graft is brought into position in the aorta over the stiff guide wire and deployed in the infrarenal aorta. The short contralateral limb of the main body of the stent graft is then cannulated from the opposite femoral access site using a guide wire. A pigtail catheter is tracked over the guide wire and spun within the stent graft to confirm intraluminal position. A second stiff guide wire is then brought through the short contralateral limb and the contralateral iliac delivery system is tracked into position through the contralateral femoral arteriotomy site. After deployment of the contralateral iliac limb, completion angiography is performed to ensure complete exclusion of the aneurysm.

Case Continued

The patient tolerates the procedure well. Completion angiography demonstrates no evidence of aneurysm perfusion or endoleak, and the patient is discharged to home on the first postoperative day. He is enrolled in a standard follow-up imaging protocol, with contrast CT scans to be obtained within 30 days, at 6 months, at 1 year, and annually thereafter. Contrast CT scans obtained at 30 days and 6 months show no aneurysm perfusion or endoleak. The 1-year follow-up scan is depicted in Figure 23-4.

■ CT Scan

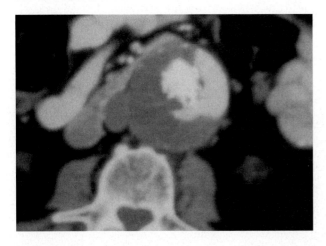

Figure 23-4

CT Scan Report

At 1-year follow up, contrast is seen perfusing the aneurysm sac.

Discussion

If surveillance imaging demonstrates arterial flow into the aneurysm sac, additional measures must be taken to determine the source of the continued perfusion. The CT scan may suggest the location of the source of the endoleak, with small endoleaks located posteriorly being suggestive of a lumbar arterial source. Endoleaks that originate from patent collateral branches of the aneurysm, including the lumbar and inferior mesenteric arteries, generate retrograde perfusion and have been classified as type II endoleaks.

Contrast that can be traced to the proximal or distal fixation sites of the stent graft may be more suggestive of an attachment site endoleak. Perfusion that originates from incomplete fixation or incomplete sealing at the attachment site results in antegrade flow into the aneurysm. These endoleaks have been classified as type I endoleaks. Antegrade endoleaks may also originate from the junction site between stent graft components. These are classified as type III endoleaks.

Antegrade endoleaks (types I and III) result in the transmission of systemic pressure to the aneurysm sac and lead to continued aneurysm expansion and rupture. Therefore, they mandate treatment at the time of diagnosis. The pressure and force generated by retrograde-collateral endoleaks (type II) is not known and their natural history is not well established. However, most investigators recommend correction if they are persistent and are associated with continued aneurysm growth.

With the appearance of a new endoleak, steps should be taken to determine its source. These may include duplex ultrasound, cine magnetic resonance imaging (MRI), and contrast angiography. Duplex ultrasound may be useful to confirm the presence of flow in the aneurysm and often may suggest the likely source of the flow. Cine MRI is a relatively novel technique that allows the gadolinium contrast bolus to be followed, to determine the source and direction of arterial flow. Definitive establishment of the source of an endoleak most frequently requires performance of a contrast arteriogram.

Angiography can also be used as a therapeutic modality, particularly in cases of retrograde endoleaks. In these cases, coil embolization or other occlusive measures may be used to thrombose the source vessel of the endoleak. Type II endoleaks frequently require both an inflow and an outflow collateral branch vessel, so efforts should be made to identify and treat these multiple aneurysm side branches. Coil embolization of type I endoleaks has also been reported; however, it is unclear that this is effective in eliminating arterial pressure or the risk of aneurysm rupture.

◼ Angiogram

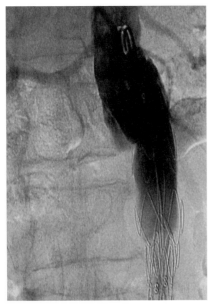 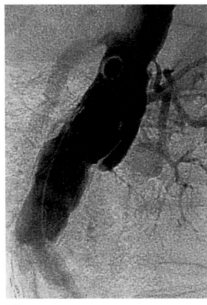 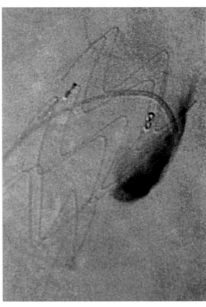

Figure 23-5(A)   **(B)**   **(C)**

Angiogram Report

Anterior-posterior (Fig. 23-5A), lateral (Fig. 23-5B), and selective (Fig. 23-5C) angiograms demonstrate continued arterial perfusion originating from the proximal attachment site, a proximal type I endoleak.

Recommendation

Antegrade endoleaks (type I and III) may be successfully treated by placement of an extension stent graft. In this case, there is sufficient undilated aorta distal to the renal ostia to allow successful placement of a proximal extension stent graft. This is the best treatment for this elderly patient with multiple comorbid illnesses. If a sufficient proximal aortic fixation region is not present, then conversion to standard aneurysm repair must be considered as the definitive treatment. Use of embolic material to seal proximal endoleaks has not been demonstrated to be effective in preventing aneurysm rupture and cannot be recommended.

This case demonstrates the importance of continued surveillance of patients after endovascular stent graft repair of AAA. When endoleaks are observed, further evaluation and intervention is necessary to prevent possible aneurysm rupture.

Suggested Readings   (see Case 24)

Peter L. Faries, MD, Rajeev Dayal, MD, Scott Hollenbeck, MD, Albeir Mousa, MD, and K. Craig Kent, MD

Presentation

The patient is a 78-year-old man who presents with 36 hours of increasingly severe pain in the left flank, radiating to the left lower quadrant. The patient states that he has undergone repair of an abdominal aortic aneurysm (AAA) 18 months previously. On physical examination, the patient is alert and oriented; he is tachycardic to 104 beats per minute with a blood pressure of 127/89 mm Hg. His abdomen is mildly distended. A large pulsatile mass is palpable with severe tenderness in the left lower quadrant. There is no flank ecchymosis. There are no abdominal incisions or scars. There are well-healed transverse groin incisions bilaterally. A computed tomography (CT) scan is recommended.

CT Scan

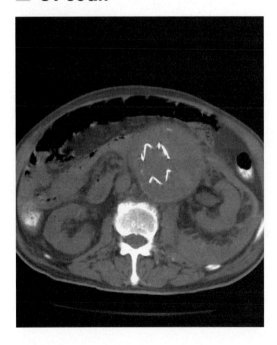

Figure 24-1 CT scan report. Large AAA with endograft inside of aorta. A large amount of retroperitoneal blood is present, suggestive of a ruptured AAA.

Differential Diagnosis

The patient presents with tachycardia, acute abdominal findings, and a pulsatile mass; however, he reports having undergone prior abdominal aortic aneurysm repair. The differential should therefore include ruptured abdominal aortic aneurysm, but should also include diverticulitis, renal lithiasis, intestinal perforation, pancreatitis, and spontaneous retroperitoneal hematoma, and may also include rare aneurysms, including splenic and other visceral artery aneurysms and para-anastomotic aneurysm with or without infection. In this instance, the physical examination is consistent with a ruptured AAA despite prior endovascular aneurysm repair.

Discussion

Endovascular AAA repair is performed transarterially through remote arteriotomy sites, most commonly in the femoral arteries. An arterial prosthesis comprised of self-expanding stents and prosthetic graft material (an endovascular stent graft) is introduced through the aneurysm, creating a new arterial lining. Success of the repair depends on exclusion of the aneurysm from the arterial circulation, and therefore from arterial pressurization.

Continued arterial perfusion of the aneurysm sac after endovascular repair has been termed an *endoleak*. Endoleaks result in continued pressurization of the aneurysm sac. The significance of the continued perfusion is determined by the source of the endoleak. Endoleaks that result in direct arterial flow into the aneurysm sac cause systemic pressurization of the aneurysm. These leaks may occur at the sites of attachment of the stent graft to the native arterial wall, the seal, or implantation zones. Direct antegrade endoleaks may also occur at junction sites between different endovascular stent graft components.

Systemic pressurization resulting from direct antegrade endoleaks has been associated with continued aneurysm expansion and rupture. As a result, radiologic imaging follow-up protocols have been used to assess the success of the endovascular repair. CT scans with intravenous contrast enhancement have been the most commonly employed follow-up study. These are typically performed 1, 6, and 12 months after the procedure and then annually thereafter.

If contrast material is visualized within the aneurysm sac by CT scan, further evaluation to determine the source of the continued perfusion may be undertaken. Although duplex ultrasound and magnetic resonance imaging have been used, the most commonly definitive test is contrast angiography. These studies may then be used to determine the most appropriate secondary intervention for correction of the endoleak. When an untreated or unrecognized endoleak results in aneurysm rupture, immediate surgical intervention is necessary to prevent exsanguination and death.

Recommendation

Immediate surgical intervention. Several approaches may be used, including placement of an occlusion balloon in the aorta proximal to the aneurysm, immediate standard surgical repair, and endovascular aneurysm repair.

▢ Surgical Approach

The patient is brought emergently to the operating room. Prior to induction of anesthesia, wide sterile preparation including the chest, abdomen, and proximal legs is performed and monitoring instrumentation is positioned. Conventional repair of elective abdominal aortic aneurysms is described in Chapter 22. Some modification may be necessary when an endovascular stent graft has been placed previously. Temporary control of the supraceliac aorta is frequently necessary. Dissection of the supraceliac aorta may be carried out by transecting the triangular ligament of the left lobe of the liver to allow its mobilization to the right. The lesser sac is entered through the lesser omentum. The right crux of the diaphragm is bluntly or sharply dissected, and the esophagus is mobilized to the left to expose the underlying aorta. An atraumatic vascular clamp is placed to establish supraceliac control of the aorta.

When the proximal or distal fixation of the stent graft is intact, or when these graft elements are fixed to the arterial wall and cannot be removed, the stent graft may be transected and the conventional graft may be anastomosed directly to the fixed portion of the stent graft. This approach provides a more rapid solution while avoiding injury to the arterial segment to which the stent graft is fixed. It also avoids the need for more extensive arterial dissection.

Placement of an occlusion balloon in the proximal abdominal aorta may provide more rapid vascular control while avoiding uncontrolled dissection of the retroperitoneum that can contribute to catastrophic hypotension. Placement may be carried out through a left brachial approach. In the operating room, on a fluorolucent table, the left arm is prepared in a sterile fashion in addition to the other anatomic areas. Dissection of the brachial artery is carried out and an introducer sheath is placed. A wire is directed into the infrarenal aorta, and the occlusion balloon is tracked over the wire into position proximal to the aneurysm. Alternatively, the contralateral femoral artery may be used for balloon access. Inflation of the occlusion balloon is performed with dilute contrast material to allow its visualization during inflation. Once aortic occlusion has been obtained, either conventional or endovascular aneurysm repair may be undertaken with greater hemodynamic control.

Endovascular repair of ruptured infrarenal abdominal aortic aneurysms may be performed in the setting of a prior endovascular repair or in a patient who has not undergone prior repair. The use of local anesthesia may avoid significant hemodynamic fluctuations that can be associated with general anesthesia; however, the anesthesiologist must be prepared to intubate if the patient should become hemodynamically unstable or if respiration ceases.

After administration of local anesthesia, dissection of the femoral arteries is performed in the typical manner. Arterial access is obtained, and a flush catheter is introduced into the abdominal aorta over a guide wire. Angiography is employed to determine the length of endovascular stent graft to be used. The choice of stent graft diameter is made on the basis of the CT scan measurements of the proximal infrarenal aorta and the iliac arteries. A bifurcated aortoiliac graft may be used if the patient is hemodynamically stable and immediate exclusion of the aneurysm is not critical. However, if the patient is hypotensive, an aortouniiliac stent graft may be placed with subsequent performance of a femorofemoral bypass. In these instances, occlusion of the contralateral common iliac artery is necessary to prevent retrograde perfusion of the aneurysm sac. If an occlusion balloon is inflated, it may be necessary to deflate the aortic occlusion balloon during placement of the stent graft to allow visualization of anatomic structures, such as the renal and internal iliac arteries and the aortic and iliac implantation zones.

In cases of endovascular treatment of ruptured aneurysms, a CT scan should be obtained within the first 24 hours to ensure that the aneurysm has been completely excluded and that no endoleak is present. The patient should then be observed using a standard radiographic protocol.

Suggested Readings

Faries PL, Bernheim J, Kilaru S, Hollenbeck S, Clair D, Kent KC. Selecting stent grafts for the endovascular treatment of abdominal aortic aneurysms. *J Cardiovasc Surg (Torino).* 2003;44:511-518.

Faries PL, Cadot H, Agarwal G, Kent KC, Hollier LH, Marin ML. Management of endoleak after endovascular aneurysm repair: cuffs, coils and conversion. *J Vasc Surg.* 2003;37: 1155-1161.

Greenberg RK, Lawrence-Brown M, Bhandari G, et al. An update on the Zenith endovascular graft for abdominal aortic aneurysms: initial implantation and mid-term follow-up data. *J Vasc Surg.* 2001;33:S157-S164.

Matsumura JS, Brewster DC, Makaroun MS, Naftel DC. A multicenter controlled clinical trial of open versus endovascular treatment of abdominal aortic aneurysm. *J Vasc Surg.* 2003;37:262-271.

May J, White GH, Ly CN, Jones MA, Harris JP. Endoluminal repair of abdominal aortic aneurysm prevents enlargement of the proximal neck: a 9-year life-table and 5-year longitudinal study. *J Vasc Surg.* 2003;37:86-90.

Ohki T, Veith FJ, Shaw P, et al. Increasing incidence of midterm and long-term complications after endovascular graft repair of abdominal aortic aneurysms: a note of caution based on a 9-year experience. *Ann Surg.* 2001;234:323-334.

Ouriel K, Clair D, Greenberg RK, et al. Endovascular repair of abdominal aortic aneurysms: device-specific outcome. *J Vasc Surg.* 2003; 37:991-998.

Vallabhaneni SR, Harris PL. Lessons learnt from the EUROSTAR registry on endovascular repair of abdominal aortic aneurysm repair. *Eur J Radiol.* 2001;39:34-41.

White GH, Yu W, May J, et al. Endoleak as a complication of endoluminal grafting of abdominal aortic aneurysm: classification, incidence, diagnosis, and management. *J Endovasc Surg.* 1997;152-168.

Zarins CK, White RA, Fogarty TJ. Aneurysm rupture after endovascular repair using the AneuRx stent graft. *J Vasc Surg.* 2000;31:960-970.

Zarins CK. The US AneuRx Clinical Trial: 6-year clinical update 2002. *J Vasc Surg.* 2003;37: 904-908.

David R. Whittaker, MD, and Marc L. Schermerhorn, MD

Presentation

A 63-year-old man presents to the emergency department with complaints of abdominal pain. He reports intermittent sharp pain over the past several months that have become increasingly more intense in character over the past several days. The pain is centrally located with radiation to his mid back. He denies alleviating or exacerbating characteristics. Further discussion reveals the presence of occasional low-grade fevers and a 5-pound weight loss. A family history of abdominal aortic aneurysms is present. He smokes heavily and has marginally controlled hypertension. His physical examination demonstrates an afebrile, hemodynamically stable male in moderate discomfort. His blood pressure is equal bilaterally and pulses are fully palpable in all extremities. His abdomen is mildly tender in the epigastric region without radiation or frank peritoneal signs. He reports mild costovertebral angle (CVA) tenderness.

Differential Diagnosis

The broad differential for these findings requires an initial focus on the potentially life-threatening possibilities. In addition to the obvious vascular system diagnoses of a ruptured abdominal aortic aneurysm (AAA) or acute aortic dissection, a perforated viscous, mesenteric ischemia, or intestinal volvulus must also be considered. Although not immediately threatening, the low-grade temperatures, CVA tenderness, and weight loss could direct the diagnosis toward a neoplastic cause. Furthermore, this constellation of symptoms is frequently seen in patients with nephrolithiasis or ureterolithiasis. An inflammatory AAA is realistically very low on the differential. Inflammatory AAAs constitute approximately 5% of all abdominal aortic aneurysms.

Discussion

This patient's presentation requires a high index of suspicion and an aggressive diagnostic work-up to rule out a potentially life-threatening diagnosis. In addition to timely laboratory studies (chemistries and complete blood count), the current speed and detail of spiral computed tomography (CT) scanners makes an intravenous contrast scan the first imaging modality of choice. An aortic catastrophe can be ruled out with reasonable certainty. If present, additional intraabdominal pathologies are often evident from these high-quality reformattable images. Although magnetic resonance arteriography (MRA) has demonstrated superiority in diagnosing periaortic inflammation, the current logistics and time required to obtain magnetic resonance imaging (MRI) scans favor obtaining a CT scan in most institutions.

◼ CT Scan

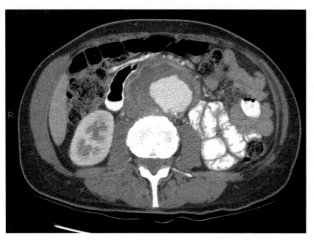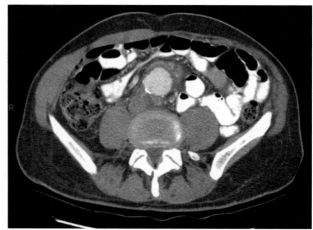

Figure 25-1 Note the eccentric reaction occurring around this inflammatory aneurysm.

CT Scan Report

CT scan demonstrates a 6-cm infrarenal AAA, with significant anterior and lateral aortic wall thickening and relative sparing of the posterior aorta. There is marked bilateral hydronephrosis and hydroureter with apparent retroperitoneal fibrotic involvement of the ureters. There is no clear evidence of aortic sac hemorrhage or extravasation.

Reports of Laboratory Tests

The patient's complete blood cell count (CBC) is normal, but he is noted to have an elevated erythrocyte sedimentation rate (101 seconds), blood urea nitrogen (34 mg/dL), and creatinine (1.8 mg/dL).

Diagnosis

Inflammatory abdominal aortic aneurysm (IAAA).

Discussion

Frequently associated back pain and abdominal tenderness with aortic palpation in patients with inflammatory aneurysms often invokes concern for a leak or rupture. The rupture rate for IAAAs, however, is actually no greater than a similar size-matched noninflammatory aneurysm. If the clinical picture or CT scan suggests leak or rupture, the work-up is complete. In the absence of an emergent situation, however, appropriate treatment requires an understanding of this variant of abdominal aneurysms.

Walker and colleagues are attributed with the first publication describing inflammatory aneurysms in 1972. It is difficult to ascertain if this pathology is an entirely separate entity or an advanced spectrum of typical aneurysms. Evidence continues to accumulate that demonstrates the involvement of an inflammatory, cytokine-mediated pathogenesis to the aorta's aneurysmal degeneration. McMillan and Pearce present a pathway of atherosclerotic accumulation with focal inflammation at the level of the intima that then shifts to an inflammatory process in the media and adventitia of the vessel wall. They suggest that this inflammation involves a trigger of some type (eg, immunologic, hemodynamic) that stimulates an imbalance between matrix metalloproteinase (MMP) and tissue inhibitors of metalloproteinase (TIMP). This imbalance then leads to aortic wall degeneration and aneurysmal formation.

There is also a growing link between inflammatory aneurysms and systemic autoimmune inflammatory syndromes. Although the erythrocyte sedimentation rate (ESR) and C-reactive protein (CRP) values may not be diagnostic, an elevated ESR or CRP level can be found in 20% to 80% of affected patients. This nonspecific test tends to be a general marker of systemic inflammation. Haug et al. found a higher incidence of autoimmune disease in patients with inflammatory aneurysms when compared to standard aneurysm control patients. Systemic lupus erythematosus (SLE), rheumatoid arthritis, polyarthritis, and giant cell arteritis were found in 19% of their patients who had inflammatory changes to their aneurysms. Furthermore, they suggest a genetic influence on the development of inflammatory aneurysms. This is supported by work from Rasmussen et al., who found a statistically significant difference in the presence of an HLA-DR allele on chromosome 6 in patients with IAAA when compared with control patients having typical degenerative aneurysms. Finally, there is a clear familial pattern of inheritance between patients with an HLA-B27 allele and ankylosing spondylitis. When aneurysmal formation does occur in these patients, the histologic structure of the aortic wall demonstrates an abundant infiltration of lymphocytes with concurrent destruction of the vessel wall's elastic fibers, similar to the changes seen in inflammatory aneurysms.

On gross examination, IAAAs have a pearly white, often densely fibrotic appearance, usually involving the anterior and lateral surface of the aorta more so than the posterior wall. This process will often involve periaortic structures including the ureters, vena cava, left renal vein, and duodenum. It is interesting that after repair of the aneurysm, the fibrosis may diminish by more than 50% when compared to preoperative thickness. Ureteral involvement often results in partial obstruction with resultant hydroureter or hydronephrosis. Fortunately, at least 40% of those patients with unilateral hydronephrosis demonstrated a significant reduction in the amount of obstruction following aneurysm repair. For the remaining 60% of patients with no change or an increase in obstruction, their post-renal obstructive picture did not have any associated deterioration in renal function at 10 months' follow-up.

Recommendation

Whether or not inflammatory aneurysms are a separate entity or an exaggerated response of the periaortic tissues, the decision to treat should be based on the same factors used to treat patients with typical degenerative-type aneurysms. The estimated rupture risk, operative risk, and life expectancy will all influence the decision to intervene. Additionally, concerning aortic characteristics such as periaortic edema, pain, and involvement of surrounding structures may prompt a more aggressive management strategy. Many inflammatory aneurysms are repaired urgently or emergently due to the inability to rule out acute expansion and imminent rupture.

This patient's CT scan and laboratory values indicate the presence of an inflammatory aneurysm with periureteral involvement and secondary hydronephrosis. Although the aneurysm does not appear to be leaking at this time, the progressive nature of his pain is a matter of concern. If all other potential sources of his pain can be ruled out, it is reasonable to recommend an urgent repair of his aneurysm.

Approach

The operative approach to this patient should have 2 primary objectives: (1) effectively replace the aneurysm with a prosthetic conduit, and (2) manage the secondary fibrotic complications. In this patient, the fibrotic complications are bilateral hydroureter and hydronephrosis.

Until the advent of endovascular AAA repair, open AAA repair was the only feasible option for aneurysm replacement. Because the periaortic reaction usually involves the anterior and lateral surface of the aorta, a retroperitoneal approach is often recommended. This theoretically allows an approach to the posterior-lateral aorta in an attempt to minimize dissection through the dense fibrotic reaction. This advantage is tempered by the limits of accessibility to the right ureter, iliac artery, and duodenum. Regardless of the approach, these aneurysms are technically demanding. This is evident by the significantly increased operating-room time and blood product utilization associated with these repairs. Furthermore, although the fibrosis may provide a good substance to the aortic wall to hold sutures, the anastomoses may require reinforcement with Teflon pledgets or polytetrafluoroethylene (PTFE) strips to prevent a late and catastrophic dehiscence. However, the overall patient mortality for open management of inflammatory aneurysms is similar to that of patients with standard degenerative aneurysms.

An endovascular repair in an appropriately chosen candidate is an inviting alternative. It obviates the need for dissection in difficult surgical planes, and removes the need for hand-sewn anastomoses to tissues of questionable quality. There are growing case reports of successful endovascular approaches to these aneurysms. Recent generations of stent grafts with improved proximal fixation devices and overall durability will likely become the approach of choice in the near future. As discussed earlier, the periaortic inflammation associated with these aneurysms has the unique characteristic of regressing in a large proportion of patients after the repair of the aneurysm. It is currently accepted that primary management of surrounding organ involvement is not necessary at the time of the aortic repair. Diligent observation will often demonstrate resolution of the inflammation and, frequently, the effects on the end organ. The resolution of fibrosis is seen after both open and endovascular repairs.

The use of perioperative anti-inflammatory medicines is controversial. The literature has several reports of trials using medications, including nonsteroidal anti-inflammatory drugs (NSAIDs), glucocorticoids, and intense immunosuppressant chemotherapeutic medications, such as cyclophosphamide and azathioprine. Although there is evidence that anti-inflammatory medications may alleviate some of the inflammatory burden, the relatively benign natural history of the inflammatory reaction associated with these aneurysms indicates that a period of observation, as mentioned earlier, is the initial recommendation. If symptoms of obstruction persist, it is then reasonable to pursue medical treatment. If this approach also fails, an additional intervention may be necessary, such as ureterolysis, stent placement, or intra-abdominal lysis of adhesions. Nitecki et al. make a point of stressing the importance of an appropriate follow-up imaging regimen to avoid long-term complications of end-organ damage, such as renal atrophy from chronic ureteral obstruction.

Surgical Approach

In the context of progressive abdominal pain, the ability to repair the aneurysm while avoiding the hostile periaortic dissection makes an endovascular repair the approach of choice. The significant bilateral hydronephrosis with concomitant decrement in renal function warrants perioperative placement of ureteral stents to relieve the acute obstruction.

This patient, however, was not a candidate for an endovascular approach secondary to anatomic considerations. Therefore, a left retroperitoneal approach was utilized to expose the aneurysm. The stented, enlarged ureters were readily recognized and avoided. No ureterolysis was performed. In the operating room, after proximal and distal control was obtained, healthy aorta was isolated to perform the anastomosis. Teflon pledgets were used to reinforce the anastomoses. The remainder of the procedure followed standard aortic surgery techniques. A supraceliac cross clamp may be utilized if the pararenal aorta is involved in the inflammatory process. In situations where acute expansion or impending rupture is suspected, an anterior approach is often the approach of choice. Because the duodenum and renal vein may be involved in the dense inflammation, it is best to perform an endoaneurysmal repair that minimizes the lateral aortic dissection and limits the hemitransection of the proximal aorta for the anastomosis.

Recommendation

Postoperative management will consist of repeat laboratory tests and CT scans at 6 and 12 weeks. Further management depends on the resolution or progression of symptoms associated with the periaortic inflammation.

Suggested Readings

Bonamigo TP, Bianco C, Becker M, Puricelli F. Inflammatory aneurysms of infra-renal abdominal aorta. A case-control study. *Minerva Cardioangiol.* 2002;50:253-258.

Deleersnijder R, Daenens K, Fourneau I, Maleux G, Nevelsteen A. Endovascular repair of inflammatory abdominal aortic aneurysms with special reference to concomitant ureteric obstruction. *Eur J Vasc Endovasc Surg.* 2002;24:146-149.

Haug ES, Skomsvoll JF, Jacobsen G, Halvorsen TB, Saether OD, Myhre HO. Inflammatory aortic aneurysm is associated with increased incidence of autoimmune disease. *J Vasc Surg.* 2003;38:492-497.

Pennell RC, Hollier LH, Lie JT, et al. Inflammatory abdominal aortic aneurysms: a thirty-year review. *J Vasc Surg.* 1985;2:859-869.

Sterpetti AV, Hunter WJ, Feldhaus RJ, et al. Inflammatory aneurysms of the abdominal aorta: incidence, pathologic, and etiologic considerations. *J Vasc Surg.* 1989;9:643-650.

Sultan S, Duffy S, Madhavan P, et al. Fifteen-year experience of transperitoneal management of inflammatory abdominal aortic aneurysms. *Eur J Vasc Endovasc Surg.* 1999; 18:510-514.

Takagi H, Mori Y, Umeda Y, et al. Abdominal aortic aneurysm with arteritis in ankylosing spondylitis. *J Vasc Surg.* 2003;38:613-616.

Teruya TH, Abou-Zamzam AM, Ballard JL. Inflammatory abdominal aortic aneurysm treated by endovascular stent grafting: a case report. *Vasc Surg.* 2001;35:391-395.

Gilbert R. Upchurch, Jr., MD, and David M. Williams, MD

Presentation

A 57-year-old man with no significant past medical history presents to an outside emergency department complaining of sharp, tearing back pain that is unrelenting in nature. The patient is found to have a blood pressure of approximately 180/95 mm Hg in both arms and is in obvious distress. He is treated with intravenous morphine, with slight improvement in his pain. The patient denies abdominal pain. He has a normal electrocardiogram (ECG). His laboratory values are remarkable for a hematocrit of 39%, a creatinine of 3.2 mg/dL, and no troponin leak. Given the significant elevation in creatinine in the setting of chest pain, the emergency department physician is concerned about an acute aortic dissection. Magnetic resonance angiogram (MRA) is not available at the small outside hospital on an emergency basis. Therefore, the patient is started on a Nipride drip and med-flighted to your institution. An emergency aortic MRA is ordered. Progressive azotemia is noted in the setting of oliguria.

▮ Aortic MRA

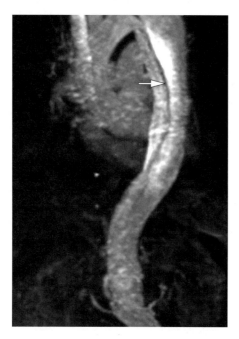

Figure 26-1

MRA Report

A Stanford B or type III aortic dissection (*arrow*) beginning just distal to the left subclavian artery and extending through the abdominal aorta. In addition, there is aneurysmal dilatation of the descending thoracic and abdominal aorta. The descending thoracic aorta measures between 3.6 and 3.8 cm. At the level of the diaphragm, the aorta measures 4 cm. In the infrarenal location, the aorta measures 4 cm with significant thrombus. The true lumen supplies the celiac artery, the superior mesenteric artery, and the right renal artery, whereas the false lumen supplies the left kidney. Both kidneys appear to be equally perfused.

Differential Diagnosis

The differential diagnosis for a patient presenting with the acute onset of sharp or ripping back pain in a patient with hypertension includes myocardial infarction, esophageal disease, gastroesophageal reflux, and aortic dissection. Given the MRA findings, the diagnosis of an acute Stanford B thoracic aortic dissection is confirmed.

Discussion

Diseases of the aorta, including aortic dissection, are the 14th leading cause of death in the United States. Knowledge of dissections is therefore important because it is one of the most serious and common diseases affecting the aorta. If unrecognized, acute aortic dissections are often fatal. Aortic dissections occur when a tear in the aortic wall is perpetuated along the length of the aorta allowing blood to forcefully separate the layers of the vessel wall. Typically, aortic dissections or tears occur from the intima into the media, creating a true and false lumen.

Aortic dissections are classified based on both their anatomic location and the time from onset. Anatomically, a Stanford A dissection involves the ascending aorta and possibly aortic valve, whereas a Stanford B dissection involves the descending thoracic aorta, distal to the subclavian artery. Aortic dissections are classified as acute (less than 14 days) or chronic (greater than 14 days) based on the time from the onset of symptoms.

Predisposing factors associated with an aortic dissection include hypertension, bicuspid aortic valve, coarctation of the aorta, and connective tissue disorders (Marfan and Ehlers-Danlos syndromes) and cocaine abuse. Intra-aortic catheterization and a history of cardiac surgery, particularly aortic valve replacement, are also associated with an increased incidence of aortic dissection.

The classic clinical presentation in a patient with an acute aortic dissection consists of the sudden onset of severe pain, often described as ripping or tearing, radiating to the interscapular or back region. Typically, this occurs in late middle-aged men, similar to the present patient.

Recommendations

Given the diagnosis of an acute type B thoracic aortic dissection in the setting of worsening azotemia, an arteriogram is indicated to better determine the exact anatomy of the dissection. More importantly, attempts at aortic fenestration or stent grafting can be performed if pressure gradients can be determined in the renal arteries. In addition, a transesophageal echocardiogram (TEE) is ordered.

TEE Report

Normal aortic valve with no wall motion abnormalities in either the right or left ventricle. A Stanford B dissection is noted just distal to the left subclavian artery.

Case Continued

Both groins were prepped and draped in the usual sterile fashion, and the skin and subcutaneous tissues over the common femoral arteries were infiltrated with 1% lidocaine for local anesthesia. Initially, the right common femoral artery was punctured. The puncture tract was dilated to a 7 French sheath over a wire. Subsequently, the left common femoral artery was punctured and the puncture tract was dilated to accommodate a 10 French sheath over a guide wire. Initially, intravascular ultrasound was performed from the arch to the iliac arteries. A selective arteriogram of the superior mesenteric artery, bilateral renal arteries, the true lumen, and false lumen of the aortic dissection was also performed. Pressure measurements were obtained at each level. A dynamic obstruction due to complete collapse of the visceral arteries was noted during the cardiac cycle. Both the celiac artery and the superior mesenteric artery originate from the true lumen of the dissection. The right renal artery comes off the true lumen as well, but the left renal artery comes off the false lumen. In addition to the aortic dissection, multiple severe stenotic lesions are demonstrated in divisional and segmental branches of bilateral renal arteries. In addition, there is aneurysmal dilatation of the distal infrarenal aorta with partial clot formation, particularly in the false lumen. The true lumen shows severe elastic recoil and collapse of the true lumen at the level of the renal arteries.

Although no significant pressure gradient was noted between the true and false lumen of the aorta, there was a curtain-type collapse of the origin of the visceral arteries. Subsequently, a fenestration was performed at the level of the superior mesenteric artery as well as at the level of the renal artery origins (Fig. 26-2A). Stenting of the completely collapsed infrarenal abdominal aorta was performed (Fig. 26-2B).

■ Angiogram

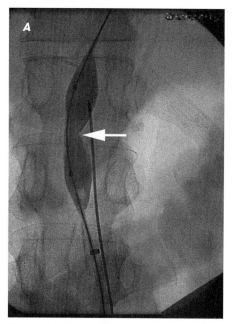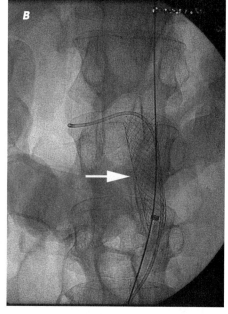

Figure 26-2A and B

Angiogram Report

Given the curtain-type collapse of the abdominal aorta at the level of the renal arteries, 2 fenestrations with 16-mm balloon dilatation catheters were performed at the level of the renal arteries (*arrow*) and at the level of the superior mesenteric artery-celiac artery (Fig. 26-2A). Following this, however, there was continued collapse of the true lumen at the level of the renal arteries. Therefore, a Wallstent (*arrow*) measuring 40 mm × 4 cm was placed in the infrarenal abdominal aorta (see Fig. 26-2B).

Diagnosis

Malperfusion of visceral and renal arteries secondary to acute Stanford B dissection.

Case Continued

Following diagnosis and treatment of malperfusion of the visceral and renal arteries, the patient was admitted to the intensive care unit and started on a beta-blocker and Nipride to control his heart rate and blood pressure. The patient was pain free following fenestration, suggesting that the acute pain he experienced was from his acute dissection, rather than from his small abdominal aortic aneurysm. The patient was discharged to home on post-fenestration day 7 on appropriate antihypertensive medications.

Recommendation

At 4-year follow-up, the patient's renal function has not worsened and remains approximately 3.5 mg/dL. The patient undergoes yearly MRAs to follow his thoracic and abdominal aortic diameter, with no significant expansion of either noted to date.

Discussion

Because malperfusion doubles the mortality of aortic dissection, prompt restoration of blood flow to critical vessels is necessary. For type A dissections, open aortic reconstruction is approximately 95% effective in reversing branch artery obstruction. However, prolonged malperfusion with evidence of end-organ ischemia may contraindicate immediate open repair. For type B dissections, medical treatment is indicated unless, as in this patient, there is malperfusion, unrelenting chest pain, or expansion of the false lumen.

Aortic dissection causes malperfusion by 2 principal mechanisms, which are determined by the relation of the dissection flap to origins of critical aortic branches, and which require different modes of treatment. When the dissection flap enters a critical branch artery and occludes the lumen (static obstruction), treatment consists of stenting the vessel open. When the dissection flap lies across a vessel origin like a curtain (dynamic obstruction), treatment consists of creating a hole (fenestration) in the flap to allow pressure equilibration and blood flow between the 2 lumens. This patient had malperfusion due to both mechanisms. The short-term outcome of these patients is determined by the ischemic damage sustained by the obstructed organ prior to restoration of flow, and to false lumen rupture in those patients whose aortic reconstruction has been delayed while recovering from the reperfusion injury.

Suggested Readings

Cambria RP, Brewster DC, Gertler J, et al. Vascular complications associated with spontaneous aortic dissection. *J Vasc Surg.* 1988;7: 199-209.

Deeb GM, Williams DM, Quint LE, Monaghan HM, Shea MJ. Risk analysis for aortic surgery using hypothermic circulatory arrest with retrograde cerebral perfusion. *Ann Thorac Surg.* 1999;67:1883-1886.

Hagan PB, Nienaber CA, Isselbacher EM, et al. The International Registry of Acute Aortic Dissection (IRAD). New insights into an old disease. *JAMA.* 2000;283:897-903.

Klompas M. Does this patient have an acute aortic dissection? *JAMA.* 2002;287:2262-2272.

Nienaber CA, Eagle KA. Aortic dissection: new frontiers in diagnosis and management. Part 1: From etiology to diagnostic strategies. *Circulation.* 2003;108:628-635.

Williams DM, Lee DY, Hamilton BH, et al. The dissected aorta. Percutaneous treatment of ischemic complications: Principles and results. *J Vasc Interven Radiol.* 1997;8:605-625.

Williams DM, Lee DY, Hamilton BH, et al. The dissected aorta: III. Anatomy and radiologic diagnosis of branch-vessel compromise. *Radiology.* 1997;203:37-44.

Omaida C. Velazquez, MD, FACS

Presentation

A 64-year-old woman presents to your office for consultation on treatment options for an asymptomatic enlarging abdominal aortic aneurysm (AAA). Five years prior, she suffered a myocardial infarction and underwent coronary artery bypass grafting. Her past surgical history also includes 3 prior laparotomies for a hysterectomy and two subsequent bowel obstructions. She has a 50-pack year history of smoking cigarettes and continues to smoke despite medical counseling on smoking cessation. She has a known AAA that was incidentally noted on plain radiographs performed for lower lumbar pain 3 years prior. Most recently, on an outside computed tomography (CT) scan the aneurysm was noted to have increased from 5.5 cm to 6.8 cm in maximum anteroposterior (AP) diameter over 6 months. She denies any symptoms of abdominal, back, or flank pain, or pain with ambulation, but she lives a sedentary life.

On physical examination, a nontender AAA can be palpated. Her femoral pulses are decreased, but palpable. Her peripheral pulses are not palpable; however, there is good capillary refill with no edema, ulceration, or tissue loss. The rest of her physical examination is unremarkable. She inquires whether she may be a candidate for a "stent-graft" repair of her AAA.

Her medical records contain results of a Persantine stress thallium test from approximately 3 weeks ago that indicate an abnormal myocardial scar involving the inferolateral region of the left ventricle, but no evidence of reversible myocardial ischemia. The laboratory examinations are normal, including blood urea nitrogen (BUN) of 14 mg/dL and creatinine level of 0.6 mg/dL.

■ CT Angiogram of the Abdomen, Axial Images

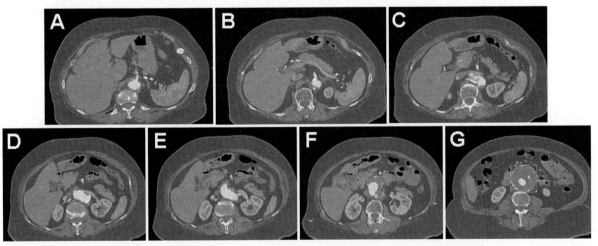

Figure 27-1 **(A)** Celiac axis **(B)** Superior mesenteric artery (SMA) **(C)** Right renal artery (R-RA) **(D)** Between R-RA and left renal artery (L-RA) **(E)** L-RA **(F)** 3 mm distal to the L-RA **(G)** Maximum AAA AP diameter; the superimposed mark measures a diameter of 6.76 cm.

CT Angiogram Report

Outside CT angiogram report suggests the presence of a pararenal AAA measuring 6.8 cm in maximum diameter. The proximal extent of the AAA appears to extend to the level of the left renal artery and distally to the aortic bifurcation. Fine cuts are not available.

Differential Diagnosis

Abdominal aortic aneurysms are often diagnosed incidentally with radiographic imaging such as plain radiographs, ultrasounds, CT scans, or magnetic resonance imaging obtained for other reasons. Patients commonly have intermittent abdominal, flank, lower back, or hip pain that prompted the imaging studies. However, such nonspecific signs and symptoms may not be specifically related to the presence of an aortic aneurysm, and therefore the diagnoses rest mostly on accurate radiographic imaging. Physical examination may also reveal a palpable pulsatile abdominal mass.

Most AAAs remain asymptomatic until they present with contained or free rupture, which is commonly associated with sudden severe abdominal or back pain and syncope. An overall mortality of close to 90% occurs in patients with ruptured AAAs. In these acute presentations, the key differential diagnoses are aortic dissection and acute myocardial infarction.

Approach

Based on the patient's history of an expanding abdominal aortic aneurysm, the films are reviewed in detail to determine whether the aneurysm is infrarenal, pararenal, suprarenal, thoracoabdominal, associated with iliac or other aortic branch aneurysms, associated with aortic dissection, or associated with arterial occlusive disease.

Recommendation

The abdominal CT angiogram suggests that the aneurysm extends cephalad to the origin of the left renal artery. The axial images also suggest significant angulation of the aorta, which may obscure a small length of normal aorta beneath the renal arteries. A repeat CT scan with 3-dimensional reconstructions and intravenous contrast is recommended.

◼ CT Scan with 3-Dimensional Reconstructions

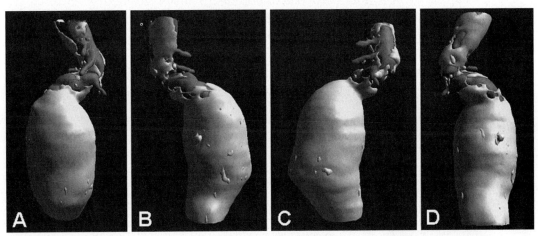

Figure 27-2 (A) Anterior-posterior, (B) Right-lateral, (C) Left-lateral, (D) Posterior-anterior

3-Dimensional CT Scan Report

Axial CT scan with 3-dimensional reconstructions (A, anterior-posterior; B, right-lateral; C, left-lateral; D, posterior-anterior) document a pararenal AAA.

◼ Approach

Because the aneurysm extends to the level of the left renal artery, the patient is not a candidate for endovascular AAA repair using any of the currently available endografts approved by the U.S. Food and Drug Administration (FDA). It is unclear whether the proximal aortic clamp can be placed between the renal arteries, suprarenally, or in the supraceliac position. Significant thrombus is present, along with calcium within the aorta (see Fig. 27-2A, B, D). Clamping above the left renal artery, but below the right renal artery, would be ideal in this case; however, you are concerned by the severe calcification (Fig. 27-2C) at this level. Calcification such as this may injure the aorta at the clamp site and pose technical difficulties with suture placement and suture-line hemostasis. Ultimately, the definitive optimal clamp site will be determined in the operating room on direct observation and palpation of the aorta.

A pararenal AAA extends to the origin of one renal artery, sometimes more, but does not include the visceral arteries. During open repair of a pararenal AAA, the optimal proximal clamp is placed below one of the renals or between the superior mesenteric artery and the highest renal artery. Distally, pararenal aneurysms may be limited to the aorta or extend to one or both iliac arteries. In addition, they may present in conjunction with an aortic dissection, aortoiliac occlusive disease, and/or renal artery stenosis. In general, the indications for surgical intervention for such associated pathology are the same as if the pathology presented in isolation.

Recommendation

Based on decreased femoral pulses on physical examination and a history of peripheral arterial disease, baseline studies of lower extremities with bilateral lower extremity pulse volume recordings (PVRs) are recommended. The imaging is completed with a noninvasive gadolinium-enhanced magnetic resonance angiography (MRA) of the abdomen and pelvis.

Gadolinium-Enhanced MRA

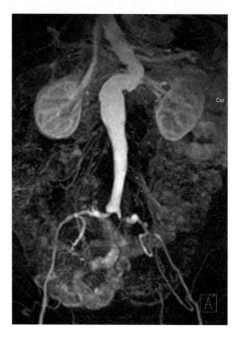

Figure 27-3

MRA Report

There are bilateral proximal common iliac artery stenoses and extremely diminutive external iliac arteries bilaterally. A short segment occlusion (potentially only a signal void from high-grade stenosis) of the left external iliac artery is also noted. Note that the gadolinium only enhances flow and not the surrounding thrombus, calcium, and dilated aortic wall.

Case Continued

The lower extremity PVRs are consistent with physical examination and the MRA findings. There is a significant gradient across the pelvic inflow vessels with decreased pressures at the proximal thighs. There is also evidence of infrainguinal arterial occlusive disease. However, there is relative preservation of pulsatile waveforms down to the ankles, with ankle-brachial indices over 0.6 bilaterally.

Diagnosis and Recommendation

You diagnose a rapidly enlarging 6.8-cm pararenal, asymptomatic abdominal aortic aneurysm. This pararenal AAA is associated with iliac occlusive disease. Prompt elective open repair is recommended.

Owing to the systemic nature of the vascular pathology present in this patient, a carotid ultrasound, echocardiogram, and pulmonary function tests are ordered, though the decision to perform these tests is surgeon-specific.

Other Diagnostic Test Reports

Carotid ultrasound: Hemodynamically significant stenoses of the cervical carotid arteries are not present.

Echocardiogram: Preservation of the myocardial function with an ejection fraction of 40%.

Pulmonary function: Severe chronic obstructive pulmonary disease (COPD) with forced expiratory volume in 1 second (FEV_1) of 33% of predicted.

Recommendation

Considering the associated COPD and the history of prior multiple abdominal operations, a retroperitoneal approach for aneurysm repair is recommended. You discuss with the patient the coexisting occlusive disease and the fact that you do not recommend concurrent iliac revascularization, unless it proves necessary. The patient has no history of claudication or rest pain and no evidence of impending tissue loss, and has relatively preserved pulsatile PVR waveforms distally. Therefore, the operation is limited to open repair of the AAA.

Approach

In this patient, who has both aneurysmal and occlusive disease with significant associated cardiac and pulmonary comorbidities, the life-threatening problem is addressed first with concurrent vascular issues followed. The plan is to repair the AAA using a retroperitoneal approach, which is associated with decreased pulmonary comorbidity. This approach also affords excellent exposure to both the infrarenal and suprarenal aorta. The patient is reassured that the iliac disease is easily amenable to percutaneous angioplasty and stenting postoperatively, if needed.

Surgical Approach

A left retroperitoneal incision starts at the lateral border of the left rectus muscle midway between the pubis and umbilicus. It extends superiorly (5 cm medial to the anterior-superior iliac spine), curving upward and laterally at the costal margin to follow the course of the 10th interspace. Incisions centered lower, onto the 11th or 12th rib, offer less exposure. Leaving the left kidney posterior hinders the degree of exposure when dealing with aortic aneurysmal disease. Therefore, cephalad exposure of the suprarenal aorta is facilitated by mobilizing the left kidney anteriorly. The left crus of the diaphragm is divided. The lumbar branch of the left renal vein can be particularly wide and short, and will require careful ligation and division to facilitate the exposure without untoward bleeding.

Discussion

In this patient, a conscious decision is made to focus on the pararenal AAA via a retroperitoneal approach. An equally effective approach might be to use a bifurcated graft with 2 distal anastomoses end-to-end onto the iliac arteries. In this case, however, because there is also a short-segment occlusion of the left external iliac artery, the surgeon would need to oversew the left common iliac artery and do an end-to-side anastomosis to the left external iliac artery or tunnel the graft under the ureter and inguinal ligament, and perform an end-to-side anastomosis to the left common femoral artery. This can technically be accomplished via a left retroperitoneal approach, sacrificing only the unavoidable increase in operative time. However, repair of occlusive disease in this asymptomatic patient is not recommended. Other technical issues associated with the use of a retroperitoneal approach include difficulties encountered when trying to expose the right renal artery and distal right iliac artery.

Suggested Readings

Cronenwett JL, Krupski C, Rutherford RB. Abdominal aortic and iliac aneurysms. In: Rutherford RB, ed. *Vascular Surgery*. 5th ed. Philadelphia, Pa: WB Saunders; 2000:1246-1280.

Goldstone J. Aneurysms of the aorta and iliac arteries. In: Moore WS, ed. *Vascular Surgery: A Comprehensive Review*. 6th ed. Philadelphia, Pa: WB Saunders; 2002:457-480.

Lederle FA. Abdominal aortic aneurysm: open repair versus watchful waiting. In: Pearce WH, Yao JST, eds. *Advances in Vascular Surgery, Current Management of Pathology of Aorta and Its Major Branches*. Chicago, Il: Precept Press; 2002:195-199.

Rutherford RB. Retroperitoneal approaches to the abdominal aorta. In: Rutherford RB, ed. *Atlas of Vascular Surgery: Basic Techniques and Exposures*. Philadelphia, Pa: WB Saunders; 1993:194-209.

Turnipseed WD. Minimal incision aortic surgery. In: Pearce WH, Yao JST, eds. *Advances in Vascular Surgery, Current Management of Pathology of Aorta and its Major Branches*. Chicago, Il: Precept Press; 2002:201-207.

Wind GG, Valentine RJ. Abdominal aorta. In: Wind GG, Valentine RJ, eds. *Anatomic Exposures in Vascular Surgery*. Philadelphia, Pa: Williams & Wilkins; 1991:211-234.

Scott A. Berceli, MD, PhD

Presentation

A 72-year-old man presents to the emergency department for evaluation of back pain. On initial questioning, he describes the onset of pain approximately 8 hours ago, with an intensity of 4/10, but over the last 2 hours the pain has increased in intensity to 8/10. The mid-lumbar pain is bilateral and continuous, and does not improve with changes in position. Specific questioning concerning an inciting traumatic event for the pain (eg, heavy lifting, recent fall) fails to identify an etiology.

His past medical history is significant for hypertension and coronary artery disease, with a previous history of myocardial infarction and coronary angioplasty 5 years ago. He denies a history of prior back pain and has not previously been evaluated for an abdominal aortic aneurysm (AAA), but reports that his brother had repair of an aortic aneurysm 3 years ago. His current medications are hydrochlorothiazide and aspirin, and he is currently smoking 1 pack per day of cigarettes, with a 60 pack-year smoking history.

Differential Diagnosis

The initial presentation of a patient with a ruptured AAA can be variable, and the differential diagnosis is developed based on their presenting constellation of symptoms. In one series, 82% of patients with aortic rupture complained of abdominal pain and 57% of back pain. With potential chief complaints involving back, abdominal, or groin pain, the diagnostic possibilities for these patients can be extensive (Table 28-1). An appropriate differential diagnosis for this patient presenting with acute onset of back pain would include paravertebral muscle spasm, vertebral fracture, lumbar radiculopathy, aortic rupture or dissection, ureteral obstruction, pyelonephritis, or pancreatitis.

Identified factors that predispose a patient to development of an AAA include male gender, increasing age, family history, hypertension, and smoking. This patient presents with all 5 of these risk factors, increasing the likelihood that his pain is secondary to a symptomatic aneurysm.

Case Continued

Vital signs on presentation are temperature 37.9°C, blood pressure 122/72 mm Hg, and heart rate 98 beats per minute. Examination of the patient's back reveals no obvious vertebral deformity and no lumbar tenderness on palpation. Abdominal examination reveals mid-abdominal tenderness with guarding, but no evidence of peritoneal irritation. Deep palpation in the periumbilical area identifies an indiscreet mass with pulsatility. No abdominal or inguinal hernias are identified, and rectal examination demonstrates no palpable masses and guaiac-negative stool. A straight leg raise, with the patient in a supine position,

Table 28-1. Differential diagnosis for back, abdominal, and groin pain in patients presenting to an emergency room

	Presenting Symptom		
	Back Pain	**Abdominal Pain**	**Groin Pain**
Gastrointestinal	Pancreatitis	Perforated viscus	Inguinal hernia
	Perforating duodenal ulcer	Mesenteric ischemia	
	Strangulated hernia		
	Acute cholecystitis		
	Ruptured appendicitis		
	Diverticulitis		
Genitourinary	Ureteral calculus		Testicular torsion
	Pyelonephritis		Epididymitis
Vascular	Ruptured AAA	Ruptured AAA	Ruptured iliac artery
	Symptomatic AAA	Symptomatic AAA	aneurysm
	Aortic dissection		
Musculoskeletal	Paravertebral muscle spasms		
	Vertebral fracture		
Neurologic	Lumbar radiculopathy		

AAA = abdominal aortic aneurysm.

can be achieved to 90 degrees without a significant increase in pain bilaterally. Femoral, popliteal, and pedal pulses are normal in both extremities.

Discussion

The clinical triad of sudden onset of abdominal (or back) pain, hypotension, and pulsatile abdominal mass is characteristic of a ruptured AAA. Unfortunately, only about 50% of the patients with ruptured AAAs present with all components of this triad. The current patient has back pain and a pulsatile abdominal mass, and may be relatively hypotensive if his systemic hypertension is poorly controlled. With this constellation of symptoms, ruptured AAA must be considered among the most likely diagnostic possibilities.

Management options at this point in the work-up are dictated by the hemodynamic stability of the patient. Patients with significant hypotension and a high degree of suspicion for a ruptured AAA should be transported emergently to the operating room for surgical intervention. For patients presenting to medical facilities unable to offer urgent surgical repair, rapid stabilization and transport to an appropriate institution should be expedited.

In a patient with stable vital signs, additional diagnostic work-up may be undertaken if immediately available. Preoperative computed tomography (CT) imaging is critical for accurate diagnosis, and may expand the surgical options to include endovascular repair of the AAA; therefore, CT imaging should be considered in the hemodynamically stable patient. Prior to proceeding, large-bore peripheral intravenous catheters should be placed, and a blood sample sent for cross matching. The abdominal/pelvic CT scan should be obtained using a

3-mm (thin)-cut protocol with intravenous contrast. The use of oral contrast will provide little diagnostic information and only further delay proceeding with surgical therapy. Continuous electrocardiographic (ECG) and automatic blood pressure monitoring, along with direct supervision of the study by a trained medical professional, is essential during this phase of the patient's care.

While retroperitoneal ultrasonography has an important role in the initial diagnosis and sequential monitoring of *asymptomatic* AAAs, ultrasound imaging has only limited utility in the diagnosis and management of *symptomatic* aneurysms. With poor sensitivity in identifying or excluding retroperitoneal hematoma, emergency ultrasound may be used sparingly in the unstable patient to confirm or exclude the presence of an infrarenal AAA, when the etiology for the hemodynamic deterioration remains uncertain.

Case Continued

The patient is alert and remains hemodynamically stable during his initial evaluation. He is immediately transported to radiology and a CT scan is obtained.

▨ CT Scan

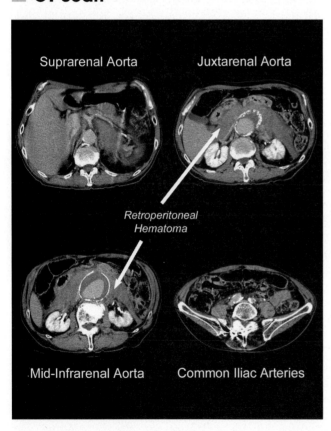

Figure 28-1

CT Scan Report

An abdominal aortic aneurysm with a maximal diameter of 6.7 cm is seen extending from the renal arteries to the aortic bifurcation. A large retroperitoneal hematoma is seen extending from the superior mesenteric artery to the aortic bifurcation. Although no contrast extravasation outside of the aorta is visualized, this appearance is characteristic for a contained aortic rupture. Detailed examination of the infrarenal aorta demonstrates a proximal neck diameter of 25 mm and a proximal neck length of 9 mm. Common iliac arteries are nonaneurysmal, with a maximum diameter of 14 mm on the right and 12 mm on the left.

Recommendation

With an inadequate infrarenal neck for placement of an aortic endograft, the patient is taken emergently from radiology to the operating room for surgical exploration and aneurysm repair.

Discussion

Although patients with a symptomatic, intact (nonruptured) AAA may be admitted to a monitored care setting for a short period of medical optimization, patients demonstrating radiographic evidence of a AAA rupture require immediate surgical intervention. Operative choices include open surgical repair and, in centers with the appropriate expertise and resources, endovascular repair. Although the role of endovascular repair in the treatment of aneurysm rupture is evolving, initial reports suggest marked improvement over the substantial mortality and morbidity of open surgical intervention.

Suitable candidates for endovascular AAA repair are primarily determined by the morphologic characteristics of the infrarenal neck of the aneurysm. Devices that are currently approved by the US Food and Drug Administration (FDA) require a neck diameter less than 28 mm and a neck length greater than 15 mm. Although this patient has an adequate neck diameter, the 9-mm neck length precludes endograft repair.

Surgical Approach

Prior to the initial arrival of the patient with a suspected ruptured AAA, the operating room and anesthesia staff is contacted to begin preparations for emergency transfer to the operating room. Preoperative preparations include type and cross matching of red blood cells, platelets, and plasma; the administration of prophylactic antibiotics; and the assembly of a cell-scavenging system in the operating room. Transport to the operating room and initiation of the operation is expedited. In centers with an established protocol for patients with suspected aneurysm rupture, triage from arrival to operation can be completed in 12 minutes.

Before induction of general anesthesia, the patient is prepped and draped from his nipples to his toes. Immediately upon induction, the operation is initiated through a vertical midline abdominal incision, extending from the xiphoid process to the pubis. With the large pararenal hematoma seen in this patient, proximal vascular control is obtained at the level of the diaphragm. Aided by placement of a nasogastric tube for identification of the esophagus, the supraceliac aorta is rapidly isolated from surrounding tissues and a vascular clamp placed in position, in case immediate aortic occlusion is required. If the retroperitoneal hematoma remains intact and the patient remains hemodynamically stable, distal control of the common iliac arteries may be performed. Following occlusion of the proximal and distal clamps, the retroperitoneal hematoma is entered and exposure of the infrarenal aorta is initiated. When an adequate infrarenal aortic neck is identified for placement of a vascular clamp, removal of the supraceliac clamp and perfusion of the abdominal viscera may be performed. The aneurysm sac is incised longitudinally along its length and the intramural thrombus removed. Bleeding lumbar arteries are ligated from inside the aneurysm with interrupted suture ligatures. The patency of the inferior mesenteric artery should be preserved for later consideration of reimplantation should colon ischemia develop. Replacement of the aorta is then begun with either a straight or bifurcated graft, depending on the presence of iliac artery aneurysms. After choosing an appropriate sized Dacron or polytetrafluoroethylene (PTFE) graft (usually 16 or 18 mm in diameter), the proximal graft is sutured to the infrarenal neck in an end-to-end fashion. The graft is then occluded and the proximal clamp (either supraceliac or infrarenal) removed. An end-to-end distal anastomosis (anastomoses) to either the distal aorta or common iliac arteries completes the repair. Upon removal of the distal clamps and reperfusion of the lower extremities, aggressive resuscitation with platelets and fresh-frozen plasma is initiated. After evaluation of the retroperitoneum to control other sites of bleeding, the aneurysm sac is re-approximated over the prosthetic graft and the abdomen closed. For patients with a large retroperitoneal hematoma and massive bowel edema, primary closure of the abdominal wall may not be possible, and temporary closure with a prosthetic patch may be required.

Case Continued

No significant aneurysmal dilation of the iliac arteries was identified, and the patient undergoes a tube graft repair of his infrarenal abdominal aorta. Estimated blood loss was 5,400 mL. Intraoperatively, he was administered 8500 mL of crystalloid, 1200 mL of cell-saver blood, 4 units of packed red blood cells, 6 units of platelets, and 2 units of fresh-frozen plasma. His abdomen was amenable to primary closure. Femoral pulses were palpable and pedal pulses were present by continuous-wave Doppler. He is transported to the intensive care unit intubated and hemodynamically stable.

Over the next 48 hours, he has intermittent episodes of hypotension that respond to the bolus administration of intravenous crystalloid solution. Since admission to the ICU, serum bicarbonate has decreased from 21 to 16 mmol/L, platelet count has decreased from 115,000 to 65,000 /mm^3, and lactic acid has increased from 1.9 to 3.4 mmol/L. Later that day, he is noted to pass 400 mL of maroon-colored stool. A sigmoidoscopy performed at the bedside demonstrates patchy areas of mucosal ischemia within the descending and sigmoid colon. He is placed on broad-spectrum intravenous antibiotics with plans for operative intervention should his condition deteriorate. Over the next 5 days, his thrombocytopenia and acidosis improve, and repeat sigmoidoscopy shows several areas of mucosal sloughing with no areas of focal necrosis.

The patient remains stable until postoperative day 9, when he becomes febrile with an elevated white blood cell count. Chest radiography reveals an infiltrate in the right lower lobe, and sputum culture is positive for *Pseudomonas aeruginosa*. He is treated with a 10-day course of antibiotics, with no further evidence of septicemia. Despite a resolving infiltrate on his chest radiograph, attempts to wean him from the ventilator are unsuccessful. On postoperative day 19, he undergoes tracheostomy placement.

Over the next 2 weeks, the patient is weaned from the ventilator, but requires the tracheostomy for frequent suctioning. As his nutritional status slowly improves, he is able to handle respiratory secretions more effectively. His tracheostomy is removed and he is discharged to a rehabilitation facility on postoperative day 42.

Discussion

Although the mortality rates for elective AAA repair range from 2% to 5%, mortality rates following operative repair of a ruptured AAA, even in high-volume centers, range from 45% to 65%. In patients who present with acute rupture and hypovolemic shock, the mortality rate approaches 95%.

Postoperative complications and the resulting mortality can be substantial. Experience from Harborview Medical Center demonstrated 61% morbidity in the intensive care unit following surgical intervention for a ruptured AAA. Most frequent postoperative complications include respiratory failure (48%), renal failure (29%), and sepsis (24%). Among the most lethal complications is ischemic colitis. Occurring early in the postoperative period, clinical findings include bloody diarrhea, metabolic acidosis, sepsis, and thrombocytopenia. Seen in 18% of patients following ruptured AAA repair, ischemic colitis resulted in a 2-fold increase in the mortality rate and was responsible for 1 out of 5 deaths in the ICU. Diagnosis is usually confirmed by flexible sigmoidoscopy, with evaluation for transmural ischemia critical in the decision-making process. Although ischemic injury isolated to the mucosa can initially be treated nonoperatively, close observation is warranted. Development of transmural ischemia, worsening sepsis, or peritoneal signs all require prompt surgical intervention with resection of involved colon.

Suggested Readings

Gloviczki P, Pairolero PC, Mucha P Jr., et al. Ruptured abdominal aortic aneurysms: repair should not be denied. *J Vasc Surg.* 1992;15:851-857.

Johansen K, Kohler TR, Nicholls SC, Zierler RE, Clowes AW, Kazmers A. Ruptured abdominal aortic aneurysm: the Harborview experience. *J Vasc Surg.* 1991;13:240-245.

Lederle FA, Wilson SE, Johnson GR, et al. Immediate repair compared with surveillance of small abdominal aortic aneurysms. *N Engl J Med.* 2002;346:1437-1444.

Meissner MH, Johansen KH. Colon infarction after ruptured abdominal aortic aneurysm. *Arch Surg.* 1992;127:979-985.

Verhoeven EL, Prins TR, van den Dungen JJ, Tielliu IF, Hulsebos RG, van Schilfgaarde R. Endovascular repair of acute AAAs under local anesthesia with bifurcated endografts: a feasibility study. *J Endovasc Ther.* 2002;9: 729-735.

Robert W. Thompson, MD, Federico E. Parodi, MD,
and Michel A. Bartoli, MD

Presentation

A 65-year-old man presents to your office after attending a community health fair, where he learned that he has an abdominal aortic aneurysm (AAA). The patient is a former cigarette smoker with mild hypertension, but has no other history of cardiovascular disease. His older brother had an aortic aneurysm repair at the age of 68. Physical examination reveals no pulsatile abdominal mass or tenderness, and there are strong bilateral femoral pulses by palpation.

Differential Diagnosis

An aneurysm is a focal or segmental enlargement of a blood vessel, most often defined as an increase in diameter to at least twice normal. Although the diameter of the abdominal aorta generally increases with age and is larger in men than women, an aortic diameter greater than 3.0 cm may be considered above the normal range expected for any age and gender. This size has therefore become the most commonly used definition of AAA in clinical practice. Asymptomatic AAAs occur in up to 9% of the population over the age of 65, and are known to be associated with atherosclerosis, hypertension, and cigarette smoking. AAAs are also more common in men than women. Approximately 15% to 20% of patients with AAAs will have a family history of aortic aneurysm.

Routine physical examination is inaccurate in detecting all but the largest AAAs, making it unsuitable in screening for this disease. In contrast, abdominal ultrasonography and other imaging studies are extremely accurate in detecting AAAs regardless of size. Ultrasonography is favored in screening for AAAs because it is noninvasive, requires no contrast enhancement, and can be done rapidly with low cost. Most health care insurers do not yet reimburse for abdominal ultrasounds performed as a screening test for AAAs; however, in many communities, such studies are available for a nominal fee as part of screening programs for cardiovascular disease. It is therefore likely that the diagnosis of AAA in this patient is accurate.

In addition to knowledge that this patient has an AAA, additional information is required to guide management. Thus, it is necessary to know the maximal size of the AAA, as well as its location with respect to the renal and iliac arteries.

Approach

A contrast-enhanced computed tomogram (CT) of the abdomen is obtained by spiral CT, complemented by post-imaging (3-dimensional) reconstruction.

Abdominal CT Scan With 3D Reconstruction

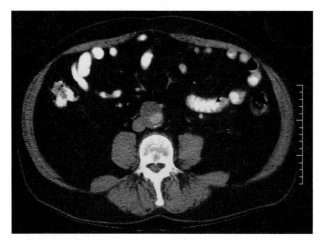

Figure 29-1

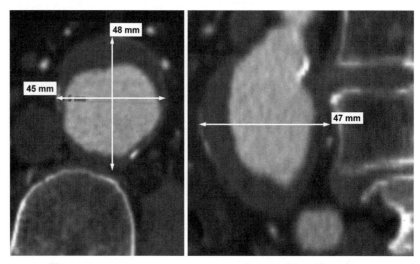

Transverse   **Longitudinal**

48 mm

45 mm

47 mm

Figure 29-2

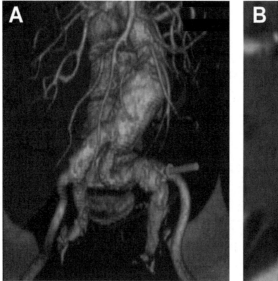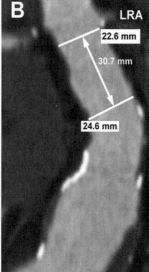

A

B

LRA

22.6 mm

30.7 mm

24.6 mm

Figure 29-3

CT Scan Report

There is an infrarenal aortic aneurysm with mural thrombus that extends into the common iliac arteries (Fig. 29-1). There is no evidence of mesenteric or renal artery stenosis, peri-aortic inflammation, or venous anomaly. Three-dimensional (3D) reconstruction of the CT images reveals maximal transverse dimensions measuring 48 mm × 45 mm (Fig. 29-2). There is mural thrombus present in the aneurysm sac, which is somewhat tortuous with extension into the common and internal iliac arteries (Fig. 29-3A). The diameter of the aorta at the level of the lowest (left) renal artery is 22.6 mm; the length of the aneurysm neck is 30.7 mm and the diameter of the aorta at this level is 24.6 mm with some angulation (Fig. 29-3B). The external iliac arteries do not exhibit occlusive atherosclerosis or aneurysmal dilatation.

Recommendation

In this case, CT imaging reveals a maximal AAA diameter of 4.8 cm. Because AAAs of this size have a relatively low risk for rupture, a strong recommendation cannot be made at this time for elective surgical repair. However, the measurements taken during CT imaging indicate that an endoluminal (stent-graft) approach would probably be feasible if elective AAA repair is selected, because there is a long infrarenal neck (more than 30 mm), the aortic diameter in this region is less than 25 mm, and there is minimal external iliac artery disease. However, there is some angulation at the neck and the left iliac artery is quite tortuous. To better inform decision making, you decide to further evaluate the patient's cardiopulmonary status and his risks for anesthesia.

Discussion

Assessment of Risk for Rupture

The principal risk of AAAs is death from rupture. Most patients with AAAs are asymptomatic prior to rupture and are unaware of their condition. The risk of aneurysm rupture is known to correlate with aneurysm size, with AAAs greater than 5.5 to 6.0 cm in diameter representing lesions with substantial risks of rupture (approximately 40% within several years of diagnosis). Although AAAs smaller than 5.5 cm carry a lower risk of rupture, their natural history is one of gradual enlargement and increasing risk of rupture over a period of several years. It is well established that elective surgical repair of large asymptomatic AAAs can prevent deaths from aneurysm rupture.

Clinical factors beyond aneurysm diameter alone may have some influence on the risk of rupture. For example, Cronenwett et al. reported increased rates of aneurysm expansion and rupture for patients with small AAAs and either severe chronic obstructive pulmonary disease (forced expiratory volume in 1 second [FEV1] < 1.0 liter) or poorly controlled hypertension (diastolic blood pressure > 110 mm Hg). Cigarette smoking is an independent risk factor for aneurysm expansion and may also influence the risk of rupture. The risk of rupture is also recognized to be greater in patients with a family history of AAAs. Recent evidence suggests that for AAAs of equal size, women may also have greater risks for AAA rupture than men.

Assessment of Risk for Repair

Any decision regarding elective repair of an asymptomatic AAA represents a balance between the estimated risk of rupture and the estimated risk of surgical repair. The risk of surgical repair is dependent on the patient's age and cardiopulmonary risk for anesthesia. It is therefore useful to have further information regarding the patient's cardiovascular status before making a final recommendation for management.

It is also important to consider the extent of aneurysm disease, because the risks of rupture and repair are considerably different for lesions extending above the renal arteries (juxtarenal or suprarenal AAAs) or into the chest (thoracoabdominal aortic aneurysms).

There is no evidence to suggest that decisions for elective repair of small AAAs should be any different for endoluminal versus open repair, because to date there is no proven difference in operative mortality rate between these two approaches for AAAs less than 5.5 cm in diameter.

Case Continued

The patient reports that he is physically active with no history of claudication, cerebrovascular disease, or myocardial infarction. He stopped smoking 2 years ago and takes no medications beyond one aspirin per day. Laboratory studies reveal total serum cholesterol and low-density-lipoprotein cholesterol levels within the normal range for age, normal fasting blood glucose, and a serum creatinine level of 0.8 mg/dL. An electrocardiogram and a plain chest radiograph are both normal, and he reports having a normal treadmill stress test within the past year.

Recommendation

The results of these tests indicate that the patient is at relatively low risk for a cardiovascular event, and would therefore be at low risk for an elective operation. He is also at low risk for aneurysm rupture. A balanced judgment must therefore be made on the benefit of elective AAA repair versus conservative (nonoperative) management with imaging surveillance to detect changes in aneurysm size.

Discussion

Two recent studies provide sound clinical evidence upon which to base this decision: the Aneurysm Detection and Management (ADAM) Trial in the US Veterans Affairs system, and the United Kingdom Small Aneurysm Trial (UKSAT). In each study, patients with AAAs less than 5.5 cm diameter were randomized to receive either early surgical repair or follow-up every 6 months with imaging surveillance, with elective repair performed if and when the AAA grew to a size greater than 5.5 cm. The results of these studies were surprisingly consistent and quite convincing: after nearly 5 years of follow-up, there was no survival benefit for early surgery compared to imaging surveillance. For the more recently completed ADAM Trial, these results were achieved even when the elective operative mortality rate for those undergoing early surgery was only 2.1%.

It is important to note that for the patients enrolled in the imaging surveillance arms of each of these trials, there was a 61% overall likelihood of having surgical repair within the follow-up period. There were also no instances of AAA rupture in these groups, and the indication for delayed repair was an observed increase in AAA size to greater than 5.5 cm. This demonstrates that imaging surveillance is a safe management strategy. In the ADAM trial, there was no increase in operative mortality for patients who underwent delayed AAA repair, countering the notion that operative risk would be higher several years after the initial diagnosis than if performed earlier. It is notable that the need for delayed repair was more likely in those with larger AAAs at the outset of surveillance: thus, 81% of patients with AAAs 5.0 to 5.5 cm in diameter eventually underwent repair.

Case Continued

Imaging surveillance is recommended and accepted by the patient, with follow-up CT scans scheduled for 6-month intervals. After 2 years of follow-up, there is no change in AAA size.

Discussion

As indicated here, current management of small asymptomatic AAAs consists largely of imaging surveillance and elective repair if and when aneurysm size reaches a diameter of 5.5 cm. There are no proven treatment approaches to reduce the rate of aneurysm expansion, nor are there means by which to accurately predict which patients will exhibit expansion. Active laboratory and clinical research efforts are currently underway to delineate the pathophysiology of AAAs, with the hope that new treatments might emerge for patients with small asymptomatic AAAs. Through these studies, it has become apparent that AAAs are characterized by a chronic immuno-inflammatory response within the aortic wall, which is accompanied by increased local production of matrix metalloproteinase and other tissue-destructive enzymes. These enzymes, in turn, are responsible for the degradation of structural proteins required to maintain aortic wall tensile strength (ie, elastin and collagen). Based on new methodology to measure aortic wall stresses, one of the approaches used in the future may involve detailed imaging-based stress analysis to identify patients at heightened risk of rupture. Another approach may be to use circulating markers of inflammation as a means to assess the risk of disease progression. It may soon be possible to attempt suppression of aneurysm growth through the use of pharmacologic agents that inhibit matrix metalloproteinases, such as doxycycline. For the present, it remains important to ensure that all patients with small AAAs receive optimal management of other cardiovascular risk factors, so as to help reduce their overall risk of adverse events even if the aneurysm itself remains clinically stable. Strong efforts to promote smoking cessation are vital and treatment with statins may also be of specific benefit. It is equally important to ensure that patients participating in an imaging surveillance program are indeed followed and monitored, because more than half can be expected to require AAA repair eventually.

Suggested Readings

Baxter BT, Pearce WH, Waltke EA, et al. Prolonged administration of doxycycline in patients with small asymptomatic abdominal aortic aneurysms: report of a prospective (phase II) multicenter study. *J Vasc Surg.* 2002;36:1-12.

Cronenwett JL, Sargent SK, Wall MH, et al. Variables that affect the expansion rate and outcome of small abdominal aortic aneurysms. *J Vasc Surg.* 1990;11:260-269.

Fillinger MF, Raghavan ML, Marra SP, et al. In vivo analysis of mechanical wall stress and abdominal aortic aneurysm rupture risk. *J Vasc Surg.* 2002;36:589-597.

Fink HA, Lederle FA, Roth CS, et al. The accuracy of physical examination to detect abdominal aortic aneurysm. *Arch Intern Med.* 2000;160:833-836.

Finlayson SR, Birkmeyer JD, Fillinger MF, Cronenwett JL. Should endovascular surgery lower the threshold for repair of abdominal aortic aneurysms? *J Vasc Surg.* 1999;29:973-985.

Greenhalgh RM, Brown LC, Kwong GP, et al. EVAR trial participants. Comparison of endovascular aneurysm repair with open repair in patients with abdominal aortic aneurysm (EVAR trial 1), 30-day operative mortality results; randomized controlled trial. *Lancet* 2004;364:843-848.

Kent KC, Zwolak RM, Jaff MR, et al. Screening for abdominal aortic aneurysm: a consensus statement. *J Vasc Surg.* 2004;39:267-269.

Lederle FA, Johnson GR, Wilson SE, et al. Prevalence and associations of abdominal aortic aneurysm detected through screening. Aneurysm Detection and Management (ADAM) Veterans Affairs Cooperative Study Group. *Ann Intern Med.* 1997;126:441-449.

Lederle FA, Wilson SE, Johnson GR, et al. Immediate repair compared with surveillance of small abdominal aortic aneurysms. *N Engl J Med.* 2002;346:1437-1444.

Lederle FA. Ultrasonographic screening for abdominal aortic aneurysms. *Ann Intern Med.* 2003;139:516-522.

MacSweeney ST, Ellis M, Worrell PC, et al. Smoking and growth rate of small abdominal aortic aneurysms. *Lancet.* 1994;344:651-652.

Powell JT. Familial clustering of abdominal aortic aneurysm: smoke signals, but no culprit genes. *Br J Surg.* 2003;90:1173-1174.

Thompson RW, Geraghty PJ, Lee JK. Abdominal aortic aneurysms: basic mechanisms and clinical implications. *Curr Prob Surg.* 2002; 39:93-232.

Wassef M, Baxter BT, Chisholm RL, et al. Pathogenesis of abdominal aortic aneurysms: a multidisciplinary research program supported by the National Heart, Lung, and Blood Institute. *J Vasc Surg.* 2001;34:730-738.

J. Gregor Modrall, MD

Presentation

A 68-year-old man with a history of alcoholic pancreatitis presents to the emergency department with right upper quadrant and epigastric abdominal pain, fevers, and chills. Vital signs include a temperature of 101.7°F, heart rate of 110 bpm, and blood pressure of 113/85 mm Hg. Abdominal examination reveals voluntary guarding in the upper abdomen. The white blood cell count is 19.7. Serum lipase, amylase, and liver function tests are normal. The patient is admitted with a presumptive diagnosis of pancreatitis. Intravenous hydration and antibiotics are initiated. Computed tomogram (CT) of the abdomen is obtained.

▧ CT Scan of the Abdomen

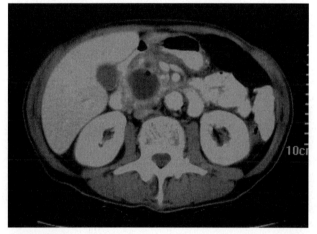

Figure 30-1

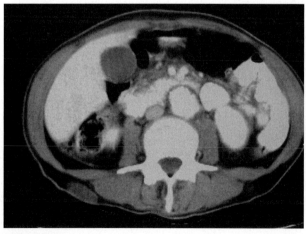

Figure 30-2

CT Scan Report

Extensive inflammatory changes surrounding the pancreas suggest pancreatitis. An 8-cm pancreatic phlegmon with loculated fluid and gas in the head of the pancreas (Fig. 30-1) is noted, suggesting a pancreatic abscess. A 3.9-cm infrarenal aortic aneurysm (Fig. 30-2) is present, which represents an interval change since the last CT scan (obtained 6 weeks earlier).

Differential Diagnosis

The CT scan findings are diagnostic for a pancreatic abscess, but the incidental finding of a new aortic aneurysm merits further discussion. The differential diagnosis for an abdominal aortic aneurysm (AAA) that develops or changes rapidly, particularly if this aneurysm is saccular in conformation, includes an infected AAA, aortic pseudoaneurysm (noninfected), aortic dissection, and noninfected atherosclerotic AAA. In a patient with a known intraabdominal or retroperitoneal infection and a newly diagnosed AAA, it must be assumed that this aneurysm represents an infected AAA until proven otherwise.

Discussion

Infected AAA refers to several pathologic conditions that lead to the presence of infection in an abdominal aortic aneurysm. Examples of infected AAAs include mycotic aneurysms due to endocarditis, microbial arteritis (from bacteremia) with aneurysm formation, infection of a preexisting AAA, and post-traumatic infected false aneurysms of the aorta. In most infected AAAs, the infection caused degeneration of the aorta to produce an aneurysm. Fewer than 5% of infected AAAs result from infection of a preexisting AAA. The most common site for an infected AAA is the infrarenal aorta (70%), but infected AAAs occasionally occur in the suprarenal or thoracic aorta.

Diagnosis of an infected AAA usually involves a high index of suspicion and imaging studies suggestive of the diagnosis. Clinical scenarios that should arouse clinical suspicion for an infected AAA include the presence of positive blood cultures in a patient with a known AAA, identification of a new AAA after a septic episode, and concurrent AAA and lumbar vertebral erosions. An antecedent history of a septic episode may be identified in approximately 61% of cases, but is not a requirement for the diagnosis. The most common presenting symptoms of an infected AAA are abdominal pain (92%), fever (77%), leukocytosis (69%), positive blood cultures (69%), palpable abdominal mass (46%), and rupture (31%).

Radiographic imaging should include both a contrast-enhanced CT scan and an arteriogram. CT findings suggestive of an infected AAA include the presence of a saccular aneurysm, evidence of partial aortic disruption or frank rupture, contiguous inflammatory changes, fluid collections, or air adjacent to an AAA. The vast majority of infected AAAs are saccular aneurysms, although infection of an existing aneurysm typically occurs in a fusiform aneurysm because most AAAs have a fusiform morphology. Arteriography often aids in the diagnosis by demonstrating saccular aneurysm morphology, and facilitates operative planning. A high-quality CT arteriogram (CTA) with 3-dimensional reconstruction may obviate the need for arteriography.

Recommendation

Arteriogram.

Arteriogram

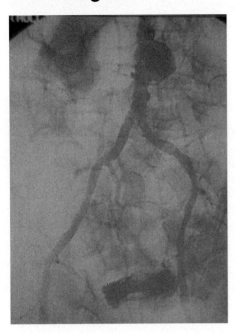

Figure 30-3

Arteriogram Report

Arteriogram reveals a saccular aneurysm of the infrarenal aorta.

Diagnosis and Recommendation

The presence of a pancreatic abscess and a saccular aneurysm is highly suggestive of an infected AAA. The high risk of rupture of an infected AAA obligates a concurrent operative approach, because neither condition may be safely delayed. The patient is advised of the need for extra-anatomic bypass for revascularization of the lower extremities via an axillobifemoral bypass, followed by resection of the infected AAA with ligation of the infrarenal AAA. Pancreatic debridement and drainage will be performed during the same operation. Potential complications of the operation include death, aortic stump blowout, amputation, and prosthetic graft infection. The patient is advised that the pancreatic abscess may require repeated debridements, and a pancreatic fistula is a possible complication.

Surgical Approach

The operative approach is dictated primarily by the clinical presentation. The classic approach in the stable patient with a nonruptured infected AAA is to perform a preemptive extra-anatomic bypass, usually via an axillobifemoral bypass, followed by excision of the infected AAA, wide debridement of the retroperitoneum, and "triple ligation" of the infrarenal aortic stump. "Triple ligation" of the aortic stump consists of a 2-layer closure of the aorta (horizontal mattress and simple running suture lines) with monofilament polypropylene suture, followed by stump coverage with a vascularized omental pedicle flap. When the diagnosis of an infected AAA is certain, the potential for bacterial seeding of the bypass graft may be minimized by completing all "clean" portions of the operation, including application of occlusive dressings, prior to initiating exposure of the infected AAA. Frank aortic rupture or uncertainty regarding the presence of infection will alter the operative sequence, as the aortic component of the operation is addressed initially in such cases. The most dramatic potential complication of aortic ligation is aortic stump blowout, which is almost universally lethal. The relatively poor long-term patency of axillofemoral bypass grafts and the potential for prosthetic graft infection are additional pitfalls of this approach.

Discussion

In situ reconstruction is an alternative approach to revascularization of the lower extremities after resection of an infected AAA. In unstable patients or those infected with a "low-grade" organism, such as *Staphylococcus epidermidis*, use of an *in situ* prosthetic graft has yielded acceptable clinical results in several series. Some authors view this approach as the treatment of choice for infected AAAs due to its relative simplicity and the absence of a ligated aortic stump at risk for blowout. Use of a rifampin-bonded Dacron graft and the liberal use of omental coverage of the graft are reasonable adjunct procedures to attempt to minimize the risk of graft infection. Rifampin bonding of a Dacron graft is accomplished by bathing the graft with rifampin (1200 mg in 20 mL normal saline) for 15 minutes prior to implantation. This approach is the mainstay of treatment for infected paravisceral or thoracic aortic aneurysms. The principal risk of this approach relates to the risk of graft infection when placing a prosthetic graft into an infected operative field. For this reason, alternative approaches may be advisable in more aggressive infections, especially those infections attributed to gram-negative or fungal species.

In situ aortic reconstruction with superficial femoral vein (SFV) offers several potential advantages over prosthetic reconstruction. As an autogenous conduit, SFV is resistant to recurrent infection and provides excellent long-term patency. In addition, SFV provides a reasonable size match to the typical infrarenal aorta. Chronic venous morbidity is minimal, as one third of patients have minor leg swelling, and no venous ulceration or venous claudication has been described after SFV harvest. However, approximately 1 in 5 limbs will require fasciotomy after SFV harvest. The principle disadvantage of using SFV for *in situ* aortic reconstruction relates to the time required for harvesting this vein (> 120 minutes or more). A detailed description of the technique for SFV harvest is provided elsewhere. Preoperative duplex ultrasonography of the SFV should be employed to confirm patency, absence of thrombus, and document adequate size (at least 6.0 mm) of this vein.

Case Continued

Due to the high probability of a polymicrobial infection of the pancreas, *in situ* reconstruction with a rifampin-bonded Dacron graft is considered suboptimal. To avoid creation of an infrarenal aortic stump at risk for blowout, *in situ* reconstruction with SFV is contemplated, but this option is eliminated after preoperative imaging of the SFV reveals evidence of a chronic thrombus. Thus, infrarenal aortic ligation and extra-anatomic bypass is the only viable option for this patient. Because the diagnosis of an infected AAA is not in question, an axillofemoral bypass is performed as the initial step in the operation. After skin closure, occlusive dressings are applied prior to proceeding with a laparotomy. At laparotomy, proximal control of the aorta is obtained initially at the supraceliac aorta, because infected AAAs are prone to disruption with excessive operative manipulation. Subsequently, the infrarenal aorta is controlled below the renal arteries, followed by distal control of the common iliac arteries. After systemic anticoagulation, clamps are applied and the infrarenal aorta is opened, debrided, and sent for culture. The aorta is debrided to healthy tissue before closing the infrarenal aortic stump in 3 layers, as described above. The origins of the common iliac arteries are closed from within the aorta. Systemic anticoagulation is reversed with protamine sulfate prior to proceeding with pancreatic debridement and drainage. Postoperative antibiotic coverage is tailored to cultures obtained at surgery. Six weeks of postoperative antibiotic coverage is advisable to prevent bacterial arteritis in the aortic stump.

Suggested Readings

Bandyk DF, Novotney ML, Johnson BL, et al. Use of rifampin-soaked gelatin-sealed polyester grafts for in situ treatment of primary aortic and vascular prosthetic infections. *J Surg Res.* 2001;95:44-49.

Muller BT, Wegener OR, Grabitz K, et al. Mycotic aneurysms of the thoracic and abdominal aorta and iliac arteries: experience with anatomic repair in 33 cases. *J Vasc Surg.* 2001;33:106-113.

Reddy DJ, Sheppard AD, Evans JR, et al. Management of infected aortoiliac aneurysms. *Arch Surg.* 1991;126:873-879.

Rosen SF, Ledesma DF, Lopez JA, et al. Repair of a saccular aortic aneurysm with superficial femoral-popliteal vein in the presence of a pancreatic abscess. *J Vasc Surg.* 2000;32: 1215-1218.

Sessa C, Farah I, Voirin L, et al. Infected aneurysms of the infrarenal abdominal aorta: diagnostic criteria and therapeutic strategy. *Ann Vasc Surg.* 1997;11:453-463.

Valentine RJ. Harvesting the superficial femoral vein as an autograft. *Semin Vasc Surg.* 2000;13:257-264.

Young RM, Cherry KJ Jr., Davis PM, et al. The results of in situ prosthetic replacement for infected aortic grafts. *Am J Surg.* 1999;178: 136-140.

case **3**

Alan Dardik, MD

Presentation*

A previously healthy 75-year-old man is referred to you for management of an abdominal aortic aneurysm (AAA). He was recently treated by his primary care physician for right lower lobe pneumonia, and on subsequent physical examination was noted to have an AAA. He was also noted to have evidence of congestive heart failure (CHF). At the time he had elevated levels of blood urea nitrogen (BUN; 95) and creatinine (Cr; 3.8), microscopic hematuria, and elevated liver function tests (LFT) including aspartate aminotransferase (AST) 120, alanine aminotransferase (ALT) 140, bilirubin 3.5, and alkaline phosphatase 120. He was treated with antibiotics, digoxin, and diuretics.

On your examination, he is afebrile with a blood pressure of 130/60 mm Hg and a pulse of 90 beats per minute. There is prominent jugular venous distention. His chest has bibasilar rales, but is otherwise clear; his heart examination is notable for an S_4 gallop and a grade III systolic ejection murmur. The abdomen appears slightly distended, but is soft; the liver is palpable, as is a large aneurysm, with a loud continuous bruit. He has bilateral pitting edema and stasis dermatitis, with palpable distal pulses. Plain radiographs show pulmonary vascular congestion, cardiomegaly, and small right pleural effusion. His computed tomography (CT) scan shows a juxtarenal abdominal aortic aneurysm, 12 cm maximal diameter, confined to the infrarenal aorta without extension to the iliac arteries. The liver and spleen are slightly, but not massively, enlarged. No other abnormality is seen.

Differential Diagnosis

The patient has a large aneurysm and signs of a large arteriovenous fistula, including an abdominal bruit and evidence of circulatory congestion (CHF, edema, venous stasis disease), hepatomegaly, and microscopic hematuria. The differential diagnoses include AAA with associated inferior vena cava (IVC) fistula, and AAA with unrelated CHF, including cardiac failure and pulmonary embolism. Previously undiagnosed congenital abnormalities, such as patent foramen ovale or central malignancies, may contribute to the circulatory overload and heart failure.

Discussion

AAA with associated IVC fistula is an unusual complication of AAAs, occurring in approximately 1% of asymptomatic and 3% to 4% of symptomatic

---

*The author thanks Dr. Richard J. Gusberg for providing the case.

aneurysms. Many documented aortocaval fistulas present as a ruptured aneurysm, and thus are repaired soon after discovery, without development of late sequelae. Thus the simultaneous presentation of AAA and CHF suggests unrelated processes, with the CHF needing treatment prior to AAA repair; unresolved CHF with treatment suggests the presence of an aortocaval fistula or another ominous finding. The importance of associating the physical findings of late sequelae of an aortocaval fistula cannot be overemphasized, as selection of additional preoperative studies can be more clearly guided if a fistula is suspected.

The initial diagnostic test is usually an imaging study, either ultrasound, CT scan, or magnetic resonance imaging (MRI), to confirm presence of the aneurysm. Occasionally, color-flow on the duplex examination demonstrates an aortocaval fistula, but this is unusual; in addition, preoperative planning is usually not performed with duplex. CT scan is more commonly used to guide preoperative planning and consideration for endovascular repair (EVAR); simultaneous opacification of the intravenous (IV) contrast in the aorta and the IVC is usually indicative of the fistula. MRI can demonstrate this finding as well, but is much less commonly used. Thus, if an aortocaval fistula is suspected prior to imaging, a CT scan with IV and oral contrast, both to diagnose the fistula and to assess the patient for possibility of EVAR is usually performed.

Other important tests include angiography, to determine the presence of and assess the extent of associated aneurysmal and occlusive disease; an aortocaval fistula is diagnosed on angiography by early filling of the IVC after intraaortic contrast injection. Measurement of central hemodynamics with a pulmonary artery (Swan-Ganz) catheter can determine the presence of a left-to-right shunt and high output cardiac failure, although this is rarely performed as an isolated preoperative diagnostic test; echocardiography can determine cardiac function and hemodynamics as well as demonstrate fistulae, including those due to a previously undiagnosed patent foramen ovale.

This patient presents with a CT scan report suggesting a large juxtarenal aneurysm unlikely to be a candidate for EVAR with current technology; early opacification of the IVC is not noted, although the use of contrast is not noted either. Because an additional CT scan is unlikely to add additional information, angiography will assess both the aneurysm neck and associated disease, and diagnose the AAA-IVC fistula, if present. A cardiac echocardiogram will determine the preoperative cardiac function, as well as check for an intracardiac fistula.

Recommendation

Cardiac echocardiogram and angiography.

Case Continued

The patient had a cardiac echocardiogram suggesting CHF, but no other abnormalities, and the following angiogram.

Angiogram

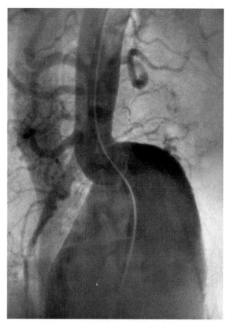

Figure 31-1

Angiogram Report

Large juxtarenal aneurysm with early opacification of the IVC.

Diagnosis and Recommendation

Juxtarenal AAA with chronic aortocaval fistula. This patient had a CT scan suggesting that an adequate neck is not present to perform EVAR, and thus aortography was used to define the surgical anatomy preoperatively as well as diagnose the aortocaval fistula.

Aneurysm repair and fistula closure is needed to prevent additional complications of the high-output shunt. Repair in the setting of CHF and renal failure has been associated with higher mortality than standard elective repair without an aortocaval fistula, at least as high as 50%; ideally aortocaval fistulae are repaired prior to permanent cardiac or renal damage. Repair is performed either from the transperitoneal or retroperitoneal approach, depending upon aneurysm configuration and surgeon preference. Although successful operation is expected with proper preoperative diagnosis and planning, complications include bleeding, infection, hemodynamic instability, impotence, colon ischemia, cardiac failure, prolonged ventilator dependence, stroke, air embolism, pulmonary embolism, acute limb ischemia, and death. Massive bleeding may occur intraoperatively. The risk of pulmonary embolism from debris within the aneurysm and the fistula also is not insignificant.

Surgical Approach

Infrarenal aneurysm repair can be performed satisfactorily from either the anterior transperitoneal approach or from the left retroperitoneal approach. It is our preference to perform all abdominal aneurysm repairs from the left retroperitoneal approach, if anatomically feasible. Repair proceeds in standard fashion, including dissection, vessel control, and heparinization. The fistula and IVC do not need to be isolated or dissected specifically. After aneurysm exclusion and opening, the back bleeding from the fistula is characteristically quite large. If a fistula is previously unsuspected, a large amount of back bleeding should prompt the surgeon to think specifically of an aortocaval fistula. The back bleeding is typically controlled proximally and distally with 2 sponge-sticks, controlling the IVC and allowing oversewing of the fistula; this method works adequately from both the transperitoneal and retroperitoneal approaches (Fig. 31-2). After fistula repair, the aneurysm is repaired in standard fashion.

Case Continued

Due to the suprarenal, and possibly supraceliac, position for the proximal clamp needed for repair of this aneurysm's neck, a retroperitoneal approach was performed. After heparinization, the aneurysm was directly clamped infrarenally prior to performance of the proximal anastomosis to allow renal perfusion during the time needed to oversew the lumbar arteries and repair of the fistula, even though this time was expected to be short. The aneurysm was opened rapidly with a Mayo scissors, and torrential back bleeding was easily and quickly controlled with sponge-sticks. The back bleeding was noted to be coming from a 2- to 3-cm chronic-appearing fistula; no patent lumbar arteries or inferior mesenteric artery (IMA) were noted. The fistula was oversewn with 3-0 Prolene suture, and, after moving the proximal aortic clamp to the suprarenal position, a bifurcation graft was placed from the infrarenal aorta to the origins of the common iliac arteries.

Discussion

The hemodynamic consequences of AAA-IVC fistula repair should be anticipated intraoperatively. The cardiac output and mixed venous oxygen content

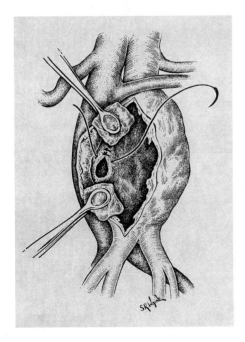

Figure 31-2 Technique for controlling bleeding from an aortocaval fistula and fistula repair via an intra-aortic suture closure. (From Dardik H, Dardik I, Strom MG, Attai L, Carnevale N, Veith FJ. Intravenous rupture of arteriosclerotic aneurysms of the abdominal aorta. *Surgery.* November 1976;80(5):647-651.)

should both fall to normal values. Continued fall in cardiac output to low values likely reflects low filling pressures that will be responsive to fluids. Mild acidosis may be present after repair as well.

Although the time to oversew a fistula is typically short, the massive back bleeding that may occur prior to fistula control may contribute to low cardiac output after repair. Therefore, some surgeons prefer to isolate and control the IVC prior to aneurysm opening; we do not perform this due to the risk of injuring the IVC, which is usually intimately adherent to the aneurysm because of the chronic inflammation of the aneurysm and the fistula.

Repair of the aneurysm with a stent graft (EVAR) may be an acceptable approach to repair of an aneurysm with an IVC fistula in selected patients. After placement of the stent graft, even though the fistula to the low-pressure IVC is unlikely to be a source of endoleak, this possibility must be considered in the presence of a persistent endoleak. Placement of a covered stent inside the caval side of the fistula may be a potential solution. However, prophylactic placement of a caval stent prior to aneurysm repair could theoretically induce aneurysm rupture through the fistula.

Case Continued

Recovery was prolonged due to pneumonia, respiratory failure, and persistent renal failure. The patient died 6 months postoperatively after refusing continued dialysis; the peripheral edema and stasis dermatitis was still present.

Discussion

Aortocaval fistula repair is associated with 50% mortality; in the presence of persistent renal failure, results are dismal. We repair aortocaval fistulae as soon as possible after discovery, to minimize the end-organ damage due to the pathophysiology of the fistula.

Suggested Readings

Bednarkiewicz M, Pretre R, Kalangos A, Khatchatourian G, Bruschweiler I, Faidutti B. Aortocaval fistula associated with abdominal aortic aneurysm: a diagnostic challenge. *Ann Vasc Surg*. September 1997;11:464-466.

Dardik H, Dardik I, Strom MG, Attai L, Carnevale N, Veith FJ. Intravenous rupture of arteriosclerotic aneurysms of the abdominal aorta. *Surgery*. November 1976;80:647-651.

Lau LL, O'Reilly MJ, Johnston LC, Lee B. Endovascular stent-graft repair of primary aortocaval fistula with an abdominal aortoiliac aneurysm. *J Vasc Surg*. February 2001;33:425-428.

McKeown BJ, Rankin SC. Aortocaval fistulae presenting with renal failure: CT diagnosis. *Clin Radiol*. August 1994;49:570-572.

Naito K, Sakai M, Natsuaki M, Itoh T. A new approach for aortocaval fistula from ruptured abdominal aortic aneurysm. Balloon occlusion technique under echogram guidance. *Thorac Cardiovasc Surg*. Feb 1994;42:55-57.

Schmidt R, Bruns C, Walter M, Erasmi H. Aortocaval fistula: an uncommon complication of infrarenal aortic aneurysms. *Thorac Cardiovasc Surg*. August 1994;42:208-211.

Ahsan T. Ali, MD, and John Eidt, MD, FACS

Presentation

A 58-year-old man with hypertension presented with complaints of a 3-day history of chills, intermittent fever with mid-abdominal pain, and a 24-hour history of vomiting bright red blood. He did not have a history of peptic ulcer disease or alcoholism. Upon examination he is found to be anxious; his pulse rate is 108 beats per minute, and his blood pressure is 110/68 mm Hg. His abdomen is soft with mild epigastric tenderness. Family history is significant for abdominal aortic aneurysm (AAA). No lesion was seen in the first or second part of the duodenum on upper endoscopy. A computed tomography (CT) scan is ordered.

■ CT Scan

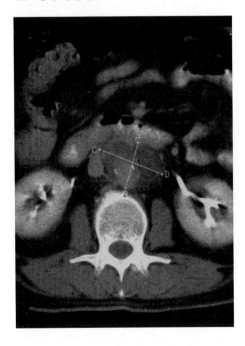

Figure 32-1

CT Scan Report

CT scan demonstrates a 4.5-cm AAA in close approximation to the duodenum with air in the aortic wall.

Differential Diagnosis

The differential diagnosis includes an upper gastrointestinal (GI) bleed from a gastric or duodenal ulcer, GI bleeding from gastritis, and primary aorto-enteric fistula (PAEF).

Case Continued

The patient begins to re-bleed, as evident from the nasogastric tube output. Esophagogastroduodenoscopy (EGD) is repeated. The bleeding appears to be coming from the fourth portion of the duodenum.

Diagnosis

Based on the history of abdominal pain, upper GI bleeding in the absence of peptic ulcer, and the CT findings of air in the aortic wall in close proximity to the duodenum, the diagnosis of primary aorto-enteric fistula is made.

Recommendation

Blood transfusion is initiated and the patient is taken to the operating room. EGD by an experienced endoscopist is very useful and should visualize the third and fourth portion of the duodenum. This will also rule out other more common causes of an upper GI bleed. High resolution CT scan with intravenous contrast will show pathology either in the aorta (aneurysm) or in the vicinity. Arteriogram does not add information, and can potentially precipitate hemorrhage. Treatment is surgical to control bleeding and establish vascular continuity.

Surgical Approach

Proximal control of the supraceliac aorta is obtained prior to mobilization of the duodenum. The PAEF is identified (Fig. 32-2). A communication of the aorta with the GI tract makes it a contaminated field. However, in an unstable pa-

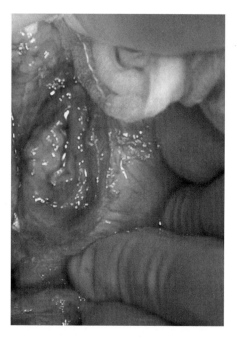

Figure 32-2 Duodenal erosion of the PAEF.

tient, time constraints do not allow for an autogenous graft or performance of an extra-anatomic bypass. An *in situ* rifampin-soaked graft is placed with omentum between the graft and the bowel. Cultures are obtained from the aortic wall. The bowel wall is debrided and closed in two layers in the standard fashion.

Discussion

PAEF is a ruptured or leaking aorta emptying into the GI tract. The communication is a result of degenerative process, which is most commonly an aneurysm, local infection, foreign body, or radiation induced. PAEFs are extremely difficult to diagnose preoperatively. In a report by Sweeny and Gadazc of 118 cases of PAEF, 97 patients died before a definitive diagnosis could be made. In another series, only one third of the patients were treated with surgical repair, with a perioperative mortality of 55%. Crucial to diagnosis is timely endoscopy with visualization to the fourth portion of the duodenum. CT scan demonstrating a loss of plane between the aorta and the duodenum with air in the aortic wall or the retroperitoneal area is suggestive of an aorto-enteric fistula. The triad of symptoms of abdominal pain, an upper GI bleed, and abdominal aneurysm together occur in only about one third of the patients. A likely scenario is that a general surgeon will discover aortic pathology at the time of celiotomy in acute circumstances. If the patient has been stable, local debridement can be attempted with extra-anatomic bypass or autogenous reconstruction. However, in an unstable patient or inexperienced hands, *in situ* replacement with rifampin-soaked graft is quite acceptable. In a review over a 15-year period, no reports of postoperative graft infections have been reported in 8 patients. If there is extensive contamination, an interval (8- to 10-day) replacement of the aorta can be performed, if possible, with the superficial femoral vein used as a neoaorta or an extra-anatomic bypass. By this time, final culture results are also available. An interval of a week also allows for surgery prior to formation of dense adhesions. Interval replacement is recommended if gram-negative or fungal infections are present, or if there is communication with the large bowel. The idea of endovascular exclusion is attractive in theory, but may depend on graft availability, advance knowledge of the diagnosis, and the logistics of surgeon/operating room training. An endovascular approach may also serve as a bridge to more definitive treatment.

Case Continued

After undergoing *in situ* tube graft replacement, a nasogastric tube is also placed in the duodenum. Diet is begun after 5 days postoperatively. Cultures do not grow any organism, but initial gram stain demonstrated a few white blood cells. The patient is discharged on a 6-week course of oral Bactrim.

Suggested Readings

Clagett GP, Hagino R, Valentine RJ. Autogenous aortoiliac/femoral reconstruction from superficial femoral-popliteal veins; feasibility and durability. *J Vasc Surg.* 1997;25:255-270.

Lemos DW, Rafetto JD, Moore TC, Menzoian JO. Primary aortoduodenal fistula: a case report and review of the literature. *J Vasc Surg.* 2003;37:686-689.

Pagni S, Denatale RW, Sweeny T, McLaughlin C, Ferneini AM. Primary aorto-duodenal fistula secondary to infected abdominal aortic aneurysm: role of local debridement and ex-

tra-anatomic bypass. *J Cardiovasc Surg.* February 1999;40:31-35.

Reiner MA, Brau SA, Schanzer H. Primary aortoduodenal fistula. *Am J Gastroenterol.* 1978;70:292-297.

Rothstein J, Goldstone J. Management of primary aortoenteric fistula. *Current Therapy in Vascular Surgery.* 4th ed. St. Louis: Mosby; 2001:277-279.

Sweeny MS, Gadacz TR. Primary aortoduodenal fistula: manifestation, diagnosis, and treatment. *Surgery.* 1984;96:492-497.

case **33**

Dennis R. Gable, MD, FACS

Presentation

A 73-year-old man with a past medical history significant for a previous myocardial infarction, atrial fibrillation, hypertension, and peripheral vascular disease, who has smoked one pack of cigarettes a day for 30 years, has just undergone an aortobifemoral bypass for aortoiliac occlusive disease and lower extremity rest pain. The operative procedure went well, without any notable technical complications and with minimal blood loss. Currently, the patient is still in the operative suite. After the operative drapes are removed, it is noted that he has a cold right lower extremity from the knee down and has a mottled right foot. On examination, there are strong palpable bilateral femoral pulses as well as a palpable left popliteal pulse. There are palpable pedal pulses on the left foot, but no palpable or Dopplerable pedal pulses on the right foot. The patient had Dopplerable pedal pulses and femoral pulses bilaterally prior to surgery.

Differential Diagnosis

The differential diagnosis for an ischemic limb immediately following aortic surgery includes atheroembolism, hypercoagulable disorder, raised intimal flap at the anastomotic site, inadequate anticoagulation during the procedure, and congestive heart failure. In this particular patient, a palpable femoral pulse bilaterally suggests patency of the newly placed aortobifemoral graft. Inability to find pulses of the right popliteal region or distally suggests a problem originating anywhere from the distal graft anastomosis to the foot, and all of the aforementioned diagnoses are a possibility.

Discussion

To optimize the outcome of patients suffering acute graft occlusion or limb ischemia after aortic surgery, and in an attempt to limit the morbidity and mortality, a prompt diagnosis is essential. An important portion of aortic surgery is to examine the patient's legs while still on the operating table at the conclusion of the procedure and to obtain Doppler or palpable distal pulses. The surgical instruments are kept sterile and the operative team remains scrubbed until these goals are met. If pulses are not found at the conclusion of a procedure and reoperation is required, then little time is wasted.

In general, when a limb salvage operation is undertaken, there is more advanced disease in the arterial tree, requiring a more complicated procedure with a higher incidence of acute thrombosis. In a series of 364 patients who underwent aortobifemoral bypass from 1973 to 1982, Ameli et al. reported an incidence of acute limb ischemia of 3.3%. Similarly, in a classic long-term evaluation of reconstructive aortic surgery, Szilagyi et al. reported a rate of graft occlusion of 8.3% in an interval from 1954 to 1963. This decreased to 2.4% in the 1964 to 1973 era, and rose slightly to 3.2% in the period between 1974 and 1983. This demonstrated the improved operative results that occur from the large experience.

Maintaining a sterile environment with the surgical team, as well as the surgical instruments, minimizes time required for reoperation, if indicated, at the end of the initial procedure. Although other imaging modalities (angiography, magnetic resonance angiography, ultrasound duplex evaluation) are used in a preoperative evaluation of a patient with chronic ischemia, these procedures also take valuable time to complete. Perioperative imaging outside the operative suite requires time to prepare for and perform the procedure, interpret the results, and return to the operative suite, if needed. When working with a time-sensitive problem, such as acute limb ischemia with the inherent possibility of limb loss if not treated promptly, this is valuable time wasted in current practice. The diagnosis of acute limb ischemia is usually made easily by careful physical examination at the end of the procedure. The exact cause of the ischemia can be diagnosed by examination of the anastomotic site or by arteriography. Within most vascular surgical practices, if acute limb ischemia is present and angiography is warranted, angiography can commonly be performed in the operative suite, on the operating table using a C-arm. If one is fortunate enough to have an operative endo-suite, a fixed fluoro unit may be used as well.

Recommendation

Proceed with interoperative arteriography and immediate reexploration.

▓ Interoperative Arteriography

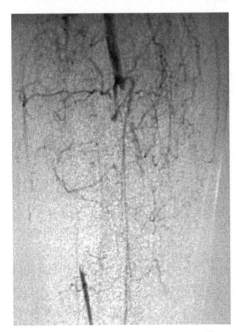

Figure 33-1

Arteriography Report

Arteriography of the right leg is shown with an isolated segment of the knee and proximal calf. A patent proximal popliteal artery is seen with abrupt occlusion of the mid-popliteal artery. Multiple small collateral vessels are seen around the knee. There is reconstitution of the proximal anterior tibial artery just distal to the origin. The posterior tibial and peroneal arteries are not visualized.

Discussion

It is important to prep the patient so that all avenues of access may be performed, including abdominal, femoral, and lower extremity access. This necessitates prepping the patient from the sternum down to, and including, circumferential prep of both legs. The easiest initial approach is to open and explore the groin region. This is especially true if there is a palpable femoral pulse, suggesting an infra-inguinal problem.

█ Surgical Approach

The patient is immediately reheparinized and anticoagulated to prevent any further thrombosis or propagation of clot up through the graft, which may involve the opposite limb and therefore cause thrombosis and ischemia of the opposite leg. Vascular clamps are applied to the femoral limb of the graft and the profunda femoris vessels and superficial femoral artery, once they are exposed. A vertical incision is made in the toe of the aortofemoral graft, if present, so as not to cross any of the suture lines. If no graft limb is present, a transverse incision is made in the common femoral artery to allow access to the profunda femoris and superficial femoral artery origins. The incision is placed so that the orifices of the superficial femoral and profunda femoris branches can be visualized clearly. If the proximal graft limb is occluded, Fogarty catheters are used to perform graft thrombectomy of the aortic graft limb. Following return of pulsatile flow, the limb of the graft is filled with heparin saline to avoid *in situ* thrombosis while the distal vascular system is cleared. At this point, the distal outflow tract to the profunda femoris artery and superficial femoral artery is examined for any evidence of a raised intimal flap, or any technical error in construction of the anastomosis that may have led to the initial thrombotic process. No technical errors are found, so the profunda femoris artery and superficial femoral artery are thrombectomized using Fogarty catheters.

Back flow is obtained, and then completion angiography is performed. In patients with a patent distal arterial tree in the lower extremity, it is especially important to examine the limb for any evidence of distal thrombosis or migration of clot, which may cause ongoing ischemia in the lower extremity, despite having a clear aortobifemoral limb.

█ Arteriogram

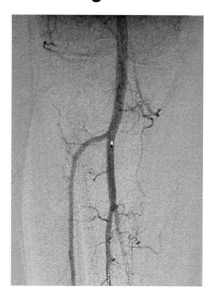

Figure 33-2

Angiogram Report

An isolated arteriogram film of the right knee and proximal calf demonstrates good flow within the popliteal artery, with three-vessel run-off to the calf via the anterior tibial, posterior tibial, and peroneal arteries. No residual thrombus is noted when compared to the arteriogram in Figure 33-1. A guide wire is seen in the tibial peroneal trunk.

Case Continued

There are strong palpable pedal pulses of both the dorsalis pedis and posterior tibial arteries following this procedure. The period of ischemia was rather short, and therefore fasciotomy is not performed; however, close observation is maintained with attention to neurologic examination of the limb postoperatively. The patient is extubated at the termination of the procedure. There are good palpable pulses in both limbs, and the patient is taken awake and alert to the intensive care unit for further monitoring. The thrombus and debris removed with thrombectomy appear to be consistent with embolization of material from the proximal aorta.

Discussion

If a distal thrombus is noted, thrombectomy is attempted from the femoral incision. On occasion, it is impossible to clear the distal popliteal artery from the arteriotomy in the groin alone. In these patients, an infrapopliteal incision may be required. Exposure is performed of the distal popliteal artery and the origin of the anterior tibial and tibial peroneal trunk. The vessels are dissected free so that the Fogarty catheter can be placed selectively in each tibial branch to obtain a complete thrombectomy, as required. The most difficult cases are those in which there is a superficial femoral artery occlusion and/or some disease of the profunda femoris outflow tract. When the profundaplasty itself is unable to sustain the patency of an aortobifemoral limb, a distal bypass procedure may be required. This is usually a bypass to the infragenicular popliteal or tibial vessels. Many times, bypass can be accomplished with prosthetic material; however, if bypass below the knee is needed for assistance in patency, the use of autogenous venous conduit will provide the patient with the best chance for long-term patency and limb salvage. Using autogenous material, however, entails a longer procedure. This must be considered, as well as the overall condition of the patient, prior to deciding which procedure would be most appropriate.

Following thrombectomy, if no technical error can be found and there is good outflow, the patient should be evaluated for a coagulation disorder. One common problem that is encountered is a heparin-induced platelet aggregation disorder. A platelet count can be obtained fairly quickly in the operative suite. If the platelet count is not markedly decreased, heparin-induced platelet aggregation is not a likely cause of any abnormal clotting disorder. At this point, more blood can be drawn for other coagulation studies, including antithrombin III, protein C, protein S, and fibrinogen studies. These studies will often take several hours or days to perform; therefore, treatment must be ongoing while awaiting results. Two units of fresh frozen plasma should be administered immediately, followed by one unit of fresh frozen plasma at least every 6 to 8 hours. Fresh frozen plasma is a "shotgun" therapy for a multitude of plasma deficiencies that can otherwise result in a thrombotic state leading to graft thrombosis. The patient is completely heparinized, and full anticoagulation is continued in the postoperative period at least until all coagulation studies are returned. Due to ongoing anticoagulation, meticulous hemostasis must be obtained prior to complete closure, to avoid any postoperative wound hematoma or bleeding, which may result in an increased incidence of wound complications and infection. Depending on the amount and duration of the lower limb ischemia, the involved limb should be examined for evidence of compartment syndrome. If there is any evidence of swelling in the calf, or a high index of suspicion of possible compartment syndrome, then four-compartment fasciotomy of the lower extremity should be considered. Fortunately, this step is only necessary in severely ischemic extremities or those that have been ischemic for prolonged periods.

Careful preoperative evaluation, preoperative monitoring, and precise operative technique have reduced the operative mortality of aortic surgery to 2% to 8% in most institutions. Starr et al. emphasized the importance of distal clamping prior to proximal clamp placement as another step in aneurysmal and aortic surgery. Other important factors in performing aortic surgery and aortobifemoral bypass include appropriate flushing with heparin saline during all anastomosis, flushing both proximally and distally prior to restoration of flow to the lower extremities, and careful selection of clamp sites on the diseased distal vessels to prevent atheromatous embolization. Imparato emphasized the importance of avoiding placement of clamps on common iliac arteries, especially in patients with aneurysmal disease, because of the frequency of aneurysmal degeneration of the common iliac artery. The common iliac artery is also often a site of calcified atheromatous plaques that can shatter on clamp placement, showering the distal circulation with debris and leading to ischemia of the pelvis, perineum, and lower extremities. Imparato recommended placing the distal clamps on the hypogastric and external iliac arteries, which in his series resulted in an incidence of postoperative limb ischemia of 0.57% in over 700 abdominal aortic aneurysm resections (the best reported rate in current literature).

Equally important as clamp placement prior to performing anastomosis is removal of the vascular clamps in an orderly process, so as to minimize the risk of embolization. The proximal clamps should be transiently released, allowing any thrombus that had developed in the cul-de-sac between the renal vessels and the proximal clamp to be removed and flushed out. Distal clamps should be sequentially removed to assure that there is back bleeding, prior to allowing antegrade flow down the lower extremities. If there is no back bleeding, minimal back bleeding, or if a thrombus is found in the iliac vessels or distal limbs of the graft prior to allowing antegrade flow, a Fogarty catheter should be inserted cautiously to remove thrombus or any atherosclerotic debris. Once the vessels are cleared of debris, flow is restored. If limb ischemia is noted following these procedures, the groin is opened to provide access to the femoral bifurcation, which permits operative angiography as well as better directed thrombectomy of the profunda femoris vessels and the superficial femoral artery.

If further atherosclerotic debris is found, or an intimal flap is noted, this must be addressed either with local endarterectomy and tacking of the plaque to the arterial wall, or a more distal bypass procedure. Raised intimal flaps at the distal anastomosis were noted to be the cause of ischemic problems in nearly 18% of the cases in a series reported by Towne et al. In a series by Ameli et al., the most common etiologic factors for graft failure were an elevated intimal flap (25%), kinking of the graft (8%), and postoperative hypotension (8%). With careful selection of the anastomotic site, attention to the site used for placement of clamps, and attention to technical aspects of anastomosis, intimal flaps are a preventable cause of limb ischemia.

Review of complications of ischemic compared to nonischemic extremities following aortic surgery generally shows an overall increase in complications of all categories, suggesting a generalized nonspecific cause leading to increased morbidity. The primary additional factor in these patients' care is that all patients with ischemic extremities require repeat induction of anesthesia or prolonged anesthesia. Therefore, prevention of limb ischemia is essential to decrease overall operative morbidity or mortality.

Suggested Readings

Ameli FM, Provan JL, Williamson C, Keachler PM. Etiology and management of aortofemoral bypass graft failure. *J Cardiovasc Surg*. 1987;28:695-700.

Brewster DC, Darling CR. Optimal methods of aortoiliac reconstructions. *Surgery*. 1978;84:739-748.

Crawford ES, Bomberger RA, Glaeser DH, Saleh SA, Russell WL. Aortoiliac occlusive disease: factors influencing survival and function following reconstructive operation over a 25-year period. *Surgery*. 1981;90:1055-1067.

Crawford ES, Saleh SA, Babb JR, Glaeser DH, Vaccaro PS, Silvers A. Infrarenal abdominal aortic aneurysm: factors influencing survival after operations performed over a 25-year period. *Ann Surg*. 1981;193:699-709.

Diehl JT, Cali RF, Hertzer NC, Beven EG. Complications of abdominal aortic reconstruction: an analysis of perioperative risk factors in 557 patients. *Ann Surg*. 1983;197:49-56.

Hicks GL, Eastland MW, DeWeese JA, May AG, Rob CG. Survival improvement following aortic aneurysm resection. *Ann Surg*. 1975;181:863-869.

Imparato AM, Berman IR, Bracco A, Kim GE, Beaudet R. Avoidance of shock and peripheral embolism during surgery of the abdominal aorta. *Surgery*. 1973;73:68-73.

Imparato AM. Abdominal aortic surgery: prevention of lower limb ischemia. *Surgery*. 1983;93:112-116.

Nevelsteen A, Suy R, Daenen W, Buel A, Stalpaent G. Aortofemoral grafting: factors influencing late results. *Surgery*. 1980;88:642-653.

Starr DS, Lawrie GM, Morris Jr GC. Prevention of distal embolism during arterial reconstruction. *Am J Surg*. 1979;138:764-769.

Szilagyi DE, Elliott JP, Smith RI, Reddy DJ, McPharlin M. A thirty-year survey of the reconstructive surgical treatment of aortoiliac occlusive disease. *J Vascular Surg*. 1986;3:421-436.

Thompson JE, Hollier LH, Patman RD, Persson AV. Surgical management of abdominal aortic aneurysm. *Ann Surg*. 1975;181:654-661.

Towne JB, Bernhard VM, Hussey C, Garancis JC. Antithrombin deficiency: a cause of unexplained thrombosis in vascular surgery. *Surgery*. 1981;89:735-742.

Volpetti G, Barker CF, Berkowite H, Roberts B. A 22-year review of elective resection of abdominal aortic aneurysms. *Surg Gynecol Obstet*. 1976;142:321-324.

case 34

Gerald B. Zelenock, MD, Steven D. Rimar, MD, and Harry Wasvary, MD

Presentation

You are called to the surgical intensive care unit (SICU) to see a 72-year-old man who had 3 episodes of watery diarrhea 8 hours after elective resection of a 6.8-cm abdominal aortic aneurysm (AAA). His AAA was initially recognized on spine radiographs obtained because of chronic back pain. A preoperative evaluation demonstrated mild chronic obstructive pulmonary disease, stable coronary artery disease, status post coronary artery bypass grafting. Formal assessment of cardiac status with an echocardiogram and Persantine thallium scan revealed no evidence of inducible ischemia and an ejection fraction of 38%.

The patient has undergone open repair of his AAA with an aorto-aortic (tube graft) reconstruction. During surgery, the neck of the aneurysm was clamped above both renal arteries right at the base of the superior mesenteric artery. Suprarenal clamp time was 28 minutes, at which time the proximal anastomosis was completed at the level of the renal arteries. The clamp was then placed across the body of the graft in the infrarenal position. The distal anastomosis was accomplished at the aortic bifurcation with an end-to-end reconstruction. A large amount of thrombus was present in the aneurysm sac. The thrombus was removed and two sets of lumbar arteries oversewn. The orifice of the inferior mesenteric artery was minimally back bleeding, and was oversewn within the aneurysm sac. Following the operation, he was extubated and transferred to the SICU. Three watery stools are noted that evening, but there was no blood detected.

Differential Diagnosis

Multiple etiologies are considered in the differential diagnosis for ambulatory patients with diarrhea. The differential diagnosis of postoperative diarrhea occurring in patients following elective general surgery procedures is also substantial. In the immediate postoperative period following open repair of an AAA, however, there is really one primary concern: intestinal ischemia. Most commonly, this is colonic ischemia.

Discussion

Occasionally, early postoperative diarrhea or a loose stool following aortic surgery can be relatively benign. Because most patients come to the hospital the morning of surgery and may have had an outpatient bowel prep, this can on rare occasion represent expulsion of retained colonic prep contents. Mechanical compression of the descending-sigmoid colon from intraoperative retraction may also stimulate an early postoperative stool. In either event, this should be self-limited and is not associated with metabolic changes. More than one loose stool, bloody diarrhea, hemodynamic instability, or metabolic changes are especially suggestive of colonic ischemia.

Case Continued

The morning after surgery (18 hours after the completion of surgery) the patient is noted on rounds to have had 3 more loose stools during the night. The last is tinged with blood. He has a stable hemoglobin and hematocrit, his blood pressure is 140/90 mm Hg, heart rate is 110 beats per minute, and respirations are 20 per minute. His metabolic panel and coagulation parameters are normal with the exception of a persistent metabolic acidosis (pH 7.28). A colonoscopy is ordered.

▇ Endoscopic Evaluation

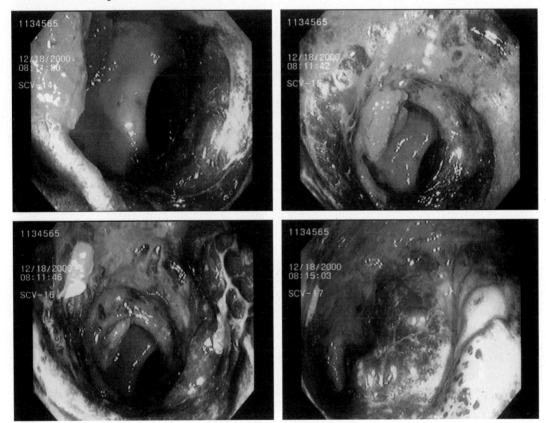

Figure 34-1

Endoscopic Evaluation Report

Advanced ischemic colitis with pseudomembranes, deep erosions, and ulceration is detected. The colonic segment has a dark, ecchymotic appearance and is noncontractile.

Discussion

No laboratory tests are pathognomonic of intestinal ischemia. However, persistent acidosis and elevated phosphorous or creatine kinase levels following aortic surgery help support the diagnosis. Fiberoptic colonoscopy is the diagnostic modality of choice to confirm the diagnosis. Precise determination of the severity of ischemia is difficult. In general, small areas of patchy mucosal erythema, pallor, or ecchymosis are consistent with mild ischemia confined to the mucosa. More extensive changes with large confluent areas of involvement indicate moderate ischemia. More advanced ischemic changes include a flaccid or rigid colonic segment with widespread discoloration, friability, ulceration, and fissures. These and other signs of advanced ischemia are suggestive of more than simple mucosal involvement. Some have recommended mucosal biopsy as an aid to quantifying the severity of ischemia, but this is not uniformly performed and may delay timely intervention. Similarly, intraluminal tonometry had a period of support, but is not frequently performed. The diagnosis in virtually all cases relies on clinical suspicion and endoscopy.

Case Continued

The patient is returned to the operating room 22 hours following the original procedure. A segmental area of the mid-sigmoid is recognized as profoundly ischemic, although no transmural infarction or soilage has occurred. A sigmoid resection with creation of a mid-descending end colostomy and a distal rectal stump (Hartmann's procedure) is performed. The patient tolerates the procedure well, and is discharged on postoperative day 10. Two months later, he has regained his preoperative weight and resumed all normal activities of daily life.

Discussion

Intestinal ischemia following aortic surgery is not rare. After elective aortic surgery, the incidence of clinically significant ischemic colitis ranges from 0.2% to 10%, with an average of 2.0%. When actively sought and objectively determined by endoscopy, the incidence of colon ischemia is 6% following elective aortic resection. In patients operated on for a ruptured AAA, serious clinical sequelae can result from even moderate ischemic changes to the intestine. These changes lead to the breakdown of the mucosal barrier function with translocation of bacteria, release of toxic waste products, and stimulation of ischemic inflammatory mediators. Loss of fluid and electrolytes can be substantial.

The clinical recognition of coexisting cardiac disease and the concomitant ability to diagnose and treat coronary artery disease, as well as better intraoperative and perioperative monitoring, has reduced mortality following elective aortic surgery. As the cause of mortality has shifted from cardiac disease to multisystem organ failure, the role of overt or subtle intestinal ischemia has become increasingly recognized as a contributing factor. There are several vulnerable areas within the intestinal circulation and several mechanisms by which intestinal ischemia can occur. A classic clinical presentation includes diarrhea, bloody diarrhea, or liquid stool in the immediate postoperative period. Persistent or progressive acidosis, unexplained hyperphosphatemia, leukocytosis, and elevation of intestinal enzymes may occur, but are sufficiently unreliable to eliminate the diagnosis.

Mechanisms of intestinal ischemia following aortic reconstruction include thrombosis of intestinal arcades secondary to hypotension; embolization of aneurysmal contents; traction injury on intestinal arcades; inappropriate technique when ligating the inferior mesenteric artery (IMA); and failure to appreciate the significance of a patent IMA serving as a major blood supply to a segment of intestine, or as a major collateral in the presence of significant celiac and superior mesenteric artery stenosis/occlusions. Unrecognized hypovolemia, use of pressor drugs intraoperatively and inadequate anticoagulation, hypercoagulable states and heparin-induced thrombocytopenia are other mechanisms contributing to postoperative intestinal ischemia-infarction. The collateral circulation to the gut is robust (Fig. 34-2), but can be compromised by normal anatomic variation, hypoplasia of intestinal arcades serving as potential collaterals, pre-existing atherosclerotic narrowing, and intraoperative injury or thrombosis.

Intestinal ischemia is usually confined to the sigmoid colon, but may involve the splenic flexure or even the right or transverse colon. On rare occasion, small bowel ischemia or extensive infarction of wide areas of the gut may occur. The latter typically occurs in the setting of pre-existing stenoses/occlusions of the celiac and superior mesenteric arteries, or as a result of injury to one or the other of these vessels. Significant rectal ischemia is also rare, and is often a result of hypotensive episodes secondary to substantial perioperative blood loss or hypogastric arterial occlusion.

At the time of aortic reconstruction, any change in status of the intestine, namely color change, hypoperistalsis or hyperperistalsis, or loss of a pulsation in the intestinal arcades, should call for Doppler assessment of the intestinal circulation. Doppler pulses should be readily apparent at the mesenteric border of the gut, and are usually detected at the antimesenteric border in properly resuscitated patients with normal perfusion.

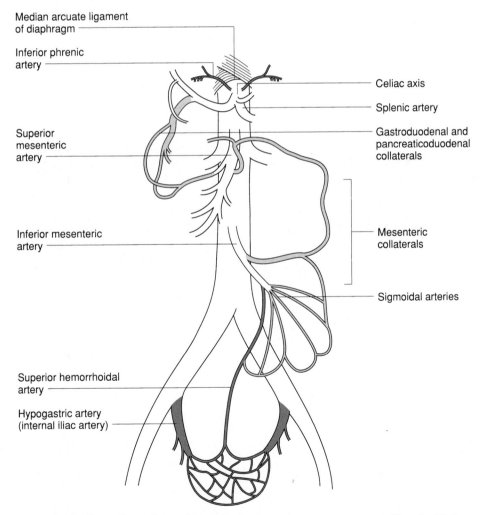

Figure 34-2 The collateral circulation to the intestine occurs at several levels. Well-recognized visceral-visceral and visceral-parietal collateral branches and anastomoses are important. Unnamed intestinal arcades and the intramural anastomoses are effective short-segment collaterals.

Some have advocated routine reimplantation of the IMA at every aortic reconstruction, whereas others do so selectively. Regardless, IMA reimplantation does not guarantee that colonic ischemia will not develop. This should not be surprising, given the multiple mechanisms that cause or contribute to colonic ischemia. Nevertheless, it is good clinical practice to assess colonic viability at the time of every aortic reconstruction, and to appropriately reimplant the IMA and/or revascularize an internal iliac artery when such is required.

When suspected intestinal ischemia is confirmed by endoscopy, an early return to the operating room for resection of the involved gut with fully diverting ostomies is favored, rather than a temporizing watchful waiting approach. Undoubtedly, some cases of relatively mild mucosal ischemia will heal; however, the possibility of missing an area of full-thickness ischemia with potential for perforation can be dangerous. Delayed return to the operating room results in fluid shifts, bacterial and toxin translocation, and progression of ischemia or hemodynamic instability. Ultimately, multisystem organ failure may develop. Return to the operating room for resection of the involved ischemic gut under these circumstances is less than ideal, and may be associated with increased mortality. Published reports regarding colonic ischemia after aortic surgery sufficient to require reoperation predict 50% mortality. Mortality increases to 75% to 80% if perforation and peritoneal/retroperitoneal contamination has occurred. At the time of re-exploration, fully diverting ostomies at the appropriate level and mucous fistula or Hartmann's pouch are preferred to primary anastomosis. In rare circumstances, an abdominal-perineal resection may be required. Consideration of colostomy closure should await full recovery from the initial surgical procedure(s), an interval that typically mandates 2 to 3 months.

Prevention of intestinal ischemia after aortic reconstruction is preferable to treatment. The problem is not rare. Diagnosis depends on endoscopy. Prompt return to the operating room for other than mild ischemic changes is advocated.

A final caveat: as endovascular techniques for aortic reconstruction continue to evolve, there is a sense that the incidence of intestinal ischemia is somewhat less than that following open repair. This issue has not been properly addressed in a prospective fashion.

Suggested Readings

Ernst CB, Hagihara PF, Daughterty ME, et al. Ischemic colitis incidence following abdominal aortic reconstruction: a prospective study. *Surgery*. 1976;80:417.

Ernst CB. Colon ischemia following aortic reconstruction. In: Rutherford RB, ed. *Vascular Surgery*. 4th ed. Philadelphia, WB Saunders; 1994; chap 99.

Mitchell KM, Valentine RJ. Inferior mesenteric artery reimplantation does not guarantee colonic viability in aortic surgery. *J Am Coll Surg*. February 2002;194(2):151-155.

Zelenock GB, Strodel WE, Knol JA, et al. A prospective study of clinically and endoscopically documented colonic ischemia in 100 patients undergoing aortic reconstructive surgery with aggressive colonic and direct pelvic revascularization, compared with historic controls. *Surgery*. 1989;106:771-780.

Zelenock GB. Visceral occlusive disease. In: Greenfield LG, Mulholland MM, Oldham KT, Zelenock GB, Lillemor KD, eds. *Surgery: Scientific Principles and Practice*. 3rd ed. Philadelphia: Lippincott-Raven; 2001:chap 82.

Thomas S. Huber, MD, PhD

Presentation

A 69-year-old man is referred for evaluation of enlarged aortic shadow detected on a routine chest radiograph. His past medical history is significant for mild chronic obstructive pulmonary disease (COPD), gout, and non–insulin-dependent diabetes. Physical examination is notable for decreased breath sounds throughout both lung fields, mild truncal obesity, a questionable abdominal aortic aneurysm, and normal femoral/popliteal/pedal pulses bilaterally. A chest/abdomen/pelvic computed tomography (CT) scan is obtained at the time of referral (Fig. 35-1).

▨ CT Scan

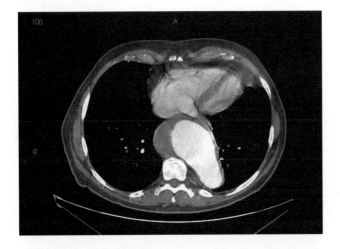

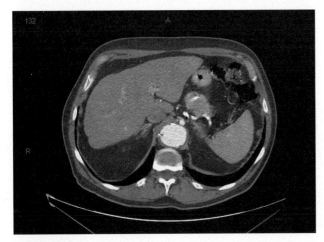

Figure 35-1

CT Scan Report

CT scan shows a 6.9-cm thoracoabdominal aortic aneurysm (TAA) that begins in the mid descending thoracic aorta and extends to the aortic bifurcation. There is no evidence of rupture, although there is a moderate amount of intraluminal thrombus throughout the abdominal component. There is some evidence of old granulomatous disease in the lung and diverticulosis in the descending colon.

Diagnosis

Type III TAA.

Discussion

TAAs are relatively uncommon and account for 2% to 5% of all aortic aneurysms with the annual volume of operative repairs in the United States less than 1000 procedures. The mean age (69 ±9 years) of patients undergoing repair is comparable to that for abdominal aortic aneurysms (AAA), although the breakdown is roughly equal by gender in contrast to the male predominance (4:1) for AAAs. The TAAs are classified by the proximal and distal extent of the aneurysmal aorta (Fig. 35-2), with most large clinical series comprised of comparable numbers of the 4 types.

Risk factors include prior aortic dissections and connective tissue disorders in addition to those traditionally reported for AAAs (family history, smoking, hypertension, aneurysms in other locations). Notably, 20% of all TAAs are sequelae of chronic aortic dissections, while the incidence of TAAs among first-degree relatives of the proband is also 20%.

The natural history of TAAs is to continue to enlarge and ultimately rupture, although the course is not as well described as that for AAAs. One clinical series reported that the 2-year survival of patients with large TAAs that did not un-

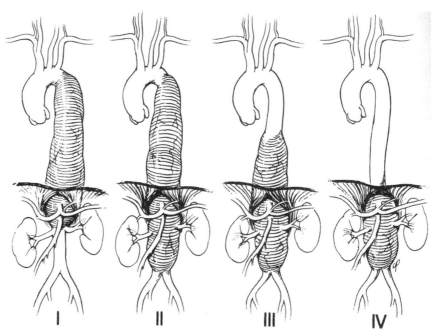

I   II   III   IV

Figure 35-2 Reprinted from Ernst CB, Stanley JC. *Current Therapy in Vascular Surgery*. 4th ed. St. Louis: Mosby; 2001:266; with permission.

dergo operative repair was only 24%, and that half of the deaths were due to aneurysm rupture. A more recent series reported that the combined annual rupture/dissection/mortality rate for TAAs larger than 6 cm was 14% and the hinge point for accelerated adverse events for the TAAs was 7 cm. The risk factors for rupture are similar to those for AAAs and include aneurysm diameter, COPD, female gender, advanced age, and renal insufficiency. The annual growth rate for aneurysms in the descending thoracic aorta is approximately 1.9 mm/y, while that for infrarenal AAAs is approximately 4 mm/y.

The treatment of TAAs is contingent upon the balance between the rupture risk and the morbidity/mortality associated with operative repair, because there are no effective nonoperative therapies. The operative mortality for intact TAAs is approximately 10% in the larger institutional series from centers of excellence, but is 22% in the country as a whole. The incidence of paraplegia/paraparesis and renal failure are approximately 10% and 15%, respectively. The predictors of operative mortality include preoperative renal failure, emergent operation, advanced age, advanced preoperative comorbidities, and postoperative complications. Notably, postoperative neurologic events and renal failure are associated with a 16-fold and 6-fold increased incidence of death, respectively. The quality of life after elective TAA repair is reasonable, with one series reporting a "good" outcome (alive/ambulatory/living at home) of 65% at 6 months. The estimated 5-year survival (Kaplan-Meier) after TAA repair is approximately 60%, and is comparable to that after AAA repair. Late aortic events and/or graft complications occur in up to 10% of individuals after TAA repair, thereby justifying lifetime surveillance. The threshold aortic diameter that merits repair remains undefined because there are no randomized trials; however, a maximal transverse measurement of 6 to 6.5 cm is likely appropriate in good-risk patients with reasonable life expectancies. A slightly smaller diameter may be appropriate for patients with chronic dissections secondary to Marfan's disease.

Recommendation

Continue preoperative evaluation and consider operative repair.

Case Continued

The patient is found to have a small area of reperfusion on an adenosine thallium study, which precipitates a cardiac catheterization. This shows some mild/moderate diffuse coronary artery disease and an estimated ejection fraction of 55%. His cardiologist "clears" him for surgery without recommendations for additional intervention. The patient's room air blood gas is within normal limits and his forced expiratory volume in 1 second (FEV_1) is 70% of the predicted value. The remaining components of his pulmonary function tests are consistent with a mild obstructive defect. His serum creatinine level is 1.2 mg/dL and the other routine serum chemistries and hematologic studies are all within normal limits. Ankle brachial indices are greater than 1.0 bilaterally.

Discussion

The decision to recommend TAA repair is contingent upon a thorough assessment of the operative risk. This entails surgeon, institution, and patient-related factors. Similar to most complex surgical procedures, the perioperative mortality rate has been reported to vary inversely with both surgeon and institutional volume. These findings and the marked disparity between the mortality rates in the larger institutional series and the country as a whole appear to justify referral to select centers of excellence. Patient evaluation includes risk stratification by the individual organ system with specific attention to the cardiac, pulmonary, and renal systems, given the older patient population and the known perioperative complications. Cardiac examination should include an assessment of left ventricular function and some type of functional study (eg, dobutamine echo, adenosine thallium), although routine cardiac catheterization is likely justifiable given the magnitude of the operative procedure. Notably, left ventricular dysfunction has been reported to be the strongest predictor of adverse cardiac events. Pulmonary assessment should include routine pulmonary function tests and room air blood gas, because pulmonary problems are the most common postoperative complication and occur in more than 25% of the patients. It is mandatory that all patients stop smoking well in advance of their procedure. A serum creatinine determination is a sufficient assessment of renal function. Similar to AAA repair, an elevated creatinine level is a significant predictor of postoperative renal failure/mortality, and some authors have contended that a creatinine level higher than 2.5 mg/dL is an absolute contraindication to TAA repair.

A thin-cut CT scan of the chest/abdomen/pelvis is the diagnostic test of choice and is usually sufficient to plan the operative procedure. The relevant CT scan findings include the proximal/distal extent of the aneurysm, size/appearance of the kidneys, the character of the aortic lumen, and the involvement/appearance of the visceral and renal vessels. Additionally, imaging with either a standard contrast or magnetic resonance arteriogram may be helpful for patients with aortic dissections and arterial occlusive diseases in the iliac/renal/visceral vessels. Notably, significant renal and/or visceral arterial occlusive disease has been reported in up to 30% of patients undergoing TAA repair.

Recommendation

Operative repair.

Surgical Approach

The patient undergoes operative repair through a thoracoabdominal incision extended through the eighth intercostal space. A spinal drain is placed for continuous drainage of the cerebrospinal fluid. A limited lateral, circumferential incision in the diaphragm is made, and the crus is taken down to facilitate aortic exposure. The patient is given Solu-Medrol, renal-dose dopamine, and mannitol prior to clamp application, although no heparin is given. The renal arteries are flushed with iced lactated Ringers after clamp application. A 22-mm Dacron tube graft is implanted from the mid-thoracic aorta to the bifurcation. The superior mesenteric artery (SMA) is perfused after the proximal anastomosis using a side-arm graft attached to the main graft and a perfusion catheter. The SMA, celiac axis, and right renal artery are reimplanted as a patch, while the left renal artery and intercostal vessels from T9 to T12 are reimplanted separately. Fresh frozen plasma and platelets are transfused after reimplanting the visceral patch and left renal artery.

Discussion

There are a variety of techniques to repair TAAs, and excellent clinical outcomes have been reported with each. Each technique has certain advantages/disadvantages and vocal proponents, although there is no consensus and it is conceivable that the most significant factor affecting outcome is the experience of the operative team/institution rather than technique itself. The common techniques include aortic occlusion and graft implantation alone ("cut and sew"), aortic occlusion and graft implantation with visceral perfusion adjuncts (sidearm graft/catheter, multiport catheter), complete circulatory arrest, and distal perfusion during graft implantation (atrial-femoral bypass with a Bio-Medicus pump, indwelling aortic shunt [Gott shunt], axillary-femoral graft). Among these, distal perfusion with atrial-femoral bypass and "cut and sew" with or without visceral perfusion adjuncts are likely the most common. Notably, endovascular repair has been reported and may represent the "next frontier" of aortic endografting, although the experience is very limited and currently experimental.

Spinal cord injury is one of the most feared complications of TAA repair. Ischemia from temporary or permanent disruption of the spinal cord blood supply is likely the most common mechanism, although other factors (including emboli and reperfusion injury) may contribute. The thoracic spinal cord is particularly susceptible to ischemic injury due to its tenuous blood supply. The artery of Adamkiewicz, a branch of one of the intercostal arteries, feeds the anterior spinal artery that supplies the lower cord and cauda equina. This artery enters the vertebral canal between the 9th and 12th vertebrae in approximately 75% of individuals. Spinal cord injury is associated with the duration of aortic cross clamp, the extent of the TAA (types I and II more than types III and IV), emergency procedures, and aneurysms associated with dissections. Strategies designed to reduce the incidence of spinal cord ischemia can be classified into those that maintain spinal cord perfusion and those that are neuroprotective. The former include identification of the critical spinal cord vessels, distal aortic perfusion, cerebrospinal fluid (CSF) drainage, and reimplantation of the intercostals vessels, while the latter include systemic/regional hypothermia and a variety of pharmacologic agents. CSF drainage and reimplantation of the intercostals are among the most widely applied techniques. Both are fairly simple and are associated with only minimal complications. Indeed, CSF drainage has been shown to reduce the incidence of spinal cord injury after TAA repair in a randomized, controlled trial. The technique is based upon the principle that reducing the CSF pressure augments spinal cord perfusion, because the spinal perfusion pressure is the difference between the arterial pressure below the aortic clamp and the CSF pressure. The intercostal vessels between T8 and L1 can be reimplanted as a patch, similar to the visceral artery patch, with large vessels and those with poor back bleeding being the most compelling.

TAA repair may be associated with significant bleeding from either technical (surgical) or coagulopathic causes. Strategies should be employed in concert with the anesthesia team to assure adequate resuscitation and to avoid developing a coagulopathy. These should include the use of autotransfusion devices, adjuncts to maintain normothermia, use of blood products as volume replacements, limiting the duration of visceral ischemia, and avoiding the use of heparin. Additionally, aggressive blood product replacement with fresh frozen plasma and platelets should be initiated after reimplanting the visceral vessels, even if the coagulation studies or platelet counts are within normal limits. Not using heparin potentially increases the risk of developing thrombi in the graft and/or outflow vessels. However, appropriate strategies for the sequence/position of the aortic clamping, liberal flushing of the graft, and prophylactic thrombectomy of the outflow vessels all reduce this potential risk.

A few technical points merit further comment. The innervation of the diaphragm should be preserved to maintain its integrity and to reduce the incidence of postoperative respiratory problems. The phrenic nerve innervates the central portion of the diaphragm and is disrupted with a radial incision. It is usually possible to obtain sufficient exposure of the aorta by incising only a small portion of the diaphragm laterally using a circumferential incision in concert with taking down the left crus. The exposure can be facilitated by placing a Penrose drain through the remaining intact portion of the diaphragm and mobilizing it as necessary to perform the various anastomoses. The extent of the visceral patch should be limited as much as possible to avoid subsequent aneurysmal degeneration. This can be accomplished by limiting the patch to the SMA, celiac axis, and right renal artery, and by placing sutures for the patch close to the orifices of the visceral vessels. The left renal artery should be bypassed or reimplanted separately, and a prosthetic limb can be sewn to the main body of the aortic graft prior to the proximal aortic anastomosis. The bypass graft to the left renal artery should be made as short as possible, because it is prone to kinking if left too long when the kidney is returned to its normal position.

Case Continued

The initial postoperative course is uncomplicated. On the second postoperative day, the patient's spinal drain becomes inadvertently dislodged and is removed. On the morning of his third postoperative day, he is weaned from mechanical ventilation and extubated. Later that afternoon, he becomes paraplegic.

Recommendation

Replace the spinal drain and optimize both hemodynamic status and oxygen-carrying capacity.

Discussion

Delayed paraplegia may develop in a small percentage of patients after TAA repair. The responsible mechanisms are outlined above and include ischemia, reperfusion injury, and cord edema. Multivariate analysis has shown that paraplegia is associated with type II repairs, chronic dissections, spinal drain complications, and hypotension. The spinal drain should be left in place for 72 hours postoperatively to optimize the spinal perfusion. Treatment strategies include replacing the spinal drain if it has been removed, and optimizing both the hemodynamic status and oxygen-carrying capacity. The latter approaches are directed at reducing the spinal cord ischemia and include volume expansion, supplemental oxygen, and liberal packed red blood cell transfusions. These maneuvers may occasionally reverse the delayed paraplegia.

Suggested Readings

Cambria RP. Thoracoabdominal aortic aneurysms. In: Rutherford RB, ed. *Vascular Surgery*. Philadelphia: WB Saunders; 2000:1303.

Chuter TA, Gordon RL, Reilly LM, Pak LK, Messina LM. Multi-branched stent-graft for type III thoracoabdominal aortic aneurysm. *J Vasc Interv Radiol*. 2001;12:391.

Coselli JS, Conklin LD, LeMaire SA. Thoracoabdominal aortic aneurysm repair: review and update of current strategies. *Ann Thorac Surg*. 2002;74:S1881.

Coselli JS, Lemaire SA, Koksoy C, Schmittling ZC, Curling PE. Cerebrospinal fluid drainage reduces paraplegia after thoracoabdominal aortic aneurysm repair: results of a randomized clinical trial. *J Vasc Surg*. 2002;35:631.

Dardik A, Perler BA, Roseborough GS, Williams GM. Aneurysmal expansion of the visceral patch after thoracoabdominal aortic replacement: an argument for limiting patch size? *J Vasc Surg.* 2001;34:405.

Derrow AE, Seeger JM, Dame DA, et al. The outcome in the United States after thoracoabdominal aortic aneurysm repair, renal artery bypass, and mesenteric revascularization. *J Vasc Surg.* 2001;34:54.

Elefteriades JA. Natural history of thoracic aortic aneurysms: indications for surgery, and surgical versus nonsurgical risks. *Ann Thorac Surg.* 2002;74:S1877.

Engle J, Safi HJ, Miller CC 3rd, et al. The impact of diaphragm management on prolonged ventilator support after thoracoabdominal aortic repair. *J Vasc Surg.* 1999;29:150.

Safi HJ, Miller CC 3rd, Huynh TT, et al. Distal aortic perfusion and cerebrospinal fluid drainage for thoracoabdominal and descending thoracic aortic repair: ten years of organ protection. *Ann Surg.* 2003;238:372.

Svensson LG, Crawford ES, Hess KR, Coselli JS, Safi HJ. Experience with 1509 patients undergoing thoracoabdominal aortic operations. *J Vasc Surg.* 1993;17:357.

case 36

David M. Williams, MD

Presentation

A 79-year-old man treated with peritoneal dialysis because of end-stage renal disease presents with asymmetric swelling of the right lower extremity after a 10-hour car trip. His dialysis management has been uncomplicated with good uremic control and stable weight. A computed tomographic (CT) examination of the abdomen and pelvis without intravascular contrast at the time peritoneal dialysis was initiated, 4 years prior, showed normal intraperitoneal distribution of contrast, a 5-cm hepatic cyst, and a 2.8-cm abdominal aortic aneurysm, but was otherwise normal for age. His medical history also includes hypertension, and gastric carcinoma status post partial gastrectomy and Billroth II reconstruction.

Differential Diagnosis

Lower extremity swelling may be due to low protein states, venous obstruction, and lymphatic obstruction. Venous obstruction may be due to right-sided heart failure, extrinsic mass or inflammation compressing venous structures, or deep vein thrombosis. Lymphatic obstruction can be congenital due to lymphatic hypoplasia, or infectious, neoplastic, or iatrogenic causes due to interruption of lymphatic channels. This patient's history of unilateral leg swelling after prolonged immobility suggests acute deep venous thrombosis (DVT).

Recommendation

Venous Doppler studies to rule out DVT are ordered.

Diagnostic Vascular Lab Report

No evidence of DVT in the right lower extremity. Doppler waveforms are abnormal in the distal external iliac, common femoral, and proximal femoral veins. Doppler waveforms in the left external iliac and common femoral veins are normal.

Clinical Follow-up

At the patient's next clinic visit, you note cold feet and some hyperpigmentation in the calves. You order a bilateral lower extremity arterial Doppler study and an abdominal aortic aneurysm scan.

Diagnostic Vascular Lab Report

Ankle-brachial indices are normal. Arterial waveforms at the ankles are triphasic. An infrarenal abdominal aortic aneurysm was imaged and measures 2.9 cm in largest transverse diameter. The common iliac arteries measure 2.1 × 2.0 cm on the right, and 1.4 × 1.3 cm on the left.

The diagnostic vascular lab report rules out deep venous thrombosis distal to the inguinal ligament as a cause of the patient's unilateral leg swelling. Obstruction of the iliac vein remains a possibility. You order a new CT examination of the abdomen and pelvis.

▨ CT Scan of the Abdomen and Pelvis

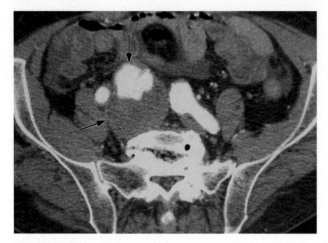

Figure 36-1

CT Scan Report

Pelvic CT examination shows a right hypogastric (or internal iliac) artery aneurysm measuring 6 × 7 cm. A large amount of thrombus is present within the aneurysm. The confluence of the right external and internal iliac veins and the adjacent common iliac vein are severely compressed.

Diagnosis and Recommendation

The patient has a large right hypogastric artery aneurysm with extrinsic compression of the ipsilateral iliac veins. The standard treatment of this lesion is aneurysmorrhaphy with debulking of the thrombus and oversewing branch arteries originating from the aneurysm. The patient's renal failure and peritoneal dialysis complicate a transperitoneal approach to the aneurysm. The large size of this aneurysm makes retroperitoneal exposure of the aneurysm and its branches a challenge. You consider the merits of open versus endovascular treatment of the aneurysm.

Open surgical treatment of hypogastric artery aneurysms requires eliminating arterial inflow and outflow to the aneurysm. Treatment depends on whether the aneurysm extends to the common iliac artery. If there is a proximal cuff of normal internal iliac artery, it is clamped and oversewn. Treatment is completed by opening the aneurysm, evacuating thrombus, and oversewing hypogastric artery branches that are back bleeding into the shell of the aneurysm. If the common iliac artery is also aneurysmal, then proximal control of the aneurysm requires construction of an iliac artery interposition graft. Debulking the aneurysm by removal of the thrombus may relieve the venous obstruction. Endovascular treatment is modeled on open surgical treatment. Control of outflow vessels requires catheterization of internal iliac branches close to their origin from the aneurysm, and proximal embolization, most often by means of metallic coils or glue. Control of aneurysm inflow is accomplished by deploying an endograft from the common to the external iliac arteries, across the internal iliac artery origin. Because the mass of the aneurysm remains, venous obstruction will persist unless it is directly addressed. Ideally, the lumen of the vein can be accessed and stented open.

■ Endovascular Approach

Intravascular ultrasound is performed through the right common femoral artery to measure the diameter and length of the common and external iliac arteries and to determine their suitability as prospective landing zones for an endograft. Then the branches of the right hypogastric artery are selectively catheterized and embolized with coils (Fig. 36-2).

Case Continued

Two days later, through a right common femoral artery cutdown, 3 endografts are deployed, including a 16-mm device in the external iliac artery, a 20-mm device in the middle, and a 24-mm device in the common iliac artery (Fig. 36-3).

The 24-mm device is placed with extreme care to avoid overlapping the origin of the left common iliac artery.

Treatment is next directed at the iliac venous obstruction due to mass effect by the aneurysm. Using punctures in the right common femoral vein and internal jugular veins, catheters are advanced to the pelvis on either side of the point

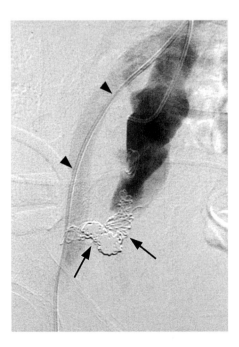

Figure 36-2. Following proximal embolization with coils (*arrow*), injection of the internal iliac artery fills a dead-end space, refluxing into the external iliac artery (*arrowheads*).

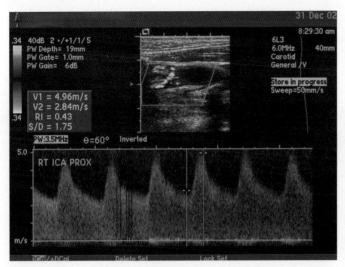

Color Plate 1   See Figure 5-1.

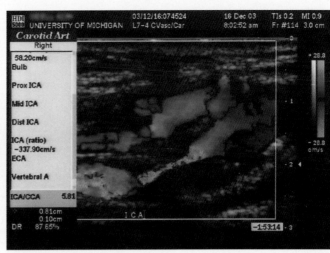

Color Plate 2   See Figure 6-1b.

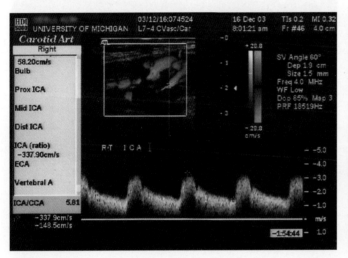

Color Plate 3   See Figure 6-1c.

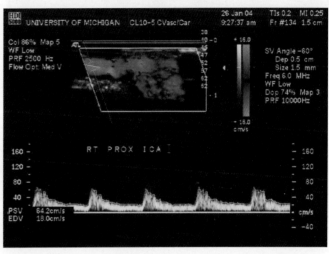

Color Plate 4   See Figure 6-2.

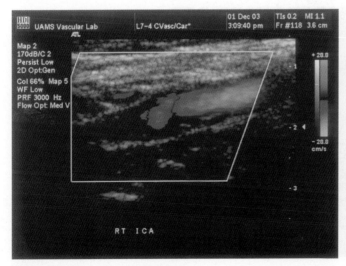

Color Plate 5   See Figure 8-1a.

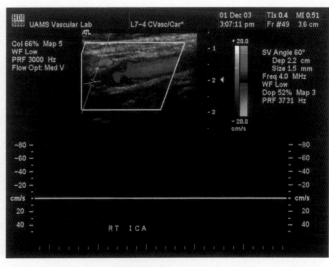

Color Plate 6   See Figure 8-1b.

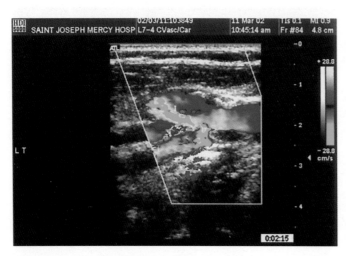

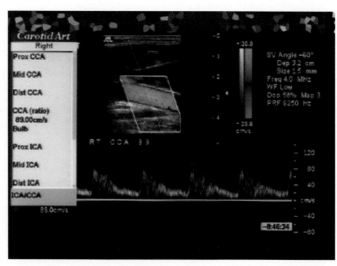

Color Plate 7 See Figure 11-1b.

Color Plate 8 See Figure 14-1a.

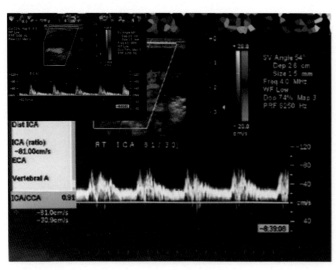

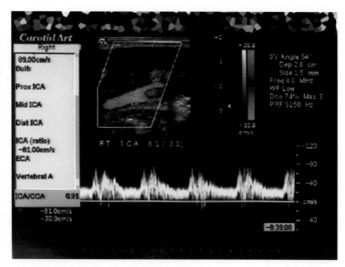

Color Plate 9 See Figure 14-1b.

Color Plate 10 See Figure 14-1c.

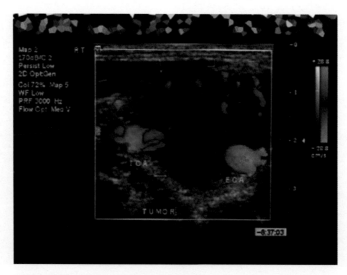

Color Plate 11 See Figure 14-1d.

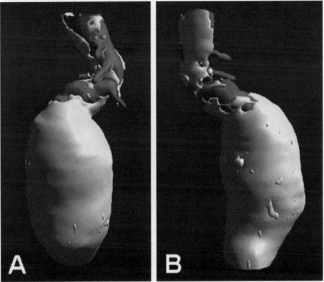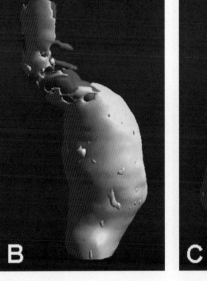

Color Plate 12 See Figure 27-2a/b.

Color Plate 13 See Figure 27-2c/d.

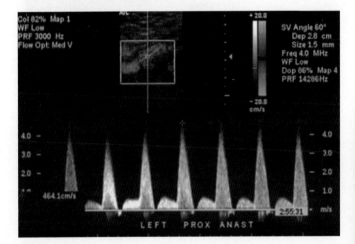

Color Plate 14 See Figure 50-1a.

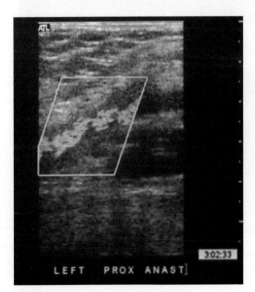

Color Plate 15 See Figure 50-1b.

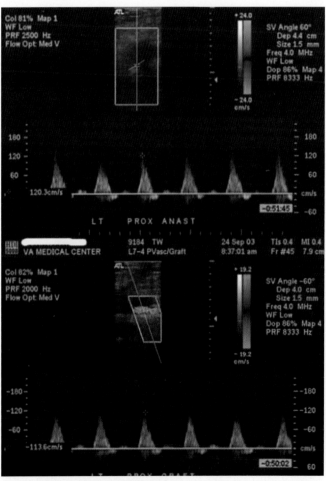

Color Plate 16 See Figure 50-3.

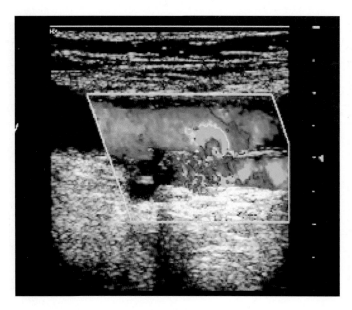

Color Plate 17   See Figure 52-1.

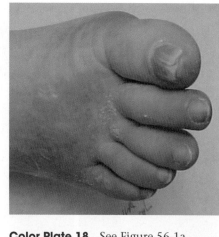

Color Plate 18   See Figure 56-1a.

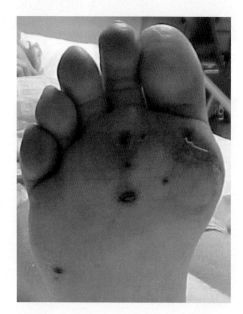

Color Plate 19   See Figure 56-1b.

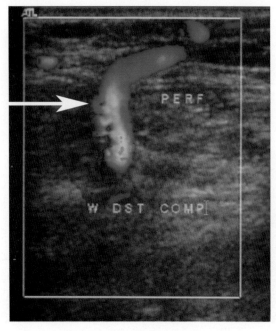

Color Plate 20   See Figure 61-3.

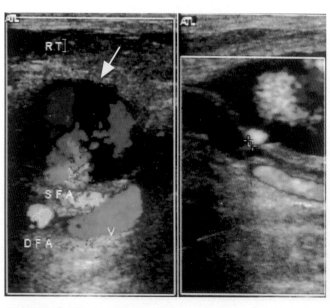

Color Plate 21   See Figure 66-1.

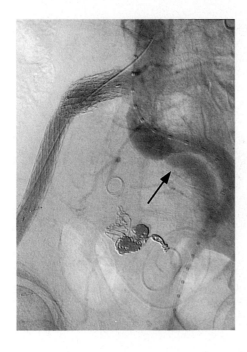

Figure 36-3. Following deployment of the AneuRx endografts, abdominal aortography with contrast injection at the bifurcation fills the left (*arrow*) but not the right internal iliac artery.

of occlusion. The pressure gradient between the femoral vein and the IVC is 12 mm Hg. The occlusion is crossed, dilated with an angioplasty balloon, and then stented using a 12 mm Wallstent in the external iliac vein and a 14-mm diameter Wallstent in the common iliac vein (Fig. 36-4).

The pressure gradient between femoral vein and the inferior vena cava (IVC) is reduced to zero.

Case Continued

The patient's leg swelling improves. He undergoes CT scans 4 months and 9 months postoperatively. These show reduction of the aneurysm mass from

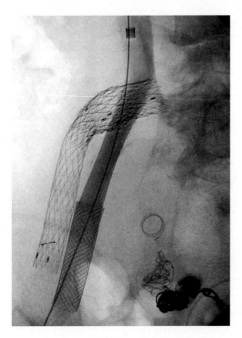

Figure 36-4. Injection of contrast material from a sheath in the right common femoral vein shows that the Wallstents have responded to balloon dilation and restored in-line venous return to the inferior vena cava.

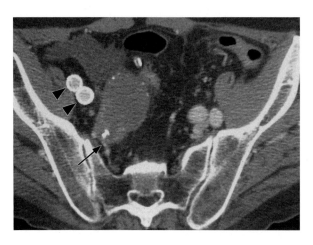

Figure 36-5. CT examination of the pelvis performed with intravenous contrast shows nearly complete thrombosis of the internal iliac artery aneurysm, except for a thin layer of contrast posteriorly (*arrow*), which appears to communicate with a small retroperitoneal branch. This appearance is highly suggestive of a type 2 endoleak. Note endoprostheses in the right external iliac artery and vein (*arrowheads*).

6.8×5.1 cm to 6.2×5.0 at 4 months, and finally 5.0×5.0 at 9 months (Fig. 36-5). In addition, a crescent of contrast material is seen pooling in the aneurysm sac, and is thought to represent back bleeding from nonthrombosed branches of the aneurysm.

Discussion

CT scan of the pelvis suggests this patient has a type 2 endoleak in his aneurysm, that is, continued blood flow from patent aneurysm branches into the aneurysm sac after endovascular treatment. There is consensus that certain endoleaks should be treated whenever possible: those arising from blood flow along the outside of the iliac endografts (type 1), or through defects in the fabric of the endograft, or through inadequate hemostasis at the junction of overlapping endografts (type 3). The urgency or even necessity of treating a type 2 endoleak such as the one in this patient is a matter of controversy. A reasonable approach to persistent type 2 endoleaks is to perform arteriography and, if the endoleak can be managed simply, to treat at the same time.

Suggested Readings

Bade MA, Ohki T, Cynamon J, Veith FJ. Hypogastric artery aneurysm rupture after endovascular graft exclusion with shrinkage of the aneurysm: significance of endotension from a "virtual," or thrombosed type II endoleak. *J Vasc Surg.* 2001;33:1271-1274.

Brin BJ, Busuttil RW. Isolated hypogastric artery aneurysms. *Arch Surg.* 1982;117:1329-1333.

Cynamon J, Prabhaker P, Twersky T. Techniques for hypogastric artery embolization. *Tech Vasc Interv Radiol.* 2001;4:236-242.

Harris RW, Andros G, Dulawa LB, Oblath RW, Horowitz R. Iliofemoral venous obstruction without thrombosis. *J Vasc Surg.* 1987;6:594-599.

Melki JP, Fichelle JM, Cormier F, Marzelle J, Cormier JM. Embolization of hypogastric artery aneurysm: 17 cases. *Ann Vasc Surg.* 2001;15:312-320.

Jonathan L. Eliason, MD, and Thomas C. Naslund, MD

Presentation

A 52-year-old man presents to your office after being seen by his primary medical doctor with a 2-week history of an enlarging left groin mass that has recently become tender. He had undergone aortofemoral bypass graft placement for severe claudication 6 years prior to presentation. On examination, the left groin incision is well healed and without erythema. There is a pulsatile mass palpable just below the groin crease that is tender to palpation. The patient's white blood cell (WBC) count is 14,000 with a left shift. A computed tomography (CT) scan is ordered.

▨ CT Scan

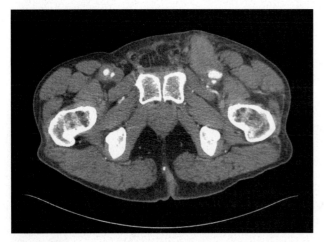

Figure 37-1

CT Scan Report

An aortobifemoral graft is present. A small amount of fluid surrounds the left limb of the graft within the pelvis. There is a pseudoaneurysm in the left groin at the anastomotic site. The majority of this appears to be thrombosed.

Differential Diagnosis

The differential diagnosis for a pulsatile mass in the groin includes aneurysms, pseudoaneurysms, and solid masses overlying the arterial structures. In this patient with an enlarging pulsatile mass in the setting of a previous prosthetic bypass to the femoral artery, a pseudoaneurysm would be considered the primary diagnosis. Also, the presence of fluid around the prosthetic graft and leukocytosis suggest that the pseudoaneurysm may be infected.

Discussion

The incidence of anastomotic femoral artery pseudoaneurysm formation in patients who have undergone prosthetic bypass procedures ranges from 2% to 5%. The pseudoaneurysms may be asymptomatic, being identified on routine physical examination; more commonly, however, patients will have pain and tenderness to palpation. Infrequently, local compression of the adjacent femoral vein or nerve can occur, resulting in deep venous thrombosis or femoral neuropathy, respectively.

The most important determination in this setting is whether or not the pseudoaneurysm is associated with prosthetic graft infection. Occult bacterial infection has been demonstrated as the etiology in as many as 60% of cases without an identifiable cause, such as trauma. Pseudoaneurysm formation can occur in the setting of noninfected prosthetic grafts, however, and is typically related to graft puncture following arteriography or anastomotic disruption, as can be seen in older prosthetic grafts where the suture or graft material has begun to degenerate. Noninfected pseudoaneurysms are amenable to direct surgical repair, such as resection of the pseudoaneurysm with primary closure or placement of a new interposition graft. The treatment of pseudoaneurysms resulting from prosthetic graft infection is typically more complex and is associated with greater morbidity and mortality.

Diagnostic testing for prosthetic graft infection should follow a careful history and examination. The history should include whether or not the patient has fevers, chills, night sweats, fatigue, weight loss, or other symptoms related to chronic infection. Examination of the groin should include inspection, evaluating for erythema or edema of the tissues, and palpation, assessing for warmth and tenderness of the pseudoaneurysm. A sinus tract in or around the groin, or hypertrophic osteoarthropathy of the ipsilateral foot, can be other subtle findings suggesting infection.

Diagnostic tests can include a complete blood count (CBC), erythrocyte sedimentation rate (ESR) or C-reactive protein (CRP), CT or magnetic resonance imaging (MRI), and tagged WBC scanning (indium scan). None of these tests are diagnostic for prosthetic graft infection by themselves; collectively, however, they provide a high sensitivity and specificity when positive. In the presence of infection, the CBC will often demonstrate a leukocytosis and/or a left shift. The ESR and CRP values, both nonspecific markers for inflammation, are typically elevated. CT or MRI usually shows fluid or inflammatory changes around the graft, while a positive tagged WBC scan will show an elevated concentration of leukocytes around the area of concern.

Recommendation

Tagged WBC scan and ESR.

Case Continued

The patient's ESR is 85 (normal value is less than 20 mm/h in men over age 50). The tagged WBC scan reveals the following.

▦ Tagged WBC Scan

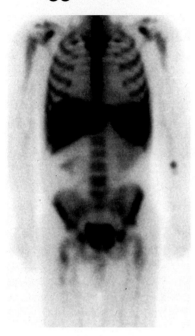

Figure 37-2

Tagged WBC Scan Report

Impression: Mildly increased activity within the left inguinal region suspicious for infection. If desired, 48-hour images could be attempted.

Diagnosis and Recommendation

This patient has a pulsatile left groin mass, elevated WBC count, elevated ESR, fluid around the left limb of an aortofemoral graft, and a tagged WBC scan positive for increased uptake in the left groin. The diagnosis is an infected left femoral artery pseudoaneurysm. The patient is offered an aortofemoral graft excision with neo-aortofemoral reconstruction using autogenous femoro-popliteal vein segments.

▦ Surgical Approach

Removal of all prosthetic graft material is essential for this type of in-line reconstruction. Harvest of bilateral femoral-popliteal vein segments is accomplished first, preferably with a two-team approach. After these surgical sites are covered with sterile dressings, the abdomen is opened and the aortofemoral graft is carefully skeletonized. Bilateral groin incisions, followed by circumferential exposure of the graft limbs and femoral arteries, are accomplished next. The patient is then heparinized, and the aortofemoral graft is excised. A neo-aortoiliac/femoral graft is then constructed from the femoral-popliteal vein segments. Aortic and bifemoral anastomoses are created next, restoring retrograde flow to the pelvis and antegrade flow to the lower extremities.

The operation described above is undertaken. The left femoral artery exposure reveals a large pseudoaneurysm. After heparinization, the pseudoaneurysm is entered, and balloon occlusion of the branches of the femoral artery is accomplished. The left limb of the graft is found to be totally disrupted from its junction with the femoral artery. The main body of the graft is also affected, with poor incorporation and an inflammatory reaction around the graft. After complete graft excision, the neo-aortofemoral graft is constructed.

The patient's hospital course is uncomplicated. He is discharged to home on postoperative day number 5, spending a total of 2 days in the intensive care unit. Intraoperative cultures from the left groin reveal the infectious organism to be *Staphylococcus epidermidis*.

Discussion

When an infected femoral artery pseudoaneurysm is the presumptive diagnosis in the setting of an aortofemoral graft, the surgical options include partial or complete graft excision and debridement, with extra-anatomic reconstruction to stay out of the infected field, or in-line reconstruction with autogenous conduit. There is considerable debate in the surgical literature as to which mode of treatment is most efficacious and carries the least risk to the patient. It is generally agreed upon, however, that graft preservation should be considered only if the following criteria are present: (1) the graft is patent, (2) the anastomoses are intact, (3) the patient does not have systemic sepsis, and (4) cultures of the wound yield bacteria other than *Pseudomonas* organisms. Therefore, if a graft infection results in a pseudoaneurysm, by definition the graft must be excised because the anastomoses are no longer intact.

Conventional treatment has typically been to combine axillofemoral bypass grafting with excision and drainage of the area of aortic infection and oversewing of the infrarenal aorta and iliac arteries. The operative mortality for this procedure had been as high as 38% prior to the 1980s; however, contemporary data reveal a perioperative mortality of less than 15%, with a better than 90% limb salvage rate at 2 years.

Replacing an infected aortic prosthesis with superficial femoral-popliteal vein was first reported in the early 1990s, and has now become a viable alternative treatment option. The advantages include long-term patency and limb-salvage rates at least as good as extra-anatomic reconstructions, as well as perioperative mortality around 10%. The drawbacks to this type of approach include a long and difficult operation, and the low but important risk of acute venous hypertension requiring a lower extremity fasciotomy.

Obviously, not all infected prosthetic-related femoral artery pseudoaneurysms arise in the setting of aortic reconstructions. The principles of removing the infected prosthetic material and reconstructing the arterial segment still apply, however. Another operation sometimes used in this setting is the obturator bypass, an in-line, extra-anatomic bypass that uses a graft tunneled from the iliac artery through the obturator foramen and between the adductor muscles to anastomose with the recipient vessel. Using this technique, the infected femoral artery pseudoaneurysm can be removed while clean tissue planes are maintained and utilized to restore flow to the lower extremity. Infected femoral artery pseudoaneurysms that don't involve an infected aortic prosthesis do not have the same morbidity and mortality of those that do. Nevertheless, they still represent a serious complication with a significant risk of limb loss.

Suggested Readings

Calligaro KD, Veith FJ, Schwartz ML, et al. Are gram-negative bacteria a contraindication to selective preservation of infected prosthetic arterial grafts? *J Vasc Surg.* 1992;16:337-346.

Calligaro KD, Veith FJ, Yuan JG, et al. Intra-abdominal aortic graft infection: complete or partial graft preservation in patients at very high risk. *J Vasc Surg.* 2003;38:1199-1205.

Clagett GP, Valentine RJ, Hagino RT. Autogenous aortoiliac/femoral reconstruction from superficial femoral-popliteal veins: feasibility and durability. *J Vasc Surg.* 1997;25:255-270.

Seeger JM, Pretus HA, Welborn MB, et al. Long-term outcome after treatment of aortic graft infection with staged extra-anatomic bypass grafting and aortic graft removal. *J Vasc Surg.* 2000;32:451-461.

Szilagyi DE, Smith RF, Elliott JP, et al. Anastomotic aneurysms after vascular reconstruction: problems of incidence, etiology, and treatment. *Surgery.* 1975;78:800-816.

Valentine RJ, Clagett GP. Aortic graft infections: replacement with autogenous vein. *Cardiovasc Surg.* 2001;9:419-425.

Yeager RA, Taylor LM Jr, Moneta GL, et al. Improved results with conventional management of infrarenal aortic infection. *J Vasc Surg.* 1999;30:76-83.

Peter K. Henke, MD, and Ruchi Mishra, BA

Presentation

A 67-year-old man presents with left lower extremity foot pain, severe in nature, that he has had for 3 hours. His prior medical history includes coronary artery disease, hyperlipidemia, past tobacco use, hypertension, but no diabetes and no prior vascular surgery. He takes an aspirin per day, plus an antihypertensive and a statin agent. His father died of an aneurysm rupture when he was 64 years old.

On examination, his heart and lungs are unremarkable, his abdomen is without palpable masses but mildly obese, and he has +2 femoral pulses. On the right side, he has an easily palpable popliteal pulse (+3) and distal pulses (+2). On his left side, only a femoral pulse (+2) is present, and no palpable popliteal or distal pulse is palpable. His left foot is cool and slightly mottled. Left foot cutaneous sensation is decreased, but motor function is intact.

Differential Diagnosis

This patient clearly has evidence of acute limb ischemia (ALI), Society for Vascular Surgery grade 2B, and requires immediate therapy to maintain limb salvage. Less likely etiologies include a primary spinal cord lesion or trauma. Significantly, because the physical examination of his right leg reveals an easily palpable popliteal pulse, a thrombosed left popliteal artery aneurysm (PAA) must be high on the differential diagnosis. Consideration of the underlying cause of ALI is important in ferreting out the best therapy. Because this patient has no evidence of a recent cardiac event, such as new-onset atrial fibrillation or a myocardial infarction, an embolic etiology for limb ischemia is not likely. It is also unlikely that the patient has thrombosis *in situ* of native circulation as a cause for his limb ischemia, because he has easily palpable pulses on the contralateral asymptomatic leg and no history of peripheral vascular occlusive disease.

Recommendation

The patient needs immediate systemic heparinization (100 to 150 U/kg administered intravenously [IV] and then 1000 U/hr IV), an aspirin if he has not taken it already, and adequate IV hydration. Consideration of immediate surgery versus arteriography is next, but because an embolic etiology of his ALI is unlikely, arteriography with possible thrombolysis is the best therapeutic route. An ultrasound technician is available, and performs a duplex ultrasound scan. The scan confirms the thrombosed left popliteal artery and evidence of aneurysm with a transverse diameter of 2.5 cm.

Duplex Scan

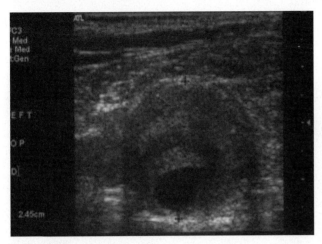

Figure 38-1

Duplex Scan Report

Duplex scan of the right leg shows a 3-cm PAA with thrombus, but patent with normal tibial outflow.

Discussion

The vast majority of patients (estimated at 96%) with PAA are male; the most common age when PAA is diagnosed is during the sixth decade. PAAs are associated with the highest rate of concurrent aneurysms, with bilaterality approaching 64%. Incidence of abdominal aortic aneurysms (AAA) with PAA is as high as 62%.

Approximately one third to one half of patients with PAA are asymptomatic. Patients may present with chronic ischemic limb symptoms from their PAA, ranging from 20% to 40%, while patients presenting with ALI related to a PAA range from 18% to 30%. The overall complication rate for PAA ranges from 18% to 77%, with limb amputation rates of up to 20%.

Three criteria predictive of complications from a PAA include diameter greater than 2 cm, the presence of intraluminal thrombus, and poor distal arterial runoff, which includes the absence of Dopplerable pulses and one vessel or less seen by angiography. However, risks of thrombolysis include bleeding, distal embolization, and lysis failures, all of which are associated with high limb amputation rates.

Approach

First and foremost is to reestablish blood flow to this patient's left lower extremity. Arteriography with thrombolysis is safe, given that he has had only approximately 3 hours of limb ischemia. Keep in mind that thrombolysis is not as fast as embolectomy for reestablishment of blood flow. There is no need to stop heparin during the endovascular interventions, except to decrease the dosage to keep the flush ports open during active thrombolysis (approximately 300 U/h). Thrombolytic agents include urokinase plasminogen activator (uPA) and tissue plasminogen activator (tPA); both agents have similar efficacy, but tPA has possibly a higher risk of hemorrhagic complications.

Arteriography

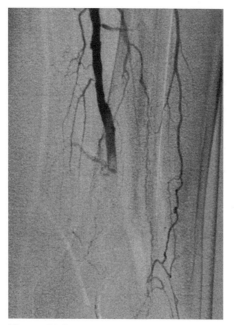

Figure 38-2

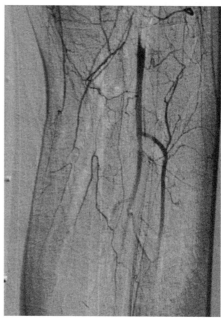

Figure 38-3

Arteriography Report

A thrombosed left PAA is confirmed with a patent SFA (Fig. 38-2) and patent below knee popliteal artery (Fig. 38-3).

Recommendation

A catheter is inserted via coaxial system to deliver tPA at a dosage of 0.5 U/h.

Case Continued

Within 4 hours, the patient has a warm left foot with improved sensation, and Doppler confirms return of pulses. Within 8 hours, he has normal blood flow to his left leg. Repeat arteriography shows full clearance of the thrombosed PAA and normal three-vessel outflow (Fig. 38-4).

Discussion

When thrombolysis is chosen, close attention to the patient's pulse status, the catheter connections, and insertion site is essential to avoid major complications such as bleeding.

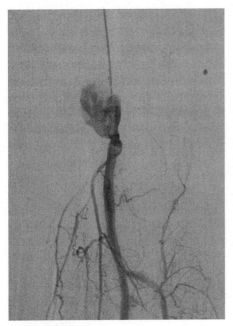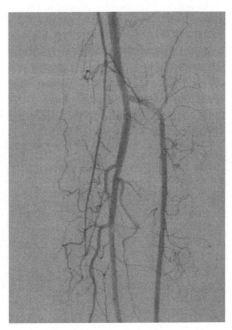

Figure 38-4

◼ Surgical Therapy

Because this patient has a symptomatic PAA, but now has normal blood flow to his left foot, the plan is to allow him to go home on low-molecular-weight heparin and return within a week for surgery. Alternatively, he could undergo elective operation during the same hospitalization. Because the arteriogram showed the femoral artery was without significant disease, the above-knee popliteal artery inflow site is chosen proximal to the PAA. In general, the shorter the bypass, the better. The approach used for this patient is exclusion of the PAA with proximal and distal ligation, combined with reversed saphenous vein bypass grafting around the affected aneurysmal segment. Most repairs are performed using the medial approach to the popliteal artery (because of technical ease, safety, and ability to preserve valuable collateral vessels). The medial approach is particularly advantageous when dealing with large PAAs that do not involve adjacent structures. The posterior approach to PAA repair is typically used when the PAA is confined to the popliteal fossa. It is associated with an increased incidence of popliteal vein and tibial nerve injury, because these structures may be adherent to the aneurysm. In multicenter studies, the range of 5- and 10-year graft patency and limb salvage rates is reported as 64% to 75%, and 90% to 95%, respectively. Studies over the past 5 years report varying rates of success with endovascular repair of popliteal artery PAAs, ranging from 47% to 75%, but the number of patients treated with endovascular grafts in these studies is small and is not the standard of care.

Follow-up

The patient returns 6 to 8 weeks later to undergo a right PAA bypass and exclusion, using the same general technique as on the left side. Patients with diffuse aneurysmal disease require long-term follow-up (duplex surveillance of the abdomen as well as the legs). The PAA may enlarge over time despite exclusion, because retrograde flow through collateral branches can re-fill the aneurysm, causing a situation similar to endotension. Because this patient has bilateral

PAAs, it is essential to get a duplex scan of his abdomen to evaluate for an AAA. Indeed, in this patient, a 4-cm AAA is confirmed by duplex. At this point, he will be followed by 6-month ultrasound examinations to assess for increases in size.

A less clear issue is what to do in a patient with a PAA and no usable autologous vein. The risks associated with the natural history of the PAA need to be balanced against the projected patency of either a composite vein bypass or a prosthetic bypass.

SUGGESTED READINGS

Ascher E, Markevich N, Schutzer RW, Kallakuri S, Jacob T, Hingorani AP. Small popliteal artery aneurysms: are they clinically significant? *J Vasc Surg.* 2003;37:755-760.

Carpenter JP, Barker CF, Roberts B, Berkowitz HD, Lusk EJ, Perloff LJ. Popliteal aneurysms: current management and outcome. *J Vasc Surg.* 1994;19:65-73.

Dorigo W, Pulli R, Turini F, Pratesi G, Credi G, Innocenti AA. Acute leg ischaemia from thrombosed popliteal artery aneurysms: role of preoperative thrombolysis. *Eur J Vasc Endovasc Surg.* 2002;23:251-254.

Ebaugh JL, Morasch MD, Matsumura JS, et al. Fate of excluded popliteal artery aneurysms. *J Vasc Surg.* 2003;37:954-959.

Mahmood A, Salaman R, Sintler M, Smith SRG, Simms MH, Vohra RK. Surgery of popliteal artery aneurysms: a twelve-year experience. *J Vasc Surg.* 2003;37:586-593.

Rutherford RB, Baker JD, Ernst C, et al. Recommended standards for reports dealing with lower ischemia: revised version. *J Vasc Surg.* 1997; 26:517-538

Whitehouse WM Jr, Wakefield TW, Graham LM. Limb-threatening potential of arteriosclerotic popliteal artery aneurysms. *Surgery.* 1983;93:694-699.

Margaret H. Walkup, MD, and William A. Marston, MD

Presentation

A 55-year-old man presents to your clinic complaining of pain in his buttocks when he walks, as well as cramping pain at night in his calves. The patient has a 40-pack year smoking history. He is currently taking medications for hypertension and elevated cholesterol. Of note, the patient also reports that he has tried various medications for his impotence without significant improvement. Upon examination, the patient's blood pressure is 155/95 mm Hg. Bilateral carotid bruits are noted. Femoral pulses are diminished bilaterally. Distal pulses are present by Doppler only.

Differential Diagnosis

The differential diagnosis of intermittent exercise-induced lower extremity pain includes arterial insufficiency; neurologic pain from lumbar disc disease; or spinal stenosis, degenerative hip disease, and diabetic neuropathy. Neuromuscular disorders may also produce muscle weakness with activity. The typical signs and symptoms of aortoiliac arterial insufficiency include hip and buttock claudication, impotence in males, and reduced femoral pulses. However, the picture may be significantly different in patients with multilevel vascular disease, where they may also have more distal symptoms including rest pain or tissue loss.

Nonvascular causes can usually be differentiated by history. Although degenerative hip disease or sciatic pain may occur with activity, they typically arise with initial movement rather than after a reproducible distance or level of activity is reached. Neuropathic pain is usually noted at rest, particularly at night, and usually improves with ambulation.

Palpation of the femoral pulses will frequently demonstrate diminished or absent pulses, but this is not a reliable method of diagnosing aortoiliac occlusive disease (AIOD). Diagnosis may be difficult in obese patients and in those with bilateral disease. If the picture remains unclear after the history and physical examination, noninvasive Doppler testing can definitively determine the hemodynamic situation in the limb, in most cases.

Diagnostic Tests and Results

The patient is referred to the peripheral vascular laboratory for arterial Doppler studies of the lower extremities.

Ankle-Brachial Index

The ankle/brachial index (ABI) is a simple test that can be performed in most clinics with a minimum of time and expense. The test requires only a blood pressure cuff and Doppler probe. The blood pressure cuff is placed just above the ankle, and is inflated while listening to the Doppler signal in the dorsalis pedis or posterior tibial artery in the foot. The Doppler signal will eventually be lost. The cuff is then deflated slowly, and the pressure where the Doppler signal returns is the pressure in the interrogated vessel at the ankle. This pressure is then divided by the higher of the two brachial artery pressures to give the ABI. An ABI of 1.0 to 1.2 is considered normal. Patients with an ABI of 0.7 to 1.0 may experience mild claudication, those with an ABI of 0.5 to 0.7 tend to have more severe claudication, and those with an ABI less than 0.5 may present with limb-threatening symptoms of rest pain or tissue loss. The ABI may be inaccurate in patients with diabetes mellitus; these patients often have severe calcification of the tibial arteries, rendering these vessels noncompressible and resulting in a falsely elevated ABI.

Doppler Waveform Analysis

Given the potential for falsely elevated ABIs in patients with AIOD, most practitioners obtain a second measure of the arterial circulation in the lower extremity. Evaluation of the Doppler waveforms obtained in the various levels of the limb can determine whether significant proximal obstruction is present. Figure 39-1 illustrates normal and abnormal Doppler waveforms. Specific measures for the presence of aortoiliac occlusive disease include the acceleration time and femoral pulsatility index. To gain further information concerning the extent of disease, the aorta and iliac vessels may be scanned with duplex ultrasonography to further determine the site(s) and severity of arterial obstruction. This technique may be limited in some patients by bowel gas, obesity, or patient tolerance.

The noninvasive vascular examination in a typical patient with aortoiliac occlusive disease will reveal an ABI of 0.5 to 0.9 (or lower, if there is multilevel disease), diminished Doppler waveforms at the groin and ankle, and a prolonged waveform acceleration time. These changes will be unilateral if the patient has unilateral iliac occlusive disease, but will be bilateral if the patient has significant aortic obstruction or bilateral iliac disease.

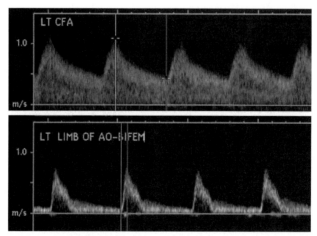

Figure 39-1 Normal Doppler waveform velocity tracings from common femoral artery (CFA) of patient with aortofemoral graft aortoiliac disease (*bottom*) compared to tracings from reported patient's CFA (*top*).

In some patients, typically those with milder symptoms, the studies described above may be normal at rest. In this situation, the patient should undergo an exercise or treadmill test. The patient ambulates until the typical claudication symptoms develop, and the studies are repeated. If there is significant arterial obstruction, the exercise ABI is decreased and waveform changes are exacerbated.

Recommendation

ABI measurements and Doppler ultrasound evaluation of the lower extremity arterial system.

Case Continued

The patient's ABIs are 0.74 on the right lower extremity and 0.68 on the left. Doppler waveform analysis reveals bilateral prolonged acceleration times in both common femoral arteries, consistent with aortoiliac occlusive disease. Based on the patient's history, physical examination, and Doppler studies, the diagnosis of aortoiliac occlusive disease resulting in claudication is made. At this point, the potential forms of treatment must be considered in relation to the severity of the patient's symptoms.

Medical Therapy

For many patients with claudication, particularly those with mild or moderate symptoms, medical therapy may be sufficient to relieve symptoms and allow increased activity. Two medications, pentoxifylline and cilostazol, are widely used for the treatment of claudication. In prospective randomized studies, both were reported to increase walking distance significantly in patients with claudication, though in some patients the benefits were relatively mild. A synergistic effect was noted with both medications when combined with an exercise-walking program. In a blinded prospective randomized trial, treatment with cilostazol resulted in a significantly greater increase (56%) in walking distance than pentoxifylline (30%) or placebo (34%).

For patients who do not respond to medical therapy or for those with more severe claudication, invasive revascularization may be necessary. Options include endovascular revascularization or surgical reconstruction. Surgical revascularization carries an increased risk of morbidity and mortality in comparison to percutaneous endoluminal techniques. However, the long-term results of surgical revascularization are better, with fewer patients returning for reintervention over time. The extent and location of aortoiliac disease must be considered, because the results for endoluminal revascularization are better in more localized areas of disease. In general, younger, healthier patients are chosen for surgical revascularization, as are those with disease that is too extensive to allow endoluminal treatment. To determine the optimal method of revascularization, a further imaging study is usually performed.

CT Angiography

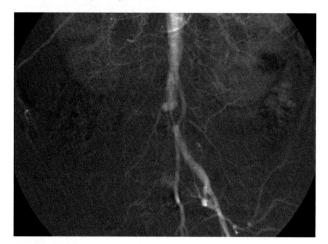

Figure 39-2

Discussion

The gold-standard modality for evaluating the aortoiliac segments for revascularization has been contrast arteriography. However, this study requires percutaneous arterial access and use of contrast that may be nephrotoxic. Other complications include significant hematoma formation (defined as than requiring surgical evacuation or transfusion), with occurrence rates around 0.5%, and pseudoaneurysm of the femoral artery, with occurrence rates of less than 1%. Recent advances in software and scanning technology have allowed finely detailed computed tomography (CT) and magnetic resonance (MR) studies to provide excellent information on the extent of aortoiliac occlusive disease. Selection of CT versus MR depends on personal preference, but we prefer CT angiography if the patient can tolerate iodinated contrast material. For patients with renal insufficiency, MR angiography with gadolinium is performed. The quality of these CT and MR studies may not match percutaneous angiography for the small arteries of the lower leg and foot; therefore, if information on the smaller vessels is required, this study is often preferred.

CT Report

The CT angiogram reveals aortic occlusion just below the origin of the renal arteries. Reconstitution of the external iliac arteries occurs through pelvic collateral vessels. The femoral vessels appear patent bilaterally.

Patient Selection

In this case, the patient is a young, otherwise relatively healthy patient with severe claudication. With 50-foot claudication, the use of medical therapy would not significantly alter his activity level, even if 100% improvement occurred. Therefore, we recommend invasive revascularization. If the CTA had revealed a limited lesion of the iliac artery or aorta, percutaneous angioplasty with possible stent insertion would have been recommended, expecting a 5-year patency of the treated vessel of 70% to 80%. However, in cases with extensive disease throughout the aortoiliac segment, the results of percutaneous techniques are usually significantly worse; therefore, surgical reconstruction is preferred in the patient who is a good surgical candidate. All patients with peripheral vascular disease must be considered also to have significant coronary artery disease, so a detailed history of any possible cardiac symptoms must be obtained, with screening studies for cardiac ischemia prior to surgery for any patients at risk.

■ Surgical Options

Multiple surgical options are available to treat aortoiliac disease. When considering the options, one must take into account the patient's comorbidities as well as the extent of their occlusive disease.

Aortofemoral Bypass

Aortofemoral bypass is considered the gold standard method of surgical repair. The procedure consists of placing a graft proximally on the infrarenal aorta and tunneling the limbs under the inguinal ligament to bypass to the femoral arteries. The patency rate is 85% to 90% at 5 years and 70% to 75% at 10 years. With proper patient selection, the operative mortality is less than 2%. Severe cardiac disease is the biggest risk factor. All patients should undergo thorough screening to evaluate cardiovascular status prior to operation. Patients with severe pulmonary disease are also at higher risk of perioperative complications. Patients with a history of multiple previous abdominal operations, intraabdominal sepsis, a diminutive infrarenal aorta, or a horseshoe kidney are not optimal candidates for aortofemoral bypass.

Thoracofemoral Bypass

Thoracofemoral bypass involves accessing the thoracic aorta through a thoracotomy and placing the proximal graft on the distal descending thoracic aorta. The graft is then tunneled from the left chest to the left suprainguinal preperitoneal space. The distal limbs are tunneled under the inguinal ligament with distal attachment to the femoral arteries. Thoracofemoral bypass is a good option for patients who are not candidates for aortofemoral repair because of a previous failed aortofemoral graft or a hostile abdomen, abnormal renal anatomy, or poorly developed infrarenal aorta. Reported patency rates for this procedure are 73% to 86%. Mortality was reported at 4% in one series. Like the aortofemoral repair, cardiovascular and pulmonary status must be evaluated before the procedure. Patients who are not candidates for infrarenal bypass secondary to their cardiac disease should be excluded from this procedure.

Options for High-Risk Patients

Axillobifemoral and femoro-femoral bypass grafting are both extra-anatomic repairs that are options for patients at high risk from their other comorbidities. Extra-anatomic bypass does not require laparotomy or thoracotomy, resulting in a lower risk of perioperative complications. Axillobifemoral bypass has patency rates from 50% to 85% at 5 years with reported mortality of 3.4%. Femoro-femoral bypass has patency rates of 60% to 80% with mortality from 0% to 5%. Despite the absence of an open thoracic or abdominal operation, these procedures have high morbidity and mortality because they are typically performed in higher risk patients with severe comorbidities.

Case Continued

Given this patient's young age and extensive aortic disease, aortobifemoral bypass is recommended. Laparotomy is performed and the infrarenal aorta is exposed. Heavy calcification of the entire aorta is found, beginning just below the renal arteries. The aorta is controlled just distal to the renal arteries and the external iliac arteries are exposed above the inguinal ligaments. We prefer to avoid groin incisions whenever possible to reduce the risk of graft limb infection. Revascularization is performed by implanting a 20 × 10-mm bifurcated Dacron graft from the infrarenal aorta to the external iliac arteries bilaterally. The graft is carefully covered with retroperitoneum or omentum prior to abdominal closure, to reduce the risk of late aortoenteric fistula.

Complications and Postoperative Course

Myocardial infarction and pulmonary complications remain the primary causes of mortality or serious perioperative morbidity. Other perioperative complications include renal failure, limb ischemia secondary to showered emboli, bleeding requiring transfusion, intestinal ischemia, spinal cord ischemia, and impotence. The uncomplicated postoperative recovery usually requires 4 to 10 days of hospital care, and typically depends on the length of postoperative ileus. Most patients are back to their usual daily activities within 6 weeks. Late complications are rare, but include graft occlusion, graft infection, or aortoenteric fistula.

Discussion

The frequency of surgical reconstruction for aortoiliac occlusive disease has decreased significantly as catheter-based procedures have improved and gained popularity. Most patients, when given a choice, would prefer a less invasive procedure with lower initial risk of complications, despite a reduced long-term benefit. Therefore, surgical reconstruction is generally reserved for patients with a long life expectancy who want the most durable revascularization, or for those who are poor anatomic candidates for percutaneous revascularization.

Suggested Readings

Brewster DC. Complications of aortic and lower extremity procedures. In: Strandness DE Jr, van Breda A, eds. *Vascular Diseases: Surgical and Interventional Therapy*. New York: Churchill Livingstone; 1994:1151-1177.

Brewster DC, Cooke JC. Longevity of aortofemoral bypass grafts. In: Yao JST, Pearce WH, eds. *Long-term Results in Vascular Surgery*. Norwalk, CT: Appleton & Lange; 1993:149-161.

Crawford ES, Bomberger RA, Glaeser DH, et al. Aortoiliac occlusive disease: factors influencing survival and function following reconstructive operation over a twenty-five year period. *Surgery*. 1981;90:1555.

Dawson DL, Cutler BS, Hiatt WR, et al. A comparison of cilostazol and pentoxifylline for treating intermittent claudication. *Am J Med*. 2000;109:523-530.

Diehl JT, Cali RF, Hertzer NR, et al. Complications of abdominal aortic reconstruction: an analysis of perioperative risk factors in 557 patients. *Ann Surg*. 1983;197:50.

Smith RF, et al. A thirty-year survey of the reconstructive surgical treatment of aortoiliac occlusive disease. *J Vasc Surg*. 1986;3:421.

Szilyagei DE, Hageman JH, Goodreau JJ, Creasy JK, Flanigan DP, et al. Rational approach to the differentiation of vascular and neurogenic claudication. *Surgery*. 1978;84:749.

Thiele BL, Bandyk DF, Zierler RE, et al. A systematic approach to the assessment of aortoiliac disease. *Arch Surg*. 1983;118:477.

Majid Tayyarah, MD, and W. Anthony Lee, MD

Presentation

A 61-year-old woman is transferred to your hospital for treatment of a "cold" left leg. At 4 AM, she awoke with pain and numbness in her left foot and later noted that it was cool. Her past history is significant for short-distance claudication, hemodialysis-dependent renal failure, a coronary artery bypass surgery, and oxygen-dependent chronic obstructive pulmonary disease (COPD). She has smoked 2 packs a day for 40 years.

On examination she has 4/5 plantarflexion and 3/5 dorsiflexion across her left ankle and diminished sensation in the entire foot. Her calf is soft and non-tender. The left foot is cooler than the right, without a clear line of demarcation. There is some venous filling at the ankle. She has no palpable femoral, popliteal, or pedal pulses in the left leg with an ankle/brachial index (ABI) of 0. On the right side she has a palpable femoral pulse, nonpalpable popliteal or pedal pulses, and an ABI of 0.6. Bilateral radial pulses are present and equal. The remainder of her examination is within normal limits. An electrocardiogram (ECG) shows normal sinus rhythm.

Differential Diagnosis

The patient has acute ischemia of the left leg. She also has significant lower extremity occlusive disease in her other leg, as evidenced by her absent popliteal and pedal pulses and abnormal ABI of 0.6. The patient likely has acute thrombosis in the setting of a critical preexisting lesion combined with chronic multilevel disease.

Acute leg ischemia is most commonly caused by either an embolus from the heart or sudden thrombosis of a major arterial inflow source, such as the iliofemoral-popliteal segment or a bypass graft. Clues indicating a thrombotic (as opposed to embolic) event include a history of claudication with an abnormal contralateral pulse examination, and lack of any history of atrial fibrillation or recent myocardial infarction that may serve as an embolic source.

Acute aortic dissection should also be considered in the differential diagnosis for acute limb ischemia. Back and/or chest pain are typically also present, and a spiral computed tomographic (CT) angiogram should be expeditiously obtained for a definitive diagnosis.

Discussion

It is helpful to classify acute limb ischemia by urgency for revascularization. One system classifies limbs as "marginally" versus "immediately" threatened. In patients without a Doppler signal at the ankle, the neurologic examination and the presence or absence of venous filling can be used to differentiate between the two states. Minimal loss of sensation in the toes with a normal motor examination and venous filling constitutes a "marginally" threatened limb. Severe sensory loss involving the entire foot, with decreased motor function and absent venous filling, constitutes an "immediately" threatened limb. In general, marginally threatened limbs can provide the luxury of a few hours to allow an expeditious workup (eg, arteriogram, vein survey, fluid resuscitation) prior to attempted revascularization, while immediately threatened limbs require prompt treatment within minutes.

Aortoiliac occlusive disease (AIOD) occurs most often in the infrarenal aorta and at the origins of the common iliac arteries. The external iliac is usually less diseased, and when present is more diffuse. Patients with isolated aortoiliac (AI) disease are usually younger and are heavy smokers. Smokers are 4 to 5 times more likely to have severe aortoiliac disease as opposed to infrainguinal disease, whereas the opposite is true for diabetics where the iliac segments are often preserved and most of the disease is localized to the profunda femoris and infrapopliteal arteries. Chronic occlusion of the infrarenal aorta may present as Leriche syndrome, defined as a constellation of buttock claudication, impotence, and absent femoral pulses.

Recommendation

This patient has an immediately threatened limb as evidenced by the loss of sensation in the entire foot and decreased motor function. Her vascular examination suggests a left iliac artery occlusion as evidenced by the absent left femoral pulse. She almost definitely has additional infrainguinal disease; however, her inflow is addressed first. The patient is given 100 IU/kg bolus of intravenous heparin and taken immediately for an intraoperative angiogram and revascularization.

Surgical Approach

The patient has been fully heparinized. The right femoral artery is percutaneously accessed using a micropuncture needle and a Seldinger technique. A 5-French sheath is inserted and an angiographic catheter is advanced into the aorta. An aortogram shows a 2-cm occlusion of the left common iliac artery, 1 cm from the aortic bifurcation (Fig. 40-1) with reconstitution of the distal left common iliac, external, and femoral arteries. As mentioned previously, this lesion is best approached from the ipsilateral femoral artery. Therefore, an image-guided left femoral artery puncture is performed using one of the following techniques: (1) in 80% to 90% of cases, the common femoral artery crosses either in the medial one third or within 1 cm from the medial cortical margin of the femoral head (Rupp method); (2) ultrasound guided; (3) direct visualization of the femoral artery, either by roadmapping or by calcifications present in the arterial wall.

After access is obtained, a retrograde iliac angiogram is obtained to confirm intraluminal access and verify distal extent of the occlusion. A left leg arteriogram is obtained. This shows a flush occlusion of the superficial femoral artery with a patent profunda femoris artery, reconstitution of a diseased popliteal artery, and two-vessel tibial runoff.

A stiff hydrophilic wire and an angled catheter are used to cross the occluded segment using digital subtraction roadmapping techniques. After the wire has entered the distal aorta, the wire is spun to verify free rotation of the angled tip, and the catheter is then advanced over the wire. Contrast is manually injected into the aorta to definitively confirm intraluminal position.

The lesion is predilated with a 5 × 40-mm balloon (Fig. 40-2). Since this is an occlusion, primary stenting is planned with a balloon expandable stent. The

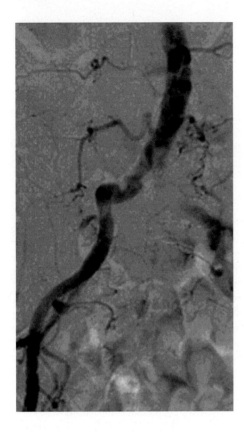

Figure 40-1 Flush aortogram showing a proximal left iliac occlusion with reconstitution of the distal common, internal, and external iliac arteries.

5-French introducer sheath is exchanged for a long 7-French sheath, which is advanced into and beyond the lesion. An 8 × 28-mm stent is delivered over the wire to the middle of the lesion using prior roadmapping. The sheath is retracted to expose the stent, and the stent is deployed. The balloon is carefully removed, leaving the wire in place, and a completion angiogram is obtained

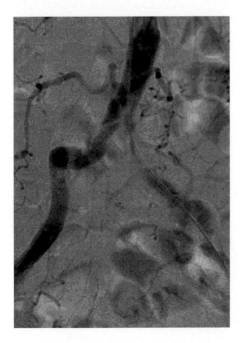

Figure 40-2 Aortogram following guidewire access across occlusion and predilation with a 5 × 40-mm balloon.

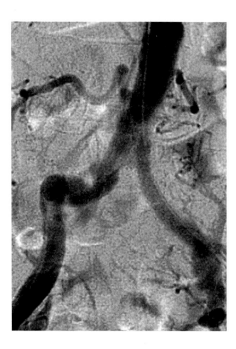

Figure 40-3 Completion aortogram showing successful recanalization of the previously occluded iliac artery.

(Fig. 40-3). The patient has resolution of her rest pain with monophasic Doppler signals in the posterior tibial and peroneal arteries. Postoperative ABI is 0.55.

Some patients with critical ischemia require inflow as well as outflow revascularization with additional endovascular or surgical therapy. There are three predictors for success after inflow revascularization alone: (1) patent profunda femoris artery, (2) identifiable inflow lesion, and (3) rest pain or minimal tissue loss.

Discussion

Percutaneous transluminal angioplasty (PTA) and stenting of aortoiliac occlusive disease have become the primary treatment modality for select lesions. Based on available evidence, Transatlantic Inter-Societal Consensus (TASC) class A and B lesions are best suited for endovascular therapy, while TASC class C and D lesions are better treated with surgery. In general, PTA with selective stenting has a technical success rate of over 90% with a primary 5-year patency of 85% and secondary patency rate of 95%. Primary stenting has shown slightly improved immediate technical success rates ranging from 97% to 100% with an assisted patency of 85% to 90% at 2 years. Complication rates range from 5% to 8%. Access site problems such as hematomas (2.9%) or pseudoaneurysms (0.5%) are the most common. Embolization (1.6%), acute thrombosis (1.9%), and arterial rupture (0.2%) are less frequent. Mortality is low at 0.2%.

A retrograde, ipsilateral approach provides the easiest route to perform PTA and stenting of common iliac and proximal external iliac lesions. Distal external iliac lesions may be too close to the ipsilateral entry site in the femoral artery and can be better approached by an "up-and-over" technique from the contralateral femoral artery. Image-guided techniques using radiographic bony landmarks or roadmapping are sometimes required to obtain percutaneous femoral access, if the ipsilateral pulse is absent or severely diminished. Use of a micropuncture needle (21 gauge) can reduce the risk of entry-related complications.

Crossing the lesion is usually the most challenging step, especially if the artery is occluded. An angled-tip hydrophilic guidewire, supported by a low-profile catheter, is ideal for crossing a tight stenosis. Close attention must be paid to the way the wire interacts with the lesion. Multiple fine forward and backward movements are made while changing the orientation of the tip. If one is crossing a long lesion, the catheter is advanced with the wire to maintain necessary control and pushability.

Chronic occlusions can be crossed in over 70% of cases. Acute occlusions can almost always be crossed. A stiffer hydrophilic wire is usually required to cross chronic occlusions. In most cases of chronic total occlusions, the wire at some point traverses in the subintimal plane. Re-entry into the true lumen must be confirmed as soon as the lesion is crossed. This is done by either spinning the wire and noting free rotation of the tip or passing a catheter and injecting contrast to visualize the lumen.

Following successful crossing of the lesion with the guidewire, PTA and/or stenting may be performed. PTA will usually suffice for simple aortic lesions and lesions in the common iliac arteries. Selective stenting is used when PTA alone is unsuccessful. In the external iliac arteries, primary stenting is typically performed, as the artery is smaller, calcified, and more prone to dissection. Success is defined as less than 10% residual stenosis, with a pressure gradient less than 5 mm Hg mean or less than 10 mm Hg systolic. Moderate stenosis or lesions with less than 5 mm Hg mean resting gradient may be assessed for hemodynamic significance with an intra-arterial papaverine challenge (30 mg). A sustained gradient of more than 10 mm Hg systolic over 2 minutes is considered significant. Occlusions and re-stenosis after prior PTA alone should be routinely stented primarily.

Bifurcation Lesions

Iliac angioplasty and stenting within 1 cm of the aortic bifurcation occasionally requires a "kissing" balloon or stent in the contralateral proximal common iliac artery. The apparent ipsilateral lesion actually represents an iliac extension of a larger plaque based at the aortic flow divider, which can be "pushed over" during an angioplasty and occlude the contralateral iliac artery. Simultaneous bilateral balloon inflation can "protect" against this event.

Postoperative Management and Follow-up

This patient is placed on lifelong anti-platelet therapy. Clopidogrel (Plavix) 75 mg/d is given for 1 month, and thereafter, aspirin 325 mg/d. Her first postoperative return visit is at 1 month, and subsequently every 6 months with serial ABI determinations in the vascular lab. Depending on the original lesion and the severity of multilevel disease, re-stenosis rates can range from 5% to 10% per year after percutaneous iliac interventions. Therefore, lifelong follow-up is mandatory. Treatment of re-stenosis is often successful with repeat angioplasty or stenting, and assisted primary and secondary patency rates can exceed 90% in 5 years.

Suggested Readings

Bosch JL. Meta-analysis of the results of PTA and stent placement for aortoiliac occlusive disease. *Radiology.* 1997;204:87-96.

Palmaz JC, et al. Stenting of the iliac arteries with the Palmaz stent: Experience from a multicenter trial. *Cardiovasc Intervent Radiol.* 1992;15:291-297.

Schneider PA. *Endovascular Skills: Guidewire and Catheter Skills for Endovascular Surgery.* 2nd ed. New York: Marcel Dekker; 2003.

Sullivan TM, et al. Percutaneous arterial dilation for atherosclerotic lower extremity occlusive disease. In: Ernst CB, Stanley JC, eds. *Current Therapy in Vascular Surgery.* 4th ed. St. Louis: Mosby; 2001; 504–509.

Tetteroo E. Randomized comparison of primary stent placement versus primary angioplasty followed by selective stent placement in patients with iliac artery occlusive disease. *Lancet.* 1998;351:1153-1159.

Lal P.K. Yilmaz, MD, and Rajabrata Sarkar, MD

Presentation

A 42-year-old woman presents to the emergency department with acute left foot pain and numbness, which have been present for the last 24 hours. She has a prior history of worsening bilateral lower extremity pain over 3 months, which she describes as calf pain after walking several blocks. Over the last 24 hours she has been having similar pain while at rest. She notes some pain now in her right leg, although not as severe as her left.

Her medical history is significant for well-controlled hypertension and mild chronic obstructive pulmonary disease. She has a 45 pack-year history of smoking. On examination she has absent femoral pulses bilaterally and early evidence of gangrene over the left toes. She also has diminished 2-point discrimination, and weak plantar and dorsal flexion and extension of both feet on neurologic examination.

Differential Diagnosis

The differential diagnoses of acute bilateral lower extremity pain and numbness include traumatic spinal cord injury, prolapsed intervertebral disk, aortic dissection, and acute aortic occlusion. In this patient with absent bilateral femoral pulses, history of worsening lower extremity pain, and cardiovascular risk factors, the primary diagnosis should be acute aortic occlusion as a result of either thrombus or embolus.

Discussion

Aortic occlusion is a vascular emergency that can be caused by either embolism (almost always cardiac in origin) or thrombosis of a severely diseased aortoiliac arterial system. The risk factors for embolic aortic occlusion are similar to those for other arterial embolism and include atrial fibrillation, prior myocardial infarction, dilated cardiomyopathy, and any prior arterial embolism. Less common causes of aortic occlusion include thrombosis of an aortic aneurysm or aortic dissection. Symptoms of embolic aortic occlusion are typical of arterial ischemia to the lower extremities and consist of the classic five Ps of limb ischemia: pain, pallor, paresthesia, pulselessness, and poikilothermia (coolness). Embolic aortic occlusion is an acute event and most patients will be able to recall exactly when the symptoms began. The ischemia and symptoms of embolic aortic occlusion are usually more severe than of thrombotic occlusion because these patients do not have preexisting collateral channels secondary to long-standing peripheral vascular occlusive disease. Thrombotic occlusion of the aorta is a more gradual process, with progression of symptoms over several days. Dehydration or decreased cardiac output predisposes to thrombotic occlusion, and thus diarrhea, vomiting, or cardiogenic or septic shock often precedes thrombotic aortic occlusion. Almost all patients with thrombotic aortic occlusion will have a prior history of symptoms of peripheral arterial occlusive disease, most commonly intermittent claudication. Unfortunately, the maxim that aortic occlusion in a patient with prior claudication is always due to thrombosis cannot be uniformly applied, because a history of claudication can be elicited in 25% of patients with embolic aortic occlusion.

The diagnosis of aortic occlusion can be based on the clinical findings of acute limb ischemia as described above and the finding of absent femoral pulses bilaterally. If there is suspicion for embolic aortic occlusion, then immediate operative thrombectomy is performed without prior angiography. If thrombosis of the aorta is suspected, then preoperative angiography is done to define the extent of occlusive disease and the sites of planned revascularization, usually aortofemoral bypass.

Patients with spinal or musculoskeletal causes of lower extremity pain or paralysis will usually have palpable femoral pulses and nonischemic extremities. Unfortunately, the diagnosis and treatment of aortic occlusion are often delayed secondary to evaluation and consideration of a neurologic cause of the symptoms. In the case of embolic occlusion with severe ischemia, this delay can be catastrophic and often results in eventual limb loss, and occasionally death.

Recommendation

Immediate angiography.

Angiograms

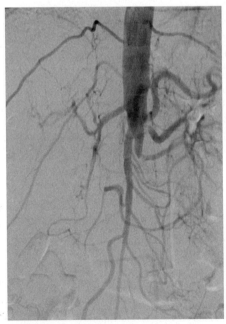
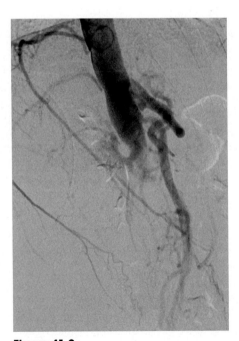

Figure 41-1   **Figure 41-2**

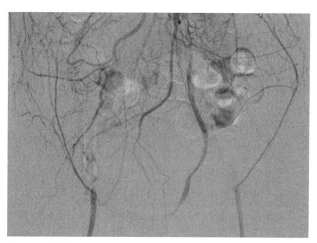

Figure 41-3

Angiogram Report

The patient underwent urgent angiography, which demonstrated complete occlusion of the infrarenal abdominal aorta (Fig. 41-1). The celiac and superior mesenteric arteries were both stenotic (Fig. 41-2). The inferior mesenteric artery was not visualized, and there was also a stenosis of the left main renal artery with occlusion of the right renal artery. The femoral arteries reconstituted via pelvic collateral vessels and the superficial femoral and deep femoral arteries were patent bilaterally (Fig. 41-3).

Diagnosis and Recommendation

Diagnosis is acute occlusion of the infrarenal aorta with celiac, superior mesenteric, and left renal artery stenoses. The patient's past medical history and the relative chronicity of symptoms, as well as the angiography findings, are consistent with atherosclerotic disease. Anticoagulation with intravenous sodium heparin is instituted to prevent propagation of thrombus and preserve collateral flow. Immediate aortofemoral bypass is recommended with mesenteric and visceral bypass. The chances of limb salvage are good with prompt surgical revascularization.

Approach

The critical decision in the approach to the patient with aortic occlusion is whether to perform preoperative angiography. In the patient with a predisposing condition for arterial embolism, no prior history of claudication, and acute symptoms of aortic occlusion, immediate surgical embolectomy is recommended without the delay associated with preoperative angiography. If there are prior symptoms of peripheral occlusive disease or if the distinction between embolic and thrombotic occlusion is not clear, then angiography is recommended. Thrombotic aortic occlusion is almost always limited to the infrarenal aorta, and is treated by aortofemoral bypass grafting or extra-anatomic bypass if the patient is a prohibitive operative risk. Perioperative mortality in the setting of acute aortic occlusion approaches 5%, and potential complications include myocardial infarction, renal failure (often secondary to myoglobinuria), and need for fasciotomy or additional distal bypass procedures.

Discussion

In cases of acute aortic occlusion, surgical treatment is based on the diagnosis of either embolic or thrombotic occlusion. If embolism is suspected, then retrograde transfemoral catheter embolectomy is performed via both common femoral arteries. Arteriotomy is made opposite the orifice of the deep femoral artery to allow distal embolectomy of this vessel as well as the superficial femoral artery. As embolism occurs most commonly in normal or minimally diseased vessels, embolectomy rapidly restores inflow. Distal thrombus in the infrapopliteal vessels, either from propagation or dislodged during embolectomy, can result in persistent ischemia of the distal leg and foot. On-table angiography is performed, followed by either catheter embolectomy of the distal popliteal and tibial arteries or infusion of operative intra-arterial thrombolytic therapy as needed.

For thrombotic occlusion of the aorta, aortobifemoral bypass is usually performed. For aortofemoral bypass grafting, care must be exercised in clamping because thrombus will usually extend to just below the renal arteries, and clamping across the thrombus can extrude thrombus into the renal arteries. We transect the unclamped aorta with an open clamp pre-positioned just below the renal arteries. The aortic pressure will blow out the remaining plug of thrombus in the juxtarenal aorta after which the clamp is applied. The distal graft limbs are often extended onto the proximal aspect of the deep femoral artery as these patients rarely have patent superficial femoral arteries.

Case Continued

Because the patient had disease of the abdominal aorta including visceral vessels, a transperitoneal approach was used to perform aortoceliac, aorto-superior mesenteric, aortorenal, aortobifemoral bypass with a Dacron graft.

Approach

For poor-risk patients with acute thrombotic occlusion of the aorta and advanced or unstable cardiopulmonary disease, an axillofemoral bypass is a lower risk option. In this younger patient with minimal to moderate co-morbid conditions, an aortobifemoral bypass provides greater durability as well as the option of treating her renal and visceral occlusive disease.

With either embolic or thrombotic aortic occlusion, care is taken during restoration of blood flow to the severely ischemic limbs to prevent metabolic and systemic complications from the toxic metabolites in the venous blood returning from the limbs. Administration of bicarbonate, mannitol, and anti-arrhythmic agents may be required, and serum potassium levels are closely monitored.

Patients with embolic occlusion of the aorta, like all patients with arterial embolism, should be treated with long-term anticoagulation. Long-term survival after arterial embolism is related to overall cardiac status but remains worse than an age-matched cohort. Aortic occlusion due to thrombosis carries a better long-term prognosis; however, a significant percentage of patients require later revascularization for distal (lower extremity) or proximal (renal or mesenteric) occlusive disease.

Suggested Readings

Babu SC, Shah PM, Nitahara J. Acute aortic occlusion: factors that influence outcome. *J Vasc Surg*. 1995;21:567-575.

Dossa CD, Shepard AD, Reddy DJ, et al. Acute aortic occlusion: a 40-year experience. *Arch Surg*. 1994;129:603-608.

Littooy FN, Baker WH. Acute aortic occlusion: a multifaceted catastrophe. *J Vasc Surg*. 1986; 4:211-216.

Surowiec SM, Isiklar H, Sreeram S, Weiss VJ, Lumsden AB. Acute occlusion of the abdominal aorta. *Am J Surg*. 1998;176:193-197.

Amy B. Reed, MD

Presentation

A 61-year-old man is referred for evaluation of right lower extremity pain. He has a longstanding history of one-block claudication; however, 2 weeks ago his right foot developed bluish discoloration after showering. Since then, he has noted increasing redness upon standing, decreased sensation, and pain in the foot at night. He reports a 60-pack year smoking history, hypertension, hyperlipidemia, and a history of myocardial infarction treated with percutaneous coronary angioplasty. On physical examination, his blood pressure is 132/80 mm Hg in both arms. The femoral pulses are weakly palpable. The right foot is cool with sluggish capillary refill and a monophasic Doppler signal in the dorsalis pedis. There are no open sores or ulcerations on either lower extremity. Laboratory studies including complete blood cell count, creatinine level, and prothrombin time are normal.

Differential Diagnosis

The differential diagnoses for unilateral lower extremity pain without ulceration include diabetic neuropathy, nerve root compression, reflex sympathetic dystrophy, venous disease, and arterial insufficiency. In this patient with a history of extensive atherosclerosis and lower extremity claudication, which has now progressed to rest pain, critical limb ischemia from atherosclerotic occlusive disease must be considered the primary diagnosis.

Discussion

Critical limb ischemia results from insufficient arterial perfusion to supply the basal metabolic demands of the toes, foot, or ankle. After taking a careful history and performing a thorough physical examination, measurement of the ankle/brachial index (ABI) is a fundamental diagnostic tool for evaluation of lower extremity arterial insufficiency. Many patients, including diabetic patients, will often have heavily calcified arteries, rendering them noncompressible and thus falsely elevating the ABI. Pulse-volume recordings (PVRs) and toe pressures are typically unaffected by calcification and should be obtained in these patients. ABIs less than 0.40, ankle pressures below 50 mm Hg, or toe pressures under 30 mm Hg with monophasic pulse volume recordings are all indicative of critical limb ischemia.

Recommendation

Noninvasive vascular laboratory studies, including ABI and PVRs, and aortography with bilateral lower extremity arteriography are ordered.

Vascular Laboratory Reports

	Right	Left
Brachial	132 mm Hg	132 mm Hg
Thigh	90 mm Hg	104 mm Hg
Calf	62 mm Hg	86 mm Hg
Posterior tibial	38 mm Hg	76 mm Hg
Dorsalis pedis	40 mm Hg	80 mm Hg
Toe	15 mm Hg	45 mm Hg
Ankle/brachial index	0.30	0.61

Pulse volume recordings: Monophasic waveforms at all levels on the right. Waveforms are biphasic at the thigh and calf level on the right, and monophasic at all infrageniculate levels on the left.

Arteriography

Aortogram with bilateral lower extremity runoff reveals the following images.

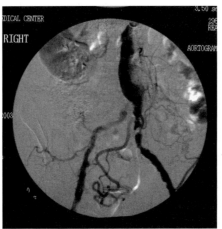

Figure 42-1

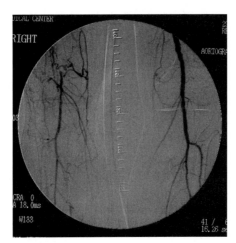

Figure 42-3

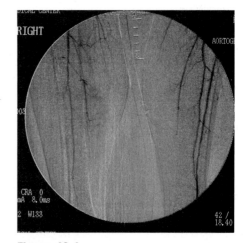

Figure 42-4

Arteriography Report

There is dilation of the infrarenal aorta, suggestive of aneurysmal disease in addition to severe aortoiliac occlusive disease bilaterally. The hypogastric arteries are heavily diseased with the appearance of a prominent middle sacral artery supplying the pelvis. The superficial femoral artery is occluded on the right with single-vessel runoff. The left superficial femoral is diseased, but patent with two-vessel runoff.

Recommendation

Ultrasonography is indicated for follow-up on the arteriographic findings, suggestive of an infrarenal abdominal aortic aneurysm (AAA). A computed tomographic (CT) study could also be used; however, this typically requires an additional dye load (150 mL of intravenous contrast) on top of the 160 mL utilized for the arteriography, and is best avoided.

Ultrasound Report

Ultrasound reveals a heavily calcified 4.0 cm AAA without iliac involvement.

Diagnosis and Recommendation

The patient has a 4-cm AAA with severe bilateral iliac arterial occlusive disease, and right superficial femoral artery occlusion with single-vessel runoff to the right foot. This patient is offered an aortobifemoral bypass with possible right femoral to popliteal artery bypass. The presence of aneurysmal disease precludes the use of percutaneous iliac angioplasty and stenting in this patient. It is explained to the patient that the right lower extremity bypass may need to be performed at a later date if the operation is lengthy or significant bleeding is encountered, but that improving the inflow will be the first step in resolution of his rest pain.

Complications mentioned include bleeding, myocardial infarction, stroke, death, and graft failure requiring further surgery and possible amputation. The patient is instructed to continue all of his preoperative medications up to the day of surgery, particularly beta blockade and aspirin. Smoking cessation and its importance postoperatively in helping to maintain graft patency is discussed with the patient.

■ Surgical Approach

Bilateral longitudinal groin incisions are performed first, taking care to dissect the profunda femoris artery to a soft, nondiseased segment if the superficial femoral artery is occluded. The aorta is dissected free from the surrounding structures at the infrarenal level through a midline incision. After systemic heparinization, the aorta and iliac arteries are clamped. Often, removal of a short segment of infrarenal aorta facilitates the lie of the bypass graft. In this patient, with a 4-cm AAA and severe aortoiliac disease with right lower extremity rest pain, an end-end configuration of the proximal anastomosis of the aorto-bifemoral bypass is necessary to deal with the AAA. A bifurcated prosthetic graft is tunneled anterior to the diseased iliac arteries, making certain the graft lies deep to the ureters. Careful closure of the retroperitoneum is required to avoid development of an aortoenteric fistula in the future.

Case Continued

Upon entering the aorta, there is a significant amount of back bleeding from the prominent middle sacral artery previously noted on arteriography. This vessel, along with several lumbar arteries, is oversewn. Heavy calcification, along with superficial femoral artery occlusion on the right, requires that the distal anastomoses be sewn to the profunda femoris artery. Inspection of the sigmoid colon at this time reveals a pale, grayish color to the serosa with no signals on Doppler insonation.

Approach

Given the extensive occlusive disease of the external and internal iliac arteries, in addition to constructing an end-end proximal anastomosis with oversewing of the middle sacral artery, pelvic and distal colonic circulation undoubtedly will be compromised. Reimplantation of the inferior mesenteric artery onto the main body of the prosthetic graft will help improve flow, not only to the colon, but also to the pelvic structures. At this time, the patient is cold and has been under anesthesia for nearly 6 hours.

Case Continued

The patient is transferred to the intensive care unit hemodynamically stable with Doppler signals in the right peroneal and dorsalis pedis (DP) arteries, as well as the left posterior tibial and DP arteries. On postoperative day 2, the patient has a guaiac-positive stool with no associated abdominal pain, fever, or leukocytosis. He remains hemodynamically stable with a systolic blood pressure of 130 mm Hg. He has another guaiac-positive stool 2 days later, prompting sigmoidoscopy, which reveals some mild patchy areas of ischemia in the mid sigmoid colon, but no areas of full-thickness necrosis. By postoperative day 6, he is able to tolerate diet advancement and all preoperative medications are resumed. His feet remain warm with Doppler signals. Repeat noninvasive vascular laboratory studies reveal ABIs of 0.60 on the right and 0.80 on the left, with complete resolution of his right lower extremity rest pain.

Suggested Readings

Criqui MH, Langer RD, Fronek A, et al. Mortality over a period of 10 years in patients with peripheral arterial disease. *N Eng J Med.* 1992;326:381-386.

de Vries SO, Hunink MGM. Results of aortic bifurcation grafts for aortoiliac occlusive disease: a meta-analysis. *J Vasc Surg.* 1997;26:558-569.

Hirsch AT, Treat-Jacobson D, Lando HA, Hatsukami DK. The role of tobacco cessation, antiplatelet and lipid-lowering therapies in the treatment of peripheral arterial disease. *Vasc Med.* 1997;2:243-251.

Marin ML, Veith FJ, Sanchez LA, et al. Endovascular aortoiliac grafts in combination with standard infrainguinal arterial bypasses in the management of limb-threatening ischemia: preliminary report. *J Vasc Surg.* 1995;22:316-325.

Prendiville EJ, Burke PE, Colgan MP, et al. The profunda femoris: a durable outflow vessel in aortofemoral surgery. *J Vasc Surg.* 1992;16:23-29.

Mark G. Davies, MD, PhD

Presentation

A 70-year-old man, who is an inpatient, complains of sudden onset of rest pain in both his legs. The pain has persisted for 2 hours and is not relieved by any measures or medications. He had been admitted with small bowel obstruction and is 15 days after a laparotomy and lysis of adhesions. This was considered a difficult operation, and the patient has developed a midline enterocutaneous fistula. He has a previous history of an extended left colectomy for Duke's stage C colon adenocarcinoma 2 years previously and has completed adjuvant chemotherapy. He has a history of bilateral lower extremity claudication at 100 yards. He has hypertension, non-insulin-dependent diabetes, and chronic renal insufficiency (serum creatinine 1.5). On physical examination, the patient is noted to be in distress and to have his legs dependent over the side of the bed. He is audibly complaining of pain. His heart rate is irregularly irregular, and he is relatively hypotensive (blood pressure 90/50 mm Hg) with oliguria (less than 10 mL/h for last the 4 hours). The peripheral pulses are absent in the right and left legs. Femoral artery pulses were documented as present, but diminished, on his admission physical examination. Both legs are cool to touch from the inguinal ligaments down. Bilateral lower extremity sensation is absent and motor function is decreased. No continuous-wave Doppler signals are identified.

Differential Diagnosis

The differential diagnosis in this case is that of a saddle embolus or acute aortic occlusion. The history of previous claudication would suggest preexisting aortoiliac disease and allow one to suspect acute aortic occlusion rather than saddle embolism. Both require emergent therapy, but with different approaches.

Recommendation

This patient is in shock and has ischemic bilateral lower extremities. An arterial blood gas and a serum chemistry panel are obtained and an angiogram is arranged. Laboratory values suggest the patient has a new-onset metabolic acidosis. This raises the suspicion of mesenteric vessel involvement. An angiogram is obtained through a left brachial artery approach, with an emphasis on defining his visceral arteries and aortoiliac anatomy.

Angiogram of the Aorta

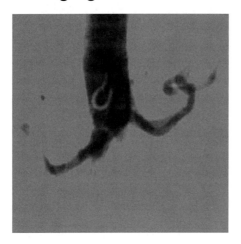

Figure 43-1

Angiogram Report

Anterior-posterior (A-P) view demonstrates infrarenal acute aortic occlusion with heavy calcifications suggestive of chronic disease. A lateral view confirmed patent celiac and superior mesenteric arteries (not pictured). There is reconstitution of the common femoral arteries bilaterally.

Case Continued

Prior to and during the angiogram, the patient is resuscitated, is prepared for surgery, and is heparinized (100 units/kg IV).

Diagnosis and Recommendation

The patient has a hostile abdomen, and as such, a direct transabdominal approach or a retroperitoneal approach would be very difficult. Options in this patient include an attempt to use endoluminal therapy to reopen one or both iliac vessels. If this fails, the patient is recommended to undergo axillobifemoral bypass grafting.

Case Continued

Under fluoroscopy, percutaneous access is gained in both common femoral arteries. Sheaths are placed and guide wires are passed retrograde into the aorta. The right guidewire passes without difficulty, but the left fails to pass into the aorta. A rheolytic thrombectomy catheter system, initially using bolus instillation of 5 mg tissue plasminogen activator in 50 mL to lace the clot with a thrombolytic agent, is followed by heparinized saline. The rheolytic thrombectomy catheter is passed over the wire multiple times without adequate restoration of antegrade flow. At this stage, it is decided to stop and pursue open intervention.

▪ Angiogram of the Aorta

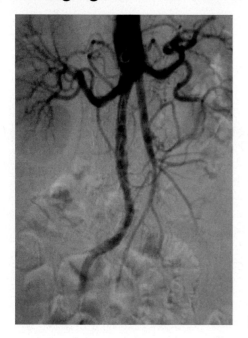

Figure 43-2

Angiogram Report

A-P view demonstrates a channel in the aorta after rheolytic catheter thrombectomy.

▪ Surgical Approach

Once informed consent has been obtained, the patient is placed under general anesthesia. The left chest, abdomen, and both legs are prepared and draped in a standard fashion to form a sterile field. An axillobifemoral bypass graft using an 8-mm EPTFE graft is performed without difficulty. Intraoperative duplex imaging confirms adequate distal outflow. The patient receives 25 mg of mannitol to induce forced diuresis prior to reperfusion of the lower limbs. Due to the severity of the lower leg ischemia, bilateral calf four-compartment fasciotomies of the lower extremities are also performed. There are continuous-wave Doppler signals in the anterior and posterior tibial arteries bilaterally.

Case Continued

The patient remains intubated and is transferred to the surgical intensive care unit (ICU). He is continued on anticoagulation with intravenous heparin. Serial serum chemistries demonstrate rising potassium levels and a metabolic acidosis. The patient also develops myoglobinuria. The patient is rehydrated with sodium bicarbonate supplemented crystalloid solutions. His hyperkalemia is aggressively treated with furosemide and an insulin glucose infusion. The patient is monitored to ensure forced diuresis. His hyperkalemia and acidosis resolve. Over the next 3 days, he is extubated and discharged from the ICU. On day 7, the patient is returned to the operating room for primary closure of his fasciotomies. He is subsequently returned to the general surgical service for management of his enterocutaneous fistula.

Discussion

Acute occlusion of the abdominal aorta due to *in situ* thrombosis is a relatively rare event with a cumulative incidence of 8% (aortic occlusion due to embolic disease has a relative incidence of 15%). However, it has a mortality rate of over 50%. The clinical presentation varies from acute limb ischemia to lower extremity neurologic symptoms suggestive of a spinal cord lesion. Acute *in situ* thrombosis and emboli to the distal aorta are the most common etiologies. In general, preexisting atherosclerosis combined with a low-flow state as a result of a low cardiac output is a relatively frequent cause of acute aortic occlusion. Hypercoagulability is also associated with acute aortic occlusion. The management of acute aortic occlusion should include immediate heparinization and resuscitation, with the goal of improving any underlying cardiac condition if it exists. Operative intervention is required whether thromboembolectomy, aortofemoral bypass, or axillofemoral bypass, in the acute neurologically impaired patient. If the lower extremity ischemia is not severe, the preferred treatment of choice should be intra-arterial thrombolytic therapy combined with mechanical rheolytic thrombectomy to rapidly debulk the clot in the iliac system. This latter method is associated with a lower mortality than operative therapy in this high-risk patient group.

Suggested Readings

Davies MG, Lee DE, Green RM. Current spectrum of thrombolysis. In: Moore W, Ahn S, ed. *Endovascular Surgery*. 3rd ed. Philadelphia: WB Saunders; 2001:255–274.

Haimovic H. Acute arterial thrombosis. In: Haimovic H, Ascher E, Hollier L, Strandness DE, Towne J, ed. *Vascular Surgery*. 4th ed. Cambridge, MA: Blackwell Scientific; 1996: 423–444.

Huber TS. Acute aortic occlusion. In: Ernst CB, Stanley JC, ed. *Current Therapy in Vascular Surgery*. 4th ed. St Louis: Mosby; 2001:395.

Presentation

A 65-year-old man underwent placement of an aortobifemoral Dacron graft for aortoiliac occlusive disease. He recovered uneventfully and was well until one and a half years later, when he developed intermittent fevers, fatigue, malaise, and weight loss. He is admitted into the hospital and worked up for fever of unknown origin. During his hospital admission, he is noted to have daily temperature spikes to 101.6°F. His examination is notable for a thin, ill-appearing man with prominent, nontender, femoral pulses. He has a well-healed abdominal incision and left groin incision; however, there is a small area of breakdown in the superior pole of his right groin incision with purulent drainage. His white blood cell (WBC) count is 7500/mm^3 and his erythrocyte sedimentation rate is 64 mm/h. His chemistry panel is normal with the exception that his albumin is 2.2 g/dL. A computed tomography (CT) scan and sinogram are ordered.

Differential Diagnosis

A pseudoaneurysm must be considered in any patient with a prominent femoral pulse and a known anastomosis in the groin. An ultrasonographic examination is a fast, safe, and reliable method of confirming the diagnosis and relates not only the size but also whether there is thrombosis within the aneurysm. An incidence of false aneurysms of 1% to 5% has been cited in the literature and is most common at the femoral anastomosis of an aortobifemoral bypass graft. The common thread among the numerous etiologic factors reported is degenerative changes in the host's arterial wall with dehiscence of the suture line. Because the anastomosis will forever be dependent on the integrity of the suture line, strict adherence to basic vascular surgical tenets, such as using nonabsorbable, monofilament suture and taking bites that include all layers of the arterial wall, are essential when sewing prosthetic material to native artery.

Any patient diagnosed with pseudoaneurysm compels the clinician to rule out graft infection. Indeed, one report suggested an infectious etiology in as many as 24% of femoral false aneurysms. Further, a pseudoaneurysm in one groin could also herald other graft problems, such as contralateral pseudoaneurysm, and mandates close scrutiny of the entire graft. Accordingly, a malnourished man presenting with fever of unknown origin and a pulsatile groin mass after aortobifemoral reconstruction has an infected graft until proven otherwise.

CT Scan

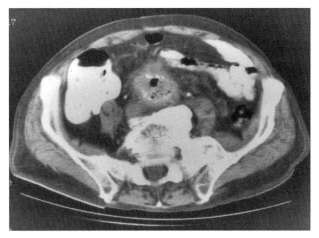

Figure 44-1

CT Scan Report

CT scan demonstrates fluid and stranding around the aortic portions of the graft extending down both graft limbs. He has bilateral pseudoaneurysms at the femoral anastomosis.

Sinogram

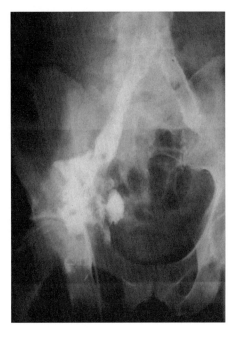

Figure 44-2

Sinogram Report

Contrast-enhanced sinogram demonstrating contrast freely flowing around the right femoral anastomosis tracking up the right limb to the bifurcation. This most certainly signifies lack of incorporation of the graft into the surrounding tissues. Gram stain from the right groin drainage revealed numerous WBCs, but no bacteria.

Diagnosis and Recommendation

The findings on the CT scan and contrast sinography confirm aortobifemoral graft infection. Findings suggestive of graft infection on contrast-enhanced CT include loss of normal tissue planes and stranding in the retroperitoneal space, abnormal collections of fluid and gas, false aneurysms, vertebral osteomyelitis, or juxta-aortic retroperitoneal abscess. Although computed tomography's diagnostic accuracy has certainly been validated in advanced graft infections, it is inconsistent in low-grade infections.

The percutaneous localization of a perigraft cavity by the injection of contrast can be a useful aid in making the diagnosis, although there is a theoretical possibility that it can contaminate an otherwise sterile graft. Culture and Gram stain of the perigraft fluid can often identify the etiologic agent, but failure to do so does not rule out graft infection. A late graft infection, often from a low-virulence microorganism, may only yield WBCs on Gram stain.

Another modality that can be used in identifying patients with aortic graft infections who do not have specific signs is radionuclide scintigraphic techniques. These include indium-labeled WBC, immunoglobin G, or technetium-labeled WBC scans. These methods identify graft infection by radioisotopic imaging of inflammatory sites. They are a useful adjunct in the nonspecific clinical presentation of low-grade graft infections; however, there have been false positives in patients with hematomas or sterile inflammatory processes around the graft.

Case Continued

The patient is taken to the operating room and undergoes an axillobifemoral bypass with a two-team approach. This is performed using externally supported, 8-mm polytetrafluoroethylene (PTFE) graft. The external draining sinus is isolated with adhesive sterile dressing. The axillary anastomosis is made through an infraclavicular incision and fashioned end to side in the first portion of the axillary artery. The PTFE graft is tunneled subcutaneously lateral to the anterior superior iliac spine. To allow a tension-free axillary anastomosis, the graft is routed adjacent and parallel to the axillary artery before passing in a gentle curve to the anastomosis. Care is taken to avoid the contaminated groin field, and the mid-profunda artery is approached through an incision lateral to the sartorius muscle. All incisions are closed and excluded with adhesive dressings before approaching the infected prosthesis.

The infected aortic graft and each limb are removed through separate groin incisions and a transabdominal incision. The distal anastomoses are disconnected first and the surrounding tissue is debrided. The arteriotomies are closed with vein patch angioplasties. The groin incisions are loosely closed and drained. The remainder of the graft is removed through the abdominal incision. The aortic stump is debrided and closed in two layers of monofilament suture. The retroperitoneal wound is debrided, cultured, and drained with closed suctioned drains brought out through separate stab incisions. The explanted graft is cultured and yielded *Staphylococcus epidermidis*.

■ Approach

Nowhere in vascular surgery is it more important to have a well thought out plan than when dealing with a patient with an infected aortobifemoral prosthesis. Consideration of current comorbidities, nutritional state of the patient, and immunocompetence all must be weighed before a definitive approach to the patient is carried out. These patients often have low albumin and low total lymphocyte counts and are anergic on skin testing. A patient with an indolent infection may have the luxury of time to be placed on total parenteral nutrition and antibiotics to improve some of these parameters prior to surgery. The patient will need an intensive care unit (ICU) bed, and the family should be prepared for a long convalescence. Diligent ICU care in the postoperative period is essential to get these critically ill patients through following a large operation.

Surgical Approach

The choices presented to the vascular surgeon contemplating reconstruction of the patient with the infected graft are many and varied. The first is whether an extra-anatomic bypass versus an *in situ* reconstruction will be performed. If an *in situ* bypass is chosen, then the choice of conduit is the next consideration. Autogenous femoral-popliteal vein, cryopreserved vein, or a new prosthetic in the same retroperitoneal bed have all been reported, and all have some merit. If an extra-anatomic choice is considered, then what will be the sequence and timing of reconstruction? Removing the infected graft followed by reconstruction may render the legs ischemic for an unnecessarily long time and can subject the patient to complications, such as compartment syndrome, paresis, or amputation. Performing an extra-anatomic reconstruction followed by immediate removal of the infected prosthesis can result in a prolonged operative time with the incumbent fluid requirements, long anesthetic time, and possibly multiple transfusions, all with the attendant physiologic stress on an already debilitated host. In our patient, we chose extra-anatomic bypass followed by immediate graft removal using the two-team approach to minimize the ischemic time to the extremities and taking advantage of the speed afforded by two teams operating simultaneously in each groin.

Case Continued

The patient tolerates the procedure well and spends 6 days in the surgical ICU. He is discharged from the hospital on postoperative day 17. Intravenous antibiotics are continued for 2 weeks following the procedure, and the patient is continued on oral antibiotics for the next 3 months. He is followed up every 3 months after discharge and undergoes clinical and noninvasive arterial evaluation (consisting of duplex ultrasonographic surveillance for graft patency). He is discharged on daily aspirin. He is alive and well 2 years after the procedure with a patent axillobifemoral bypass graft.

Discussion

The reported incidence of aortofemoral graft infection is 0.5% to 3%, making it a rare, but dreaded, complication of reconstructive aortic surgery. Graft infections have been divided at 4 months into early and late. Although less common, early graft infections are caused by more virulent microorganisms such as *Staphylococcus aureus* or one or more of the gram-negative organisms. These patients are toxic and they present septic, and the diagnosis is straightforward. The imaging modalities (eg, CT scan) routinely used are more accurate at making the diagnosis in these early infections, and often have classic features such as perigraft abscess or fluid collection.

However, the vast majority of patients with graft infections often present late. Late infections are subtler, often delaying diagnosis and definitive surgical management in a patient who already may be nutritionally and immunologically compromised. For instance, infection several years after implantation or infections caused by less virulent microorganisms may present with nonspecific constitutional symptoms such as malaise, abdominal pain, or intermittent gastrointestinal bleeding.

Historical information such as abdominal pain, recent medical procedures, or illnesses that may result in hematogenous or lymphatic spread should be investigated. Recent nonhealing wounds, foot infections, or urologic manipulations all can contribute to transient bacteremia and possible graft infections. On examination, any pulsatile groin mass should alert the clinician to possible graft infection. Delayed healing incisions, cellulitis and/or a perigraft mass, or graft cutaneous sinus tract all can be harbingers of an infected graft. The extremities should be carefully examined for septic emboli, which can appear as a cluster of petechiae downstream from the infected anastomosis.

Although several potential etiologic sources of prosthetic infection exist, it is likely from contamination at the time of implantation due to a break in sterile technique. The source can be from the graft itself, the surgical instruments, or from the host or a member of the surgical team. The graft itself is an inert material, and once contaminated will harbor organisms indefinitely. The porous nature of the woven Dacron fabric may allow sequestration of bacteria in a privileged place, unable to be penetrated by WBCs. The superficial location of the graft in the groin increases its chance of contamination, especially if there is a wound complication or need for re-exploration. Great care must be exercised to avoid contact with the graft and the patient's dermis, especially in the groin areas.

S. aureus, *S. epidermidis*, and *Escherichia coli* are the causative organisms in 80% of graft infections. Less frequently implicated organisms include *Klebsiella*, *Proteus*, *Enterobacter*, *Pseudomonas*, and nonhemolytic streptococci. The *S. epidermidis* species is especially difficult to detect. Accordingly, the graft infection that is produced includes a sterile exudate, absence of graft incorporation, and a normal WBC count. Methods of tissue culture have been described in graft infections with organisms of low virulence, such as *S. epidermidis*, which improve the chances of identifying the etiologic agent. Culture of explanted bioprosthetics in a tryptic soy broth yielded more isolates over traditional blood agar methods. Further, when using biofilm disruption, either by sonication or a mechanical grinding process, the yields of recovering an isolate were even greater.

The surgical goals of managing a patient with infected aortobifemoral prosthesis are twofold: preserve limb viability and function and remove the infected graft. Complete excision of the infected graft and revascularization through a noninfected bed has been the standard treatment of graft infection. However, some advocate newer *in situ* reconstruction using autogenous, prosthetic, or allograft conduits as a safe and durable alternative. Proponents of this method report that the operation can be performed in selected patients with low-grade infections in whom signs of sepsis are absent with sufficiently low mortality (7.9%) and lower extremity amputation rate (5%). Although these results were encouraging, there was still a sufficiently high complication rate (12.5%) for lower extremity compartment syndrome and recurrent infection rate (10%) to warrant caution. Patient characteristics for which this treatment may be appropriate include presentation of infection months to years after implantation, no clinical signs of infection, sterile blood cultures, and inability to culture bacteria from perigraft fluid. These infections are usually found to be due to coagulase-negative staphylococci on graft-biofilm culture.

In contrast, contemporary series of extra-anatomic bypass followed by graft explantation report a mortality rate of 12.5% and a 7% amputation rate. A second operation was required to maintain axillofemoral patency in 14 of 48 survivors (29% incidence), and an aortic stump dehiscence occurred in 1 out of 55 patients. Although these results are sobering, they represent a tremendous improvement over results published just a decade ago and reflect improvements in operative technique, anesthetic care, postoperative ICU care, and infectious disease science.

Few other diseases encountered in vascular surgery can test the creativity and ingenuity of the surgeon like an infected aortobifemoral graft infection. Clearly, no single approach is suitable for all patients, and the contemporary vascular surgeon must be proficient at each of these to tailor the operation to the patient.

Suggested Readings

Bandyk DF, Berni GA, Thiele BL, et al. Aortofemoral graft infection due to *Staphylococcus epidermidis. Arch Surg.* 1984;119:102-107.

Bandyk DF, Novotney ML, Back MR, et al. Expanded application of in situ replacement for prosthetic graft infection. *J Vasc Surg.* 2001;34:411-419.

Fiorani P, Speziale F, Rizzo L, et al. Detection of aortic graft infection with leukocytes labeled with technetium 99m-hexatazime. *J Vasc Surg.* 1993;17:87-97.

Kwaan JHM, Dahl RK, Connolly J. Immunocompetence in patients with prosthetic graft infection. *J Vasc Surg.* 1984;1:45-50.

Reilly LM, Stoney RJ, Goldstone J, et al. Improved management of aortic graft infection: the influence of operation sequence and staging. *J Vasc Surg.* 1987;5:421-432.

Szilagyi DE, Smith RF, Elliott JP, et al. Anastomotic aneurysms after vascular reconstruction: problems of incidence, etiology, and treatment. *Surgery.* 1975;78:800-816.

Yeager RA, Taylor LM, Moneta GL, et al. Improved results with conventional management of infrarenal aortic infection. *J Vasc Surg.* 1999;30:76-82.

Joss D. Fernandez, MD, and Marc A. Passman, MD

Presentation

A 66-year-old woman, who underwent aortobifemoral bypass grafting for claudication from aortoiliac occlusive disease 3 years ago, presents to the emergency department after an episode of hematemesis. She relates a history of low-grade fevers and fatigue over the past 2 weeks, and intermittent melena over the past 2 months. Physical findings are significant for orthostatic hypotension, tachycardia, temperature of 38.6°C, mid epigastric discomfort without peritoneal signs on abdominal palpation, and a guaiac-positive rectal examination.

Differential Diagnosis

The diagnosis of aortic graft-enteric fistula should be suspected in any patient with symptoms of gastrointestinal bleeding and prior aortic bypass graft. Aortic graft-enteric fistula is rare, with a reported incidence after aortic bypass grafting of 0.6% to 4%. Secondary aortic graft-enteric fistula occurs following aortic bypass using prosthetic graft, either along the suture line of the anastomosis, or along the main body-limb of the graft.

The pathogenesis of aortic graft-enteric fistula is unknown, but technical problems at initial aortic operation, repetitive mechanical trauma from aortic pulsation leading to erosion of the graft into the intestine, suture or graft material fatigue, and delayed indolent graft infection have been implicated. Prevention of aortic graft-enteric fistula at the time of initial aortic graft placement consists of strict aseptic technique, perioperative antibiotics, hemostasis at the suture line, and complete covering of prosthetic material with retroperitoneum. Leaving the duodenum intraperitoneal by reapproximating the lateral edges of the peritoneum and additional graft bolstering over the suture line has also been suggested to reduce fistula formation. A retroperitoneal approach may also decrease the potential for aortic graft-enteric fistula.

Symptoms and signs of aortic graft-enteric fistula are varied, but include gastrointestinal bleeding (84%), sepsis (35%), abdominal pain (33%), back pain (20%), abdominal pulsatile mass (7%), and groin mass (5%). Of those with gastrointestinal bleeding, presenting symptoms include hematemesis (47%), melena (41%), herald bleeding (37%), shock (27%), hematochezia (9%), and bright red blood per rectum (7%).

Once aortic graft-enteric fistula has been excluded, other more common causes of upper gastrointestinal hemorrhage should be considered. The complete differential diagnosis of upper gastrointestinal hemorrhage includes peptic ulcer disease (50%), erosive gastritis (5% to 25%), esophageal varices (9% to 21%), Mallory-Weiss tear (11% to 14%), malignancy (3%), and esophagitis (2% to 8%).

Case Continued

Fluid resuscitation is administered, and the patient's heart rate and blood pressure normalize. Blood laboratory studies reveal anemia (hematocrit 24%) and leukocytosis (white blood cell count 14.5 thousand/uL). Blood cultures are pending, but the initial Gram stain reveals gram-positive cocci. Esophagogastro-duodenoscopy is performed to the fourth portion of the duodenum, revealing no source of bleeding. Computed tomography (CT) scan with intravenous contrast and with oral contrast is obtained of the abdomen and pelvis.

Serial CT Scan

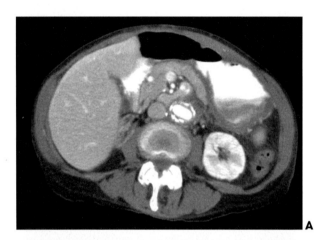

A

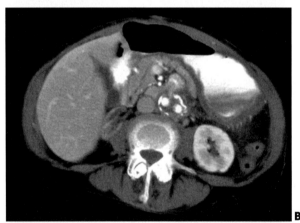

B

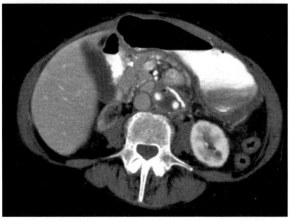

C Figure 45-1

CT Scan Report

Serial CT scan (abdomen) images reveal abutment of the fourth portion of the duodenum near the main body and limbs of the graft, periaortic fat stranding, and fluid around the graft with air adjacent to right limb of bifurcated graft.

Diagnosis

Aortic graft-enteric fistula.

Discussion

Serum laboratory studies including complete blood cell (CBC) count, erythrocyte sedimentation rate (ESR), and blood culture with Gram stain are often nonspecific, but with the clinical history may be suggestive of potential aortic graft-enteric fistula. Lack of diagnostic yield with blood cultures may reflect a noninfectious etiology with only half of eventual operative cultures being positive, in part due to systemic antibiotics started empirically. When positive, operative cultures usually contain mixed organisms. Common organisms include gram-positive cocci (*Streptococcus* and *Staphylococcus* species) (36%), *Escherichia coli* (11%), *Klebsiella* (2%), *Enterobacter* (2%), and *Candida* species (2%).

Aortic graft-enteric fistula can occur at any level of the gastrointestinal tract: duodenum (74%), small bowel (19%) (jejunum, 65%; ileum, 8%; and unspecified, 27%), colon (5%), and appendix (1%). Given the most common location of aortic graft-enteric fistula in the third or fourth portion of the duodenum, and the need to consider other more common causes of upper gastrointestinal bleeding, the preferred initial diagnostic test should be esophagogastroduodenoscopy (EGD). EGD should be performed by an experienced endoscopist and in an operating room setting. If an active bleeding source is seen in the third or fourth portion of the duodenum, direct and emergent operative treatment should be undertaken. If clot is visualized in the third or fourth portion of the duodenum, it should be left intact because any attempt to remove the clot can lead to fatal hemorrhage. However, failure to find a bleeding source does not eliminate aortic graft-enteric fistula from the differential. Although most common in the third and fourth portion of the duodenum, aortic graft-enteric fistula can occur in other locations of the gastrointestinal tract below the ligament of Treitz, and additional endoscopy may be required.

CT scan of the abdomen and pelvis with intravenous contrast and no oral contrast should follow if EGD is nondiagnostic. Water as an alternative to oral contrast may improve visualization of the fistula. Fluid surrounding the graft, fat stranding, bowel wall edema, or air outside the bowel wall suggests graft infection and possible fistula. Intravenous contrast entering the bowel is diagnostic. CT scanning has the additional advantage of evaluating other potential causes for the patient's symptoms.

Angiography is usually a nondiagnostic test, but is helpful for operative planning. Angiographic documentation of extravasation of intravenous contrast into the bowel is rarely seen, but when present is diagnostic. Other findings suggesting aortoenteric fistula include aortic-graft pseudoaneurysm and bowing of the graft. Selective mesenteric angiography may demonstrate bleeding from the bowel wall, which may be the source of hemorrhage in aortic graft-enteric erosion. Angiography also may define the fistula site, proximal/distal aortic-graft anastomosis, juxtarenal and suprarenal aortic anatomy, and lower extremity runoff. As magnetic resonance angiography (MRA) and CT angiography (CTA) technology improve, these modalities may eventually replace conventional angiography.

There is no longer a role for fluoroscopic interrogation of the upper gastrointestinal tract with oral contrast for diagnosis of aortic graft-enteric fistula. Although diagnostic accuracy is similar to endoscopy, its use affects the ability to perform CT scan or angiography. Findings include a sinus tract from the bowel wall, contrast material around the graft, defect in the bowel wall, partial intestinal obstruction, and bowel displacement.

Nuclear white blood cell scanning is not useful for diagnosing aortic graft-enteric fistula, but is sensitive for aortic graft infection. Indium 111-labeled leukocyte scans have less nonspecific bowel uptake and a greater target-to-background ratio than gallium 67 scans. These scans are useful in the stable patient with questionable aortic graft infection. A positive scan suggests infection, but is not diagnostic of aortic graft-enteric fistula.

Recommendation

Operative repair.

Discussion

Nonoperative interventions carry 100% mortality. If the patient is hemodynamically unstable and/or active bleeding is present, operative repair should be performed immediately. If the patient is stable, operative repair should not be delayed, but careful preoperative planning needs to be in place. Although the initial cause of aortic graft-enteric fistula may be noninfectious, once present, clinical decision-making should be based on the assumption that the aortic graft is infected. Important surgical tenets include timing of operative repair, optimal and timely control of the aorta above the graft, complete removal of devitalized aortic tissue and prosthetic graft material, consideration of aortic and bowel reconstruction and lower extremity revascularization options, and prevention of future secondary aortic problems.

Surgical Approach

Preoperative broad-spectrum antibiotics are initiated and the patient is taken to the operating room. Bilateral femoral veins are harvested for autologous reconstruction of the aorta with closure of the lower extremity incisions prior to abdominal incision. Laparotomy is performed, and reveals a fistula between the fourth portion of the duodenum and the proximal anastomosis of the prior aortic graft. There is turbid fluid around the graft, and intraoperative cultures are taken. The enteric portion of the fistula is repaired primarily with a serosal patch. The entire bifurcated aortic prosthetic graft is removed. The femoral veins are inverted to allow direct valve lysis. Neo-aortic reconstruction is performed from the infrarenal aorta to the bilateral common femoral arteries using the femoral veins, which are reconstructed into a bifurcated graft configuration. A pedicle omental patch is placed over the abdominal portion of the neo-aortic reconstruction.

Discussion

Several options exist for repair of secondary aortic graft-enteric fistula. If the patient is hemodynamically unstable, exploration begins with early proximal control of the supraceliac aorta. Preoperative endoluminal balloon tamponade and endovascular aortic stent grafts for actively bleeding fistula may be an option for aortic control, if technically feasible and expeditious. Because the objective is immediate control of bleeding, emergent operative treatment may include direct repair of the fistula and primary aortic graft repair, if the aorta will allow secure repair. However, this is just a temporizing solution to allow for stabilization of the patient and definitive treatment should only be delayed 1 to 2 days. If the extent of devitalized and infected tissue precludes immediate direct repair, then definitive treatment will need to be performed on an emergent basis with removal of infected aortic graft preceding reconstruction.

When the patient is hemodynamically stable, definitive operative planning should include preparation for revascularization prior to aortic exposure and removal of infected aortic graft. Extra-anatomic bypass using axillofemoral bypass, either staged or immediately prior to aortic graft resection, has been the traditional approach. The decision of a staged or sequential interval is based on the clinical setting, with the former reserved for patients with occult bleeding or with significant co-morbidities. The technique for axillofemoral bypass may involve use of a unilateral axillary artery with a crossover femoral-to-femoral bypass or separate grafts from bilateral axillary arteries. Use of the distal descending thoracic aorta has been described as an alternative to the axillary artery as an inflow source. The femoral exposure may also need to be modified so as not to expose any potentially infected aortofemoral graft at the groin level. Distal anastomosis is to the common femoral arteries if there has been no prior prosthetic material in the groins. Otherwise, exposure of the superficial femoral artery, lateral approach to the profunda femoral artery, or exposure of the popliteal artery may be required. Once extra-anatomic bypass is completed, incisions are closed prior to proceeding with aortic graft excision and bowel repair. Thorough debridement of retroperitoneal tissue, perigraft tissue, and infected aorta is critical to successful outcome. The infrarenal aortic segment is usually adequate to allow closure at this level; however, if the devitalized infected aortic tissue extends to the suprarenal level, hepatorenal and splenorenal bypass may be required prior to removal of the aortic graft. The aortic stump is closed with a tension-free, double layer of monofilament suture. Coverage of the aortic stump with anterior spinal ligament, omental pedicle flap, or jejunal serosal patch can also be utilized. The disrupted bowel is treated with aggressive debridement of devitalized tissue and with primary closure or segmental resection with primary bowel anastomosis.

More recently, neo-aortic reconstruction with femoral vein, as described for treatment of aortic graft infection, has become an alternative to the traditional approach for treatment of aortic graft-enteric fistula, and was the surgical choice in this case presentation. The advantage of neo-aortic reconstruction with femoral vein is the use of autologous tissue, avoidance of aortic stump-related problems, and reported decreased potential perioperative mortality and limb loss. However, there are technical challenges and a potential extended operative time course, which may limit its widespread application.

Other options for repair of aortic graft-enteric fistula include *in situ* replacement using cryopreserved allograft or antibiotic-impregnated prosthetic material. Cryopreserved allografts and antibiotic-impregnated prosthetic grafts have the disadvantages of being nonautologous, increasing cost, and lack of immediate availability. Delayed graft rupture, aneurysm formation, graft calcification, and recurrent graft infection have also been described.

It is difficult to compare results of the above approaches based on the small, historical, nonrandomized, usually single-center experiences reported in the literature. Reported mortality and amputation rates are 26% and 25% for graft excision followed by extra-anatomic bypass, 18% and 11% for extra-anatomic bypass followed by aortic graft excision, 27% and 17% for *in situ* graft repair, and 10% and 10% for neo-aortic graft reconstruction with femoral vein, respectively.

Case Continued

Postoperatively, the patient is admitted to the intensive care unit for continued supportive care with extubation on postoperative day one. Intraoperative Gram stain reveals gram-positive rods, gram-positive cocci, and gram-negative rods. Cultures demonstrated growth of mixed gram-positive bacteria with no predominant organism. Antibiotics are continued for a 2-week course. Upper gastrointestinal contrast study is performed on postoperative day 5; with no evidence of duodenal leak, she resumes a normal diet. She is discharged from the hospital at one week.

Suggested Readings

Burks JA Jr, Faries PL, Gravereaux EC. Endovascular repair of bleeding aortoenteric fistulas: a 5-year experience. *J Vasc Surg.* 2001;34: 1055-1059.

Champion MC, Sullivan SN, Coles JC, et al. Aortoenteric fistula: incidence, presentation recognition, and management. *Ann Surg.* 1982;195:314-317.

Clagett GP, Bowers BL, Lopez-Viego MA. Creation of a neo-aortoiliac system from lower extremity deep and superficial veins. *Ann Surg.* 1993; 218:239-249.

Connolly JE, Kwaan JHM, McCart PM, et al. Aortoenteric fistula. *Ann Surg.* 1981;194: 402-412.

Gilbert DA, Silverstein FE, Tedesco FJ, et al. The national ASGE survey on upper gastrointestinal hemorrhage. Part III. Endoscopy in upper gastrointestinal bleeding. *Gastrointest Endosc.* 1981;27:94.

Kieffer E, Bahnini A, Koskas E, et al. In situ allograft replacement of infected infrarenal aortic prosthetic grafts: results in forty-three patients. *J Vasc Surg.* 1993;17:349–355.

Kuestner LM, Reilly LM, Jicha DJ, et al. Secondary aortoenteric fistula: contemporary outcome using extra-anatomic bypass and infected graft excision. *J Vasc Surg.* 1995;21: 184-196.

Loftus IM, Thompson MM, Fishwick G, et al. Technique for rapid control of bleeding from an aortoenteric fistula. *Br J Surg.* 1997; 84:1114.

Pipinos II, Carr JA, Haithcock BE, et al. Secondary aortoenteric fistula. *Ann Vasc Surg.* 2000;14:688-696.

Towne JB, Seabrook JR, Bandyk D, et al. In situ replacement of arterial prosthesis infected by bacterial biofilms: long-term follow-up. *J Vasc Surg.* 1994;19:226–233.

Debabrata Mukherjee, MD, FACC

Presentation

A 66-year-old man with a history of type II diabetes mellitus, hypertension, hyperlipidemia, and a pack/day smoking history presents with lifestyle-limiting exertional leg pain. The leg pain has been present for over a year and is predictably based on walking distance. Physical examination reveals normal heart and lungs, bilaterally diminished pedal pulses, and a right femoral bruit.

Differential Diagnosis

The most likely cause for his symptoms is atherosclerotic narrowing of the lower extremity arteries resulting in intermittent claudication (IC). IC should be distinguished from a different entity, so-called pseudoclaudication, which is secondary to lumbar spinal canal stenosis. Features that distinguish true claudication from pseudoclaudication are shown in Table 46-1. Other conditions that may mimic IC include chronic compartment syndrome, symptomatic Baker's cyst, venous claudication, and muscle spasms.

Discussion

The symptoms of peripheral vascular occlusive disease (PVOD) of the lower extremities usually begin quite gradually. In fact, individuals with PVOD may often be unaware of subtle symptoms. Some patients do not seek medical care until the disease is at an advanced stage because the symptoms are so insidious and gradual. The most typical symptom of patients with PVOD is IC, which is usually described as an aching or cramping sensation associated with walking, but

Table 46-1. Differences Between True Claudication and Pseudoclaudication

	Claudication	Pseudoclaudication
Onset	Exertion	Standing, walking
Character	Crampy, ache	Paraesthetic, sharp
Bilateral	+/-	Usually
Walking distance	Constant	Variable
Etiology	Vascular	Spinal
Relief	Standing	Sitting, leaning forward

should diminish abruptly with rest. This symptom typically occurs in the muscle group distal to an arterial obstruction. For example, symptoms of calf IC result from superficial femoral artery occlusion. The most common site of superficial femoral artery occlusive disease is in the distal thigh at the adductor canal. Symptoms may occur in the thigh, hip, and buttock if PVOD involves the aortoiliac segment or internal iliac arteries.

Recommendation

The patient receives amlodipine and hydrochlorothiazide. He is referred for exercise ankle/brachial index (ABI) testing to assess for significant PVOD.

Ankle-Brachial Index Report

Bilateral resting ABIs are indicative of moderate PVOD, and the resting segmental pressures and waveforms are suggestive of aortoiliac disease. The patient is exercised at the standard elevation at 1.5 MPH for 5 minutes, at which time the patient complains of leg pain and cramping. The post-exercise ABIs dropped to the severe PVOD range and failed to return to within 10% of the post-exercise ABIs after 5 minutes.

Diagnosis and Recommendation

Based on the typical symptoms and abnormal ABIs, the clinical diagnosis is PVOD. Because the patient has lifestyle-limiting IC, he may be considered for potential revascularization. Prior to revascularization, he should receive a trial of optimal medical therapy incorporating a structured exercise regimen of ambulation to claudication, rest, and restart for 30 minutes 4 to 5 times per week.

Discussion

All patients with PVOD should also receive evidence-based medical therapy to reduce future cardiovascular morbidity and mortality. Angiography remains the gold standard to determine the severity and extent of PVOD. By using digital substraction technology, high-quality images can be obtained using a small amount of contrast material. However, angiography is an invasive procedure and is indicated only in patients in whom revascularization is being considered. Revascularization is indicated for lifestyle-limiting claudication, rest pain, ischemic ulceration, gangrene, and diabetic patients with IC. It is appropriate to have a lower threshold for performing revascularization in diabetic patients because of higher incidence of limb loss. Diabetic patients also may not have the same degree of claudication as nondiabetic persons because of neuropathy. Revascularization may be performed either percutaneously or surgically.

Recommendation

The patient is started on aspirin, clopidogrel, and atorvastatin. An echocardiogram reveals an ejection fraction of 30%; therefore, he is not a candidate for cilostazol, because this agent may precipitate congestive heart failure. He is asked to completely stop smoking and is enrolled in an exercise program.

Case Continued

After 8 weeks of a structured exercise regimen and medical therapy, the patient's symptoms improve, but he continues to have IC, affecting his functional ability with occasional rest pain. Because of inadequate control of symptoms with medical therapy, he is referred for angiography of the lower extremities.

Discussion

Appropriate risk factor modification and optimal medical therapy is an integral component of the treatment of patients with PVOD. Complete cessation of tobacco use should be the goal in these patients. Stopping smoking can reduce the 5-year amputation risk tenfold and decrease the mortality rate by 50%. All patients should be on lipid-lowering therapy with a target low-density lipoprotein (LDL) level of less than 100 mg/dL. Antiplatelet agents reduce both the risk of limb loss and the need for surgical revascularization in patients with IC. Antiplatelet therapy also substantially reduces the risk of myocardial infarction, stroke, or death in patients with PVOD. All patients should be on aspirin unless contraindicated. Dual antiplatelet therapy with aspirin and clopidogrel has significant incremental beneficial effects in patients with PVOD. Cilostazol may significantly increase claudication distance in some patients. However, this drug is a phosphodiesterase inhibitor, and is contraindicated in patients with congestive heart failure and ejection fraction less than 40%. A regular walking regimen may significantly improve symptoms. The best program is a stop-start walking regimen and includes regular daily walks, 30 to 45 minutes/day, at least 3 times/week, for at least 6 months. Individuals should walk as far as possible, using near maximal pain as a signal to stop, and resume walking when pain goes away.

◼ Angiogram of the Aortoiliac System

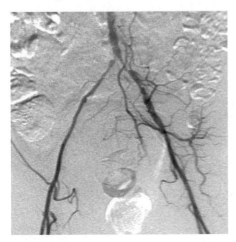

Figure 46-1

Angiogram Report

Angiogram reveals bilateral severe common iliac artery stenosis with a pressure gradient greater than 50 mm Hg across both sides. There is mild superficial femoral artery (SFA) stenosis and two-vessel runoff in both lower extremities.

Discussion

Endovascular Approach

Percutaneous transluminal angioplasty (PTA), with or without stenting, is the procedure of choice for focal stenosis involving the distal abdominal aorta, common iliac, and external iliac arteries (less than 5 cm in the iliac artery). Initial technical success for stenosis is greater than 95% in most series, with long-term patency exceeding 70% at 2 years and 60% at 5 years. The overall complication rates are less than 5% (usually access site-related and minor), and the mortality rate is less than 1%. Iliac artery occlusions demonstrate similar long-term patency, provided that they are recanalized successfully. Although PTA may be applied selectively in short lesions without the need for adjunctive stenting, it is generally accepted that stenting improves initial technical success and has extended the ability to treat bilateral aortoiliac lesions. Selected patients with severe IC in the setting of femoropopliteal disease may also be considered for endovascular treatment. Predictors for successful outcome include absence of diabetes, short focal lesions, good distal runoff, and lack of residual lesions. Indications for stenting in the femoropopliteal arteries include complications such as extensive dissection or thrombosis. Initial studies with drug-eluting and covered stents in the femoropopliteal arteries appear promising.

Surgical Approach

Results for surgical bypass for aortoiliac disease are excellent, with operative mortality rates of less than 3% and long-term patency rates of more than 90% at 5 years and more than 70% at 10 years for both aortofemoral bypass and aortic endarterectomy. The aortobifemoral bypass (AFB) is considered the reference standard for treatment of aortoiliac disease, because it consistently offers the most reliable results. The prosthetic material used most commonly is Dacron, and a bifurcated graft measuring 18 × 9 mm is most often employed. The size may be reduced to 14 × 7 mm in the female patient. The limb length is adjusted to match the femoral arteries or those of the SFA. Patency rates do not seem to differ with an end-to-side versus an end-to-end proximal anastomosis. Distal anastomosis may be to the common femoral artery (CFA) in patients with widely open profunda femoris artery (PFA) and superficial femoral arteries (SFA). Alternatively, the hood of the graft may be extended to the proximal SFA in patients with stenosis involving the origin of the SFA, but with patent distal SFA and PFA, or to the PFA (provided the caliber of the PFA is at least 3 mm and the length is at least 15 to 20 cm). The graft may be extended to the PFA alone, for example, when the SFA and the CFA are extensively obliterated or the hood of the graft may be split to patch proximal stenosis involving the SFA and PFA.

Case Continued

The patient undergoes successful stenting of bilateral common iliac arteries with complete resolution of the gradient across the stenoses. There is also significant improvement in bilateral ABIs and resolution of his IC after the procedure.

■ Post-procedure Angiogram

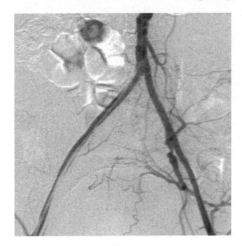

Figure 46-2

Suggested Readings

Bosch JL, Hunink MG. Meta-analysis of results of percutaneous transluminal angioplasty and stent placement for aortoiliac occlusive disease *Radiology*. 1997;204:87-96.

de Vries SO, Hunink MG. Results of aortic bifurcation grafts for aortoiliac occlusive disease: a meta-analysis. *J Vasc Surg*. 1997;26:558-569.

Hiatt WR. Medical treatment of peripheral arterial disease and claudication. *N Engl J Med*. 2001;344;1608-1621.

Intermittent Claudication in Transatlantic Inter-Society Consensus (TASC). Management of peripheral arterial disease. *J Vasc Surg*. 2000;31:S54-S122.

Mukherjee D, Lingam P, Chetcuti S, et al. Missed opportunities to treat atherosclerosis in patients undergoing peripheral vascular interventions: insights from the Michigan Peripheral Vascular Disease Quality Improvement Initiative (PVD-QI2). *Circulation*. 2002;106:1909-1912.

Mukherjee D, Yadav SJ. Update on peripheral vascular diseases: from smoking cessation to stenting. *Cleve Clin J Med*. 2001;68:723-734.

Weitz JI, Byrne J, et al. Diagnosis and treatment of chronic arterial insufficiency of the lower extremities: a critical review. *Circulation*. 1996;94:3026-3049.

case 47

Leslie D. Cunningham, MD, PhD, and Michael S. Conte, MD

Presentation

A 78-year-old woman with a history of hypertension and hypercholesterolemia presents to your office with one month of worsening left foot pain that localizes to the base of the toes. She describes it as a "burning pain." The pain is present at rest, improves with dependency, and worsens when lying in bed or with foot elevation. She also notes a consistently reproducible "tightening" or "ache" of the left calf that occurs after one block of walking and is relieved by rest. She is not diabetic. She has a remote, 15-pack year history of cigarette smoking. She denies a history of stroke or myocardial infarction (MI). She has never had deep venous thrombosis. Her left second toe was amputated in the remote past following a minor traumatic injury complicated by infection. On examination, she has no carotid or abdominal bruits and no palpable abdominal masses. Her femoral pulses are easily palpable and equal. She has no other palpable pulses below this level on the left, but has a palpable right popliteal pulse. Doppler signals are insonated at both the dorsalis pedis and posterior tibial arteries (DPA and PTA, respectively) on the right and the PTA on the left. Her left foot demonstrates rubor when dependent and pallor on elevation. There is a marked absence of hair on the leg, and the skin appears atrophic, dry, and scaly.

Differential Diagnosis

The differential diagnosis of ischemic rest pain includes the pain and paresthesias of diabetic peripheral neuropathy, gout, rheumatologic disorders, osteoarthritis, and common foot conditions such as plantar fasciitis, bone spurs, and benign muscle cramps. The influence of dependency and elevation on this patient's foot pain and color are nearly pathognomonic of severe chronic ischemia and would not be typical of these other conditions. Ischemic rest pain is typically localized to the forefoot (toes, instep) and is usually severe enough to require narcotics for adequate management. Benign nocturnal muscle cramps in the calf or thigh are a common condition not associated with circulatory disease. Trophic changes of the skin and loss of dermal appendages over the leg and foot are characteristic of chronic ischemia. In this setting, it is important to examine the feet for ulcers that occur at points of friction (eg, between the toes). A history of poor healing or infection that leads to amputation following minor trauma is also suggestive of severe ischemia or poorly controlled diabetes. The reproducible association of calf pain with ambulation and relief with rest in this patient is characteristic of arterial occlusive disease with calf claudication, and lends further support to the presumption that her pain has a vascular etiology.

Discussion

Atherosclerosis is a systemic disease. This obligates one to assess other vascular beds (cerebral, coronary, mesenteric, renal, and aortoiliac) for ischemic symptoms when evaluating a patient for complaints of infrainguinal arterial insufficiency. Recognized risk factors for atherosclerosis include tobacco use, male gender, diabetes, hyperlipidemia, hypercholesterolemia, and hypertension. Patients initially presenting with calf claudication are at increased risk for cardiovascular death, but at relatively low risk for limb loss (approximately 5% and 1% per year, respectively). In contrast to patients with claudication, reported 5-year mortality rates for patients with critical limb ischemia (CLI; rest pain or gangrene) requiring bypass range from 30% to almost 90%. Factors associated with higher mortality rates are diabetes, renal insufficiency, and renal failure. The goal of revascularization procedures in this patient population is limb salvage. Vein bypass grafts performed for CLI have reported patency rates of up to 80% at 5 years and limb salvage rates that approach 90%. Patients presenting with CLI are increasingly older and female. The prevalence of symptomatic atherosclerotic disease is greater in males than females at younger ages (40 to 60 years old), but it should be recognized that cardiovascular death is the leading cause of death for women as well as men.

Initial objective testing for lower limb ischemia is done in the noninvasive vascular laboratory. Studies performed include an ankle/brachial systolic pressure index (ABI), segmental Doppler pressure (SDP) measurements, and pulse volume recordings (PVR). These are helpful in distinguishing ischemic pain from other causes of limb pain and aid in the assessment of the level (aortoiliac versus femoropopliteal versus tibial) and severity of the occlusive disease. The ABI is a ratio of ankle systolic pressure to the higher brachial artery pressure, and is easily performed in the clinic or at the bedside with the use of a handheld Doppler. An index of less than 0.7 variably correlates with symptoms of calf claudication. An ABI of less than 0.4 is often associated with a history of rest pain or ulcer on physical examination. SDP measurements assess the drop-off in systolic blood pressure due to occlusive disease. These are measured by inflating blood pressure cuffs at several locations along the length of the leg. The systolic pressure at which a continuous wave Doppler signal insonated at the ankle returns is compared to the higher of the brachial artery pressures measured. The difference in the pressures measured is attributable to occlusive disease proximal to the blood pressure cuff. Pressure drops of greater than 20 mm Hg are generally considered physiologically significant. PVR are obtained with blood pressure cuffs inflated to 60 to 70 mm Hg placed along the leg in locations similar to SDP measurements. These partially inflated cuffs transmit changes in leg volume that occur with cardiac systole. The waveforms obtained indirectly correlate to the arterial pressure waves generated by the heart during systole. Damping (decrease) of the waveform is related to the presence and severity of occlusive disease proximal to the measuring cuff. PVR are particularly useful in settings where cuff measurements of systolic pressure may be artificially elevated by arterial calcification. Examples include the arteries of patients with longstanding diabetes or hemodialysis-dependent renal failure. Cuff measurements of digital arterial pressures can also be useful, as these arteries are not frequently calcified. However, digital pressures do not permit assessment of the level of disease afforded by PVR.

Diagnosis

Severe arterial occlusive disease of the left leg.

Recommendation

Noninvasive arterial testing: SDP measurement, ABI determination, and PVR.

▉ Noninvasive Laboratory Workup

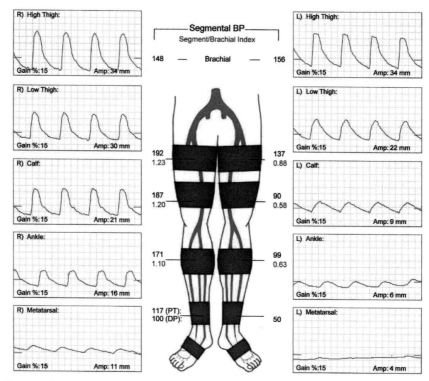

Figure 47-1

Results of Noninvasive Testing

The ABI of 0.32 and severely depressed waveform of the PVR at the metatarsal level on the left are consistent with critical ischemia of the left foot. The reduction in SDP (greater than 20 mm Hg) and damping of the PVR at the low thigh and ankle are consistent with two levels of significant arterial occlusive disease (superficial femoral artery and tibioperoneal system). There is a marginal pressure drop in the left thigh, suggestive of mild iliac disease.

Recommendation

The patient has noninvasive arterial tests consistent with critical left leg ischemia. A left lower extremity arteriogram for operative planning is appropriate.

Arteriogram

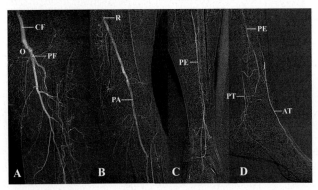

Figure 47-2

Arteriogram Report

There is no significant stenosis of the distal aorta, left common iliac artery, or external iliac artery (not shown). There is mild stenosis of the left common femoral artery. Arteriogram shows a patent common femoral artery (CF), occluded superficial femoral artery origin (O), and patent profunda femoris artery (PF) (Fig. 47-2A). The left superficial femoral artery is occluded at its origin and reconstitutes (R) the above knee popliteal artery (PA) via profunda femoris artery collaterals at the level of Hunter's canal (Fig. 47-2B) with single-vessel runoff to the ankle via the peroneal artery (PE) (Fig. 47-2C). The tibioperoneal trunk is severely diseased. The peroneal artery (PE) fills the anterior tibial (AT) and dorsalis pedis artery and posterior tibial artery (PT) via collaterals (Fig. 47-2D).

Diagnosis and Recommendation

This patient requires a bypass of the occluded SFA, diseased tibioperoneal trunk, and proximal peroneal artery. The patient is offered a common femoral artery (CFA) to mid-peroneal artery bypass with autogenous greater saphenous vein for relief of rest pain and limb salvage. She is told that her risk of perioperative myocardial infarction is less than 5% and that the likelihood of early graft failure (30 days) is approximately 5%. Between 60% and 70% of similarly constructed bypass grafts last 5 years without intervention, and patency approaches 80% with revisions. The limb salvage rate for patients having a successful bypass approaches 90% at 5 years.

The patient should expect to have follow-up visits with a vascular surgeon for the remainder of her life. This follow-up includes routine surveillance of the bypass graft by duplex ultrasonography. The goal of surveillance is to detect grafts that are failing due to the development of anastamotic intimal hyperplasia or progression of occlusive disease proximal to the graft or in the runoff bed. Close follow-up permits revision of the graft before it fails, and is an implicit part of the entire operative strategy for successful lower extremity bypass surgery.

The 5-year mortality rate for patients initially presenting with critical limb ischemia is high. It is reiterated to the patient that atherosclerosis is a systemic disease and that control of blood pressure, hypercholesterolemia, blood sugar for diabetics, and smoking cessation are of paramount importance for both preservation of her limb as well as her life. Her preoperative cardiac assessment is initiated, and is focused primarily on functional status. A history of significant coronary artery disease (prior MI, abnormal electrocardiogram, or revascularizations), valvular heart disease, diabetes, and advanced age are important risk factors to identify. Because of her CLI and limited exercise capacity, some type of provocative cardiac stress testing (dobutamine echocardiography or persantine-thallium imaging) may be indicated. She is started on aspirin and a beta-blocker preoperatively to reduce her perioperative cardiac morbidity and mortality. The potential complications of the procedure discussed with the patient include wound infections, MI, bleeding, graft failure, limb loss, renal failure, stroke, and death.

Surgical Approach

The selection of an appropriate conduit for the bypass is critical to its long-term success. The best conduit is a single segment of ipsilateral greater saphenous vein (GSV) followed by contralateral GSV. Cephalic and basilic (arm) vein as well as lesser saphenous vein, as either a single piece or as a composite graft, is preferred to synthetic conduits of Dacron or polytetrafluoroethylene (PTFE). The vein is utilized in an antegrade fashion after lysis of the valves, or it can be reversed. The vein is studied preoperatively by duplex ultrasonography to ensure adequate diameter (greater than 2 mm undilated) and to identify major braches, duplicated venous systems, sclerotic areas, and congenital absence. Tunneling of the infrainguinal bypass grafts is done either superficially in the subcutaneous space or beneath the sartorious muscle and through the popliteal space to the infrageniculate target. The superficial graft tunnel has the advantage of being more readily accessible for revision, if needed. The advantage of the deeper tunnel is that the graft is protected in the event of a wound infection or dehiscence. The proximal and distal anastomoses, as well as the graft throughout its course, are imaged by either arteriography or duplex ultrasonography in the operating room to identify any technical problem that would result in early graft failure. Arteriography has the advantage of more easily imaging the native vessels and their collaterals that make up the runoff for the bypass.

Case Continued

The bypass is performed between the CFA and the mid-peroneal artery with ipsilateral GSV. The graft is tunneled subsartorially, though the popliteal fossa and into the distal wound. The distal anastamosis is fashioned, while a proximal tourniquet is used to control bleeding from the open peroneal artery. A completion arteriogram is obtained.

Arteriogram

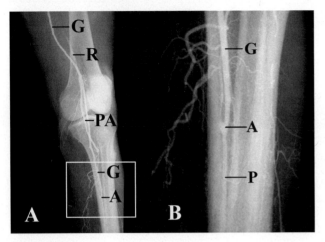

Figure 47-3

Arteriogram Report

Arteriogram shows the course of the vein bypass graft (G), the reconstituted superficial femoral artery (R) filling the popliteal artery (PA), the location of distal anastomosis (A), and the distal native peroneal artery (P) runoff and DPA runoff (not shown). Excellent filling of the dorsalis pedis artery and arch collaterals is demonstrated (not shown). Detail of the arterial anastomosis is shown in Fig. 47-3B.

Case Continued

The patient is discharged from the hospital on postoperative day 5. Follow-up is scheduled for a wound check in the office one week after discharge. Her first graft surveillance duplex ultrasound is scheduled for one month after the operation.

Suggested Readings

Chew DKW, Conte MS, Belkin M, et al. Arterial reconstruction for lower limb ischemia. *Acta Chir Belg*. 2001;101:106-115.

De Frang RD, Edwards JM, Moneta GL, et al. Repeat leg bypass after multiple prior bypass failures. *J Vasc Surg*. 1994;19:268-277.

Edwards JE, Taylor LM, Porter JM. Treatment of failed lower extremity bypass grafts with new autogenous vein bypass grafting. *J Vasc Surg*. 1990;11:136-145.

Grayburn PA, Hillis LD. Cardiac events in patients undergoing noncardiac surgery: shifting the paradigm from non-invasive risk stratification to therapy. *Ann Intern Med*. 2003;138:506-511.

McDaniel MD, Cronenwett JL. Basic data related to the natural history of intermittent claudication. *Ann Vasc Surg*. 1989;3:273-277.

Poldermans D, Boersma E, Bax JJ, et al. The effect of bisopropolol on perioperative mortality and myocardial infarction in high-risk patients undergoing vascular surgery. *N Engl J Med*. 1999; 341:1789-1794.

Taylor LM, Hamre D, Dalman RL, et al. Limb salvage vs amputation for critical ischemia: the role of vascular surgery. *Arch Surg*. 1991;126:1251-1258.

Veith FJ, Gupta SK, Samson RH, et al. Progress in limb salvage by reconstructive arterial surgery combined with new or improved adjunctive procedures. *Ann Surg*. 1981;194: 386-401.

Audra S. Noel, MD

Presentation

A 54-year-old woman with left calf claudication for 40 years has developed similar right-sided symptoms in the past year. Symptoms occur after walking 4 to 5 blocks. She has hypertension and hypercholesterolemia. On physical examination, she has 1+ (out of 4) femoral pulses and 3+ popliteal pulses bilaterally. Pedal pulses are 1 to 2+ bilaterally. She has no foot ulcers.

Differential Diagnosis

In a patient with risk factors for atherosclerosis, occlusive disease should be considered first as the etiology for claudication. However, the duration of this patient's symptoms suggests a potential congenital diagnosis, including aortic coarctation, embryological arterial abnormalities, or cardiac lesions causing peripheral emboli. In a patient with a stronger pulse at the popliteal level compared to the femoral artery, persistent sciatic artery (PSA) should be suspected.

Diagnostic Tests and Results

Noninvasive vascular studies demonstrate ankle/brachial indices of 0.68 and 0.74 on the right and left, respectively, decreasing to 0.4 and 0.71 after 1 minute of exercise. She is able to exercise for 5 minutes, completing the 283-yard protocol with right calf weakness.

■ CT of the Abdomen and Pelvis

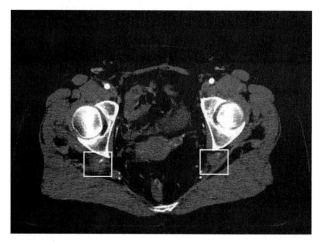

Figure 48-1

CT Scan Report

Computed tomography (CT) scan of the abdomen and pelvis demonstrates bilateral thrombosed 2-cm PSA aneurysms (*white boxes*) from the pelvis to the popliteal arteries.

▉ Abdominal Aortogram

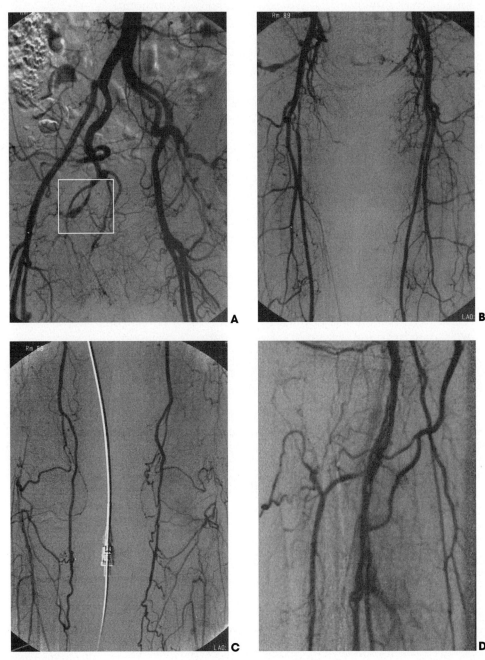

Figure 48-2

Aortogram Report

Abdominal aortogram with bilateral lower extremity runoff shows a right remnant sciatic artery (*white box*) that is thrombosed as it exits the pelvis, refilling a tiny fragment at the lesser trochanter level (Fig. 48-2A). No evidence of the left sciatic artery is noted on arteriogram. The distal bilateral superficial femoral arteries (Fig. 48-2B) end at the adductor hiatus and the popliteal arteries refill via two collateral arteries (Fig. 48-2C). There are luminal irregularities in both popliteal arteries indicative of partially recanalized thrombus (Fig. 48-2D).

Diagnosis and Recommendations

This 54-year-old woman has bilateral persistent sciatic arteries with aneurysmal degeneration and stable claudication. She has evidence of prior embolic events, but has little to no flow within the aneurysms on the present examination. Although femoral-popliteal reconstruction could be considered, as she has adequate external iliac and common femoral arteries, the patient did not feel that her symptoms were lifestyle limiting and no operation was performed. Serial CT scans were recommended on a yearly basis to assess aneurysm size.

▇ Approach

Management of PSA with or without aneurysmal changes depends on the degree of symptoms. No intervention is required if PSA is found incidentally or if the patient has stable mild ischemic symptoms, such as the described patient. PSA aneurysm rupture has not been reported, but aneurysm size should be followed serially with ultrasound or CT angiogram.

▇ Surgical Approach

A PSA aneurysm alone, without significant distal ischemic disease, can be successfully managed with percutaneous embolization. If catheter-based techniques are unsuccessful, open ligation with or without concomitant arterial revascularization has been described. Interposition grafting, with either prosthetic or vein conduit, from the normal femoral, external iliac, or hypogastric artery to the popliteal artery may be performed in conjunction with aneurysm ligation or endoaneurysmorrhaphy via a retroperitoneal approach. Excision of the aneurysm should be avoided, as it is often adherent to the sciatic nerve, and footdrop has been reported in open aneurysm repair. The limb loss rate has been reported as high as 18%, but this includes many patients with primary amputations due to embolic events.

Discussion

Fewer than 100 cases of PSA have been reported in the literature since Green first described this congenital anomaly in 1832. In normal embryological development, the sciatic or axial artery is evident at the 6-mm stage and supplies blood flow to the lower limb. The femoral and sciatic arteries are approximately equal in caliber by the 14-mm stage, but the sciatic artery then involutes, leaving the femoral artery as the dominant vessel. If any of these developmental stages are abnormal, both the femoral and sciatic arteries may be present, in either complete or incomplete segments, and may occur unilaterally or bilaterally.

The incidence of a PSA is estimated to be 0.01% to 0.05%, with bilateral PSAs occurring in 12% of cases.

Clinical findings in PSA are related to thrombosis, embolization, or local effects from the aneurysm. The risk of aneurysm in a PSA is at least 50%. Concomitant findings of varicose veins, persistent sciatic veins, arteriovenous malformations, and abdominal wall capillary hemangiomas have been reported. On physical examination, the presence of pedal pulses with the absence of femoral pulses should raise the suspicion of PSA.

Diagnostic imaging includes ultrasound, CT, and arteriography, which can be accomplished with spiral CT arteriography in one study. Magnetic resonance arteriography can be used in patients with renal insufficiency.

Surgical and endovascular approach to PSA treatment has been outlined above and is used for symptomatic patients with patent aneurysms or ischemic disease. Patients with PSA should also be treated carefully if undergoing hip operations due to the surgical proximity of the aberrant artery, or if undergoing renal transplantation to the ipsilateral hypogastric artery.

Suggested Readings

Brantley SK, Rigdon EE, Raju S. Persistent sciatic artery: embryology, pathology, and treatment. *J Vasc Surg.* 1993;18:242-248.

Calleja F, Jimenez MAG, Roman M, Canis M, Concha M. Operative management of a persistent sciatic artery aneurysm. *Cardiovasc Surg.* 1994;2:281-283.

Green PH. On a new variety of the femoral artery. *Lancet.* 1832;1:730-732.

Parry DJ, Aldoori MI, Hammond RJ, Kessel DO, Weston M, Scott DJA. Persistent sciatic vessels, varicose veins, and lower limb hypertrophy: an unusual case or discrete clinical syndrome. *J Vasc Surg.* 2002;36:396-400.

Savov JD, Wassilev WA. Bilateral persistent complete sciatic artery. *Clin Anat.* 2000;13:456-460.

Shutze WP, Garrett WV, Smith BL. Persistent sciatic artery: collective review and management. *Ann Vasc Surg.* 1993;7:303-310.

Sultan SAH, Pacainowski JP, Madhavan P, et al. Endovascular management of rare sciatic artery aneurysm. *J Endovasc Ther.* 2000;7:415-422.

Kristopher Deatrick, BS, and Peter K. Henke, MD

Presentation

A 23-year-old woman with no significant past medical history visits your office complaining of aching pain in her right leg with running, lifting weights, or strenuous exercise of her lower extremities. She is otherwise healthy, and exercises regularly as a member of her university's swimming team. She does not smoke, takes no medications, and has no family history of premature cardiac or vascular disease. On examination, no obvious trauma or injury to her extremities is present. Musculoskeletal examination shows intact ligaments and no limitation in range of motion. Dorsalis pedis pulses at rest are 2+ bilaterally.

Differential Diagnosis

Claudication is usually fairly stereotypical in its quality, frequency, and reproducibility. The diagnostic challenge lies in not missing a classic history in a young, otherwise healthy patient. In a young patient, rare etiologies of vascular claudication must be considered. Thromboangiitis obliterans, commonly known as Buerger's disease, is characterized by multiple segmental thrombotic occlusions of distal small and medium arteries. Although an exact cause is unknown, it is exclusively seen in smokers, and thus is effectively ruled out in this case. Fibromuscular dysplasia, characterized by alternating segments of stenosis and dilatation, can also result in arterial occlusion in younger non–high-risk patients. However, the popliteal artery is a relatively uncommon site of dysplastic change, and this condition is approximately nine times more common in women than in men. Another possibility includes popliteal adventitial cystic disease. In this condition, the growth of cysts in the subadventitial tissue gradually encroaches on the lumen of the vessel.

The most likely diagnosis in a young athlete with claudication is popliteal artery entrapment. It is caused by an aberrant course of the popliteal artery in relation to the muscles (primarily the gastrocnemius) in the popliteal fossa. Prior to obtaining definitive invasive imaging studies, documentation of functional artery occlusion by noninvasive means is possible. This can be accomplished on physical examination by palpating distal pulses as the patient actively plantar flexes his or her foot. Recording pulse waveforms with Doppler flow analysis and calculating ankle/brachial indices (prior to and during contraction) increase the sensitivity of this maneuver.

Case Continued

The pulses on the right side are palpable at rest. The unilateral foot pulses are palpable but diminished with plantar flexion. Noninvasive Doppler studies are obtained.

Doppler Studies

```
Doppler:
RIGHT                           LEFT
  Femoral      Triphasic
  Sup. Femoral Triphasic
  Popliteal    Biphasic
  Post. Tibial Biphasic      Post. Tibial    Triphasic
  Dors. Pedis  Triphasic     Dors. Pedis     Triphasic


Segmental Limb Pressures:
RIGHT                           LEFT
  Brachial:    115           Brachial:       111
  High Thigh   155 - 1.35
  Low Thigh    154 - 1.34
  Calf         99 - 0.86
  Ankle (PT)   90 - 0.78     Ankle (PT)      132 - 1.15
  Ankle (DP)   94 - 0.82     Ankle (DP)      136 - 1.18


  Digits                     Digits:
  First        67 - 0.58     First           100 - 0.87
```

Figure 49-1

Doppler Ultrasound Report

It is evident that the patient likely has a segmental blockage of the right popliteal artery. There is no evidence of occlusive disease on the left. With forced flexion, the gastrocnemius compresses the popliteal artery, attenuating the pulse waves, and this is evident with plantar flexion on the left. Although this test is not absolutely diagnostic, it is highly suggestive of popliteal entrapment.

Recommendation

Because popliteal entrapment is bilateral in up to one third of patients, a positive examination in the asymptomatic leg would be highly suggestive of this condition. Definitive diagnosis requires an imaging study that provides more accurate localization and mapping of the anatomy in the popliteal fossa, specifically, the relation of the neurovascular structures to the musculoskeletal elements. Both computed tomographic scanning and magnetic resonance imaging provide excellent resolution and anatomic detail of this compartment, but are not as accurate for defining arterial anatomy as an arteriogram. With a suspicion of popliteal entrapment and a known right popliteal artery occlusion, a lower extremity arteriogram is requested.

▨ **Arteriography**

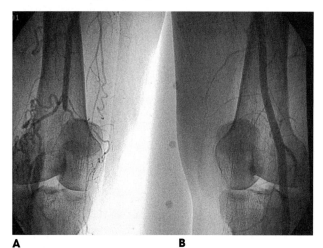

A **B**

Figure 49-2

Arteriography Report

This study suggests a chronic right popliteal occlusion (A) and mild medial deviation of the left popliteal artery (B). Other findings on arteriography that are considered diagnostic of popliteal entrapment consist primarily of three distinct findings: medial deviation of the proximal mid-popliteal artery, segmental occlusion of the mid-popliteal artery, and poststenotic dilatation.

Discussion

Popliteal artery entrapment is due to one of several possible developmental abnormalities in the relationship of the popliteal artery to the other structures of the popliteal fossa, most notably the gastrocnemius and plantaris muscles. There are four basic types of anatomic popliteal entrapment. In type I entrapment, the popliteal artery passes medial to the medial head of the gastrocnemius as it originates on the femur. In type II entrapment, the popliteal artery follows a more direct course (less medial deviation) than it does in type I entrapment, but still passes medial to the medial head of the gastrocnemius. In type III entrapment, the popliteal artery itself maintains its normal position between the medial and lateral heads of the gastrocnemius, but is compressed by an accessory muscular or fascial band originating from the medial head of the gastrocnemius, and attaching to the femur. In type IV entrapment, the artery passes deep to the popliteus muscle or a fibrous band in the same location. In this type of entrapment, the popliteal artery itself may pass either medial or lateral to the medial head of the gastrocnemius. Approximately 18% of the cases of popliteal artery entrapment are of other types, which cannot be grouped into these classes.

Diagnosis

Popliteal artery entrapment syndrome with symptomatic right popliteal artery occlusion.

Recommendations

Although most patients (especially those in younger age groups) have structurally normal arteries at the time of diagnosis of popliteal entrapment, surgery is universally recommended for those patients with a demonstrated anatomic entrapment. Even if the patient has not experienced an acute thrombotic event prior to the diagnosis, the natural history of vascular entrapment is fairly aggressive occlusion. Over time, repeated vascular trauma and thrombosis lead to progressive fibrosis of the vessel wall. The lumen of the vessel therefore becomes a thrombogenic environment, which may lead to an acute occlusion. The goal of surgery in this condition is the restoration of the normal relationship between the popliteal artery and the muscles of the popliteal fossa.

In light of your findings at arteriography, you recommend a surgical exploration and bypass of the occluded segment on the right.

▉ Surgical Approach

In popliteal artery entrapment uncomplicated by acute occlusion or an anticipated graft, the posterior approach is generally considered superior. This allows the clearest visualization and recognition of the structures in the popliteal fossa, and facilitates reconstruction. In all cases, the essential principle of repair is the same: division of the structure causing the entrapment, and restoration of the normal relationship of the artery and muscles. In type I or II entrapment, it may be necessary to divide the gastrocnemius at its origin. In this case, reconstruction of this muscle is necessary to restore function. In type III entrapment, simply dividing or excising the band causing compression will relieve the obstruction. Correction of the type IV abnormality requires division of the popliteus muscle, or the compressive band, as the case dictates. In the worst case, a bypass is performed for the occluded segment via a medial above and below-knee approach.

Discussion

Although popliteal artery entrapment is a relatively rare phenomenon, present in only 1.6% to 3% of the general population, at least two studies have suggested that in a young athlete with signs and symptoms of a vascular occlusion, the incidence may be as high as 60%. Therefore, it is important to consider this possibility in young patients who present with pain typical of an ischemic limb, even though they may not have the other classic signs of acute or chronic ischemia. Pulses in the affected leg may be absent in up to 63% of patients, and diminished in 10%. Although it is possible to induce absence of the pulse by passive plantar flexion, this is possible in only approximately 11% of cases. Extremes of dorsiflexion and plantarflexion, such as may occur with running, are both capable of replicating the symptoms of pain that prompt patients to seek medical attention.

Apart from anatomic entrapment, there are documented cases of young patients with normal popliteal anatomy suffering from the popliteal entrapment syndrome. This is known as functional popliteal entrapment; as its name implies, it is almost purely related to an active functional compression of the popliteal artery. Although it has been theorized that this type of occlusion is due to overtraining and hypertrophy of the gastrocnemius muscle, it has also been demonstrated that approximately 50% of the normal population may be capable of inducing an obstruction of the popliteal artery with knee extension and plantarflexion of the foot. The occlusion in both symptomatic and asymptomatic patients seems to be due to lateral compression of the popliteal artery at the level of the soleal sling. The gastrocnemius, plantaris, and popliteus muscles may all play a role in this type of occlusion.

Case Continued

This patient undergoes a successful above-knee to below-knee reversed saphenous vein bypass (Fig. 49-3).

Postoperatively, she has an unremarkable course. Intraoperative arteriogram shows a technically good result. Recovery time is allowed for several months, and then she opts for gastrocnemius release for her less symptomatic left leg, as no significant popliteal artery narrowing is present. Long-term graft surveillance is essential. No specific activity limitations are prescribed.

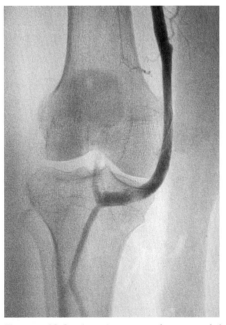

Figure 49-3. Arteriogram of successful above-knee to below-knee bypass with reversed saphenous vein.

Suggested Readings

Di Marzo L, Cavallaro A, Mingoli A, Sapienza P, Tedesco M, Stipa S. Popliteal artery entrapment syndrome: the role of early diagnosis and treatment. *Surgery.* July 1997;122:26-31.

Erdoes LS, Devine JJ, Bernhard VM, Baker MR, Berman SS, Hunter GC. Popliteal vascular compression in a normal population. *J Vasc Surg.* December 1994;20:978-986.

Flinn WR, Benjamin ME. Popliteal vascular entrapment syndrome. In: Stanley JC, Ernst CB, eds. *Current Therapy in Vascular Surgery.* St. Louis: Mosby; 2000.

Levien LJ, Veller MG. Popliteal artery entrapment syndrome: more common than previously recognized. *J Vasc Surg.* October 1999; 30:587-598.

Lambert AW. Wilkins DC. Popliteal artery entrapment syndrome. *Br J Surg.* November 1999;86:1365-1370.

Persky JM, Kempzinski RF, Fowl RJ. Entrapment of the popliteal artery. *Surg Gynecol Obstet.* 1991;173:84.

Turnipseed WD. Popliteal entrapment syndrome. *J Vasc Surg.* May 2002;35:910-915.

Peter K. Henke, MD

Presentation

A 75-year-old man is seen for routine follow-up after undergoing reoperation on left femoral to below-knee popliteal bypass with reversed saphenous vein, which was done 6 months ago for rest pain. The patient had a prior femoral to above-knee popliteal bypass with prosthetic, and this had failed within 1 year. Past medical history includes diabetes, tobacco use times 30 years (and currently), hypertension, and hyperlipidemia. Medications include aspirin, an angiotensin-converting enzyme (ACE) inhibitor, and a multivitamin. The patient has no current symptoms and is ambulating more than half a mile without claudication. Physical examination shows a well-healed incision in his left groin and below-knee calf incision. The patient has a faintly palpable dorsalis pedis pulse with an excellent biphasic Doppler signal.

Recommendation

Follow-up protocols should be instituted for surveillance of lower extremity bypass grafts to assess for stenosis of the graft that could lead to thrombosis, which may not be detected by the patient symptomatically or by ankle/brachial index change. The patient's ankle brachial indices are 0.75 on the right and 0.85 on the left (no change from initial postoperative values) with biphasic Doppler waveforms.

Graft Scan

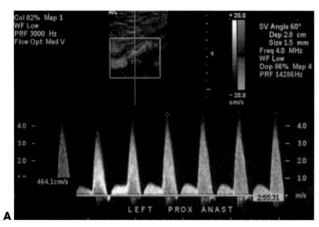

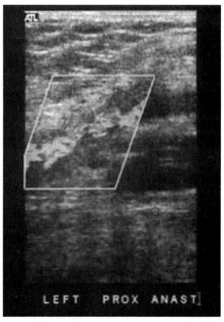

Figure 50-1

Graft Scan Report

Graft scan shows an unexpected high-grade proximal lesion with evidence of greater than 75% stenosis, based on velocities (Fig. 50-1A) and gray scale imaging (Fig. 50-1B).

Discussion

Duplex graft surveillance is a well-established technique proven to significantly improve graft patency and limb salvage by 30% to 50% over 5 years and decrease early graft thrombosis by more than 50%. The concept is that a hemodynamically significant stenosis in the graft can be found and corrective treatment carried out before the patient becomes symptomatic secondary to a thrombosed graft. Salvage techniques such as graft thrombolysis and revision are much less successful than if treated electively. Most graft stenoses occur within the first 2 postoperative years, and thus more frequent early scanning is recommended (about every 3 months for the first year, every 6 months for the second year, and then yearly). Graft duplex velocities increase at the region of stenosis, and comparison between the highest velocity and proximal velocity is essential. Example of risk stratification for velocities is shown in Table 50-1.

Recommendation

Patients can undergo direct graft repair based on the duplex ultrasound, but arteriography is recommended to determine the extent of the proximal stenosis, as well as to determine if there are any distal stenoses not seen with duplex interrogation.

Table 50-1. Stratification of Risk of Graft Thrombosis by Surveillance Data

Risk of Thrombosis	HVC		LVC		Change in ABI
Category I (highest risk)	PSV >300 cm/sec **Or** Vr >3.5	**and**	GFV <45 cm/sec	**and**	>0.15
Category II	PSV >300 cm/sec **Or** Vr >3.5	**and**	GFV >45 cm/sec	**and**	<0.15
Category III (intermediate risk)	180 <PSV >300 cm/sec **Or** Vr >2.0	**and**	GFV >45 cm/sec	**and**	<0.15
Category IV (low risk)	PSV >180 cm/sec **And** Vr >2.0	**and**	GFV >45 cm/sec	**and**	<0.15

HVC, High-velocity criteria; *LVC,* low-velocity criteria; *ABI,* ankle brachial index; *PSV,* peak systolic velocity; *Vr,* velocity ratio (from Wixon CL, Mills JL, 2001 in *Current Therapy in Vascular Surgery,* with permission)

▨ **Arteriography**

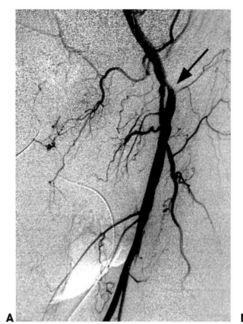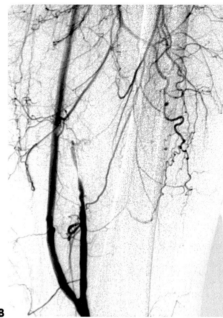

A   **B**

Figure 50-2

Arteriography Report

The arteriogram confirms a 2-cm proximal stenosis (Fig. 50-2A) with the remaining graft and outflow (Fig. 50-2B) not significantly diseased.

Discussion

Either endovascular or open patch angioplasty are reasonable options. Because the lesion is proximal and can be easily anatomically accessed, as well as the likely better durability of open patch angioplasty as compared with endovascular therapy, this option is chosen. Other surgical options include a vein segmental interposition graft, which is often the best option for a distal stricture where reoperation may be very hazardous. Endovascular angioplasty has mixed results, but is reasonable to use in patients who have distal stenosis, which may be difficult to access surgically through dense scar tissue, or in patients with large limbs. The use of cutting balloon angioplasty has significant promise in this setting (anecdotal).

The surgical technique is straightforward, but care and patience are essential. Standard reoperative dissection techniques should be used for surgical exposures. Sharp knife dissection, wide exposure, and alternating between difficult and easier areas of dissection decreases frustration, which may lead to impulsive moves (and more misery). The best material to use for the patch is autologous vein, either a saphenous vein or arm vein segment. Alternatively, the author has had good success with bovine pericardium. Intraoperative duplex is then obtained to confirm that the repair is adequate and that stenosis is rested (Fig. 50-3).

Case Continued

This patient does well and is discharged on postoperative day 2.

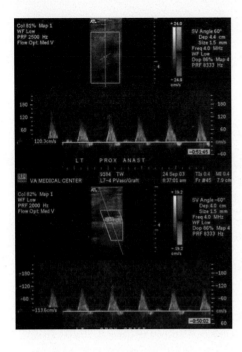

Figure 50-3

Recommendation

This patient needs management of atherosclerotic risk factors, including emphasis on smoking cessation. Programs utilizing a combination of medical therapy such as Wellbutrin with counseling are most effective and therefore are recommended. Consideration is given to starting the patient on an HMG co-reductase inhibitor (statin), as statins have been shown to significantly increase graft patency and limb salvage independent of factors such as graft type, operative indication, and patient demographics. The graft scanning protocol is resumed as if a new graft was placed, because repaired areas are prone to restenosis.

Suggested Readings

Alexander JQ, Katz SG. The efficacy of percutaneous transluminal angioplasty in the treatment of infrainguinal vein bypass graft stenosis. *Arch Surgery.* 2003;138:510-513.

Bergamini TM, George SM Jr, Massey HT, et al. Intensive surveillance of femoropopliteal-tibial autogenous vein bypass improves long-term graft patency and limb salvage. *Ann Surg.* 1995;221:507-516.

Henke PK, Blackburn S, Proctor MC, et al. Patients undergoing infrainguinal bypass for atherosclerotic vascular disease are underprescribed cardioprotective medications: effect in graft patency, limb salvage, and mortality. *J Vasc Surg.* 2003 (in press).

Mills JL, Bandyk DF, Gahtan V, Esses GE. The origin of infrainguinal vein graft stenosis: a prospective study based on duplex surveillance. *J Vasc Surg.* 1995;21:16-25.

Mills JL Sr, Wixon CL, James DC, Devine J, Westerband A, Hughes JD. The natural history of intermediate and critical vein graft stenosis: recommendations for continued surveillance or repair. *J Vasc Surg.* 2001;33:273-280.

Nehler MR, Moneta GL, Yeager RA, Edwards JM, Taylor LM Jr, Porter JM. Surgical treatment of threatened reversed infrainguinal vein grafts. *J Vasc Surg.* 1994;20:558-565.

Sullivan TR Jr, Welch HJ, Iafrati MD, Mackey WC, O'Donnell TF Jr. Clinical results of common strategies used to revise infrainguinal vein grafts. *J Vasc Surg.* 1996;24:909-919.

case 5

Amy B. Reed, MD

Presentation

A 42-year-old man arrives in the emergency department complaining of a one-week history of a cool, painful left foot. He had previously undergone an aorto-bifemoral bypass graft at an outside institution. He is now one year out from a left femoral to posterior tibial artery bypass graft with greater saphenous vein, which you performed for rest pain after his prosthetic femoral above-knee popliteal artery bypass graft had occluded. On examination, the femoral pulses are palpable bilaterally. The left foot is cool and slightly mottled with a monophasic Doppler signal over the posterior tibial artery. The bypass graft is nonpalpable. His motorsensory examination is normal, except for slight numbness over the plantar arch.

Differential Diagnosis

The differential diagnosis for acute lower extremity ischemia typically includes arterial thrombosis secondary to underlying atherosclerotic arterial occlusive disease, atheromatous embolization from a more proximal unstable plaque, or thromboembolism from an aortic aneurysm or cardiac source. Early deep vein thrombosis can present in a similar manner; however, the leg will typically be swollen. Other less common causes of acute limb ischemia, such as thrombosed popliteal artery aneurysm, popliteal entrapment, and severe vasospasm, must also be kept in mind. In this patient with a previous history of peripheral bypass surgery, graft thrombosis must be considered the primary diagnosis.

Recommendation

After systemic heparinization, the initial diagnostic test in this patient is an aortogram with left lower extremity arteriogram. Acute limb ischemia is stratified into four categories based on severity and limb threat: Class I—limb viable; Class IIa—limb marginally threatened; Class IIb—limb immediately threatened; and Class III—irreversible limb changes. Patients with Class I or IIa ischemia often have time for angiography and possible thrombolytic therapy, whereas patients with Class IIb and early III typically require immediate revascularization. This patient has Class IIa ischemia, and would be best served by arteriography with possible thrombolysis of the suspected graft thrombosis.

Arteriography Report

Aortogram with left lower extremity runoff reveals a patent aortobifemoral bypass graft with occlusion of the superficial femoral, popliteal, and anterior tibial arteries. The stump of the bypass graft at the proximal anastomosis is visualized;

however, the remainder of the graft is occluded. The posterior tibial artery is re-constituted in the proximal third of the calf.

Discussion

Catheter-directed thrombolysis for Class I or IIa limb ischemia has several poten-tial advantages, including more gentle clot lysis, the ability to clean out the in-volved segment as well as the distal vessels, and potentially revealing the underly-ing stenotic lesion. The decision to proceed with angiography and possible thrombolysis is dictated by the severity of the ischemia and perceived limb threat.

Approach

A Teflon-coated wire is used to select the stump of the proximal anastomosis, and is able to be manipulated into the mid-portion of the occluded bypass graft. An infusion catheter is advanced over the wire, followed by a 250,000-U uroki-nase pulse spray into the graft. A continuous infusion of urokinase is begun at 250,000 U/h for 6 hours, followed by 125,000 U/h overnight. A repeat arteri-ogram the following morning reveals reperfusion in the proximal half of the graft. The infusion continues for an additional 24 hours, with notable improve-ment in the distal Doppler signals. A repeat arteriogram is ordered.

Arteriogram

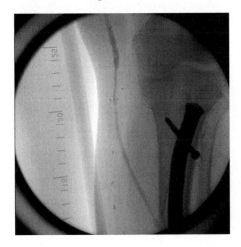

Figure 51-1

Arteriogram Report

The bypass is able to be visualized after thrombolysis, and reveals an area of nar-rowing and subtotal occlusion just below the knee.

Approach

This area of narrowing will need to be addressed and revised in order to preserve long-term patency of the bypass graft. Though the graft is now palpable and dis-tal Doppler signals improved, a Duplex graft scan is necessary to uncover ele-vated velocities in the region of the graft below the knee, which appears abnor-mal on arteriography. The scan reveals proximal and mid-portion graft velocities of 50 to 70 cm/s with elevation to 300 cm/s below the knee for a segment ap-proximately 4 cm in length. Velocity at the distal anastomosis is 42 cm/s.

Diagnosis and Recommendation

Successful lysis of occluded femoral to posterior tibial artery bypass with underlying graft stenosis uncovered in the distal third of the bypass graft. The patient is offered graft revision using a short segment of distal greater saphenous vein from the ipsilateral extremity. It is explained to the patient that long-term graft patency is diminished, given the need for thrombolytics and graft revision, and that possible complications include graft failure as well as possible need for amputation, in addition to bleeding and infection.

Discussion

If thrombolytic therapy is successful, correction of the underlying graft lesion or distal runoff will be necessary. Intimal hyperplasia at valve sites and anastomoses are often the main culprits, and may be amenable to balloon angioplasty if focal. Long areas of stenosis are best treated with open patch angioplasty or an interposition graft. Construction of a new distal anastomosis will often require a jump graft with vein to a more distal tibial vessel in a nonoperated site.

Surgical Approach

The bypass graft is dissected free from surrounding soft tissue and scar via the previous medial incision. A segment of distal greater saphenous vein is harvested and is of excellent caliber. After systemic heparinization, proximal and distal control of the vein graft is achieved, followed by excision of the atretic segment of graft. End-to-end spatulated anastomoses are performed to interpose the harvested piece of greater saphenous vein. There is an excellent pulse in the vein graft with a palpable posterior tibial pulse at the ankle. Intraoperative Duplex interrogation of the bypass graft shows complete resolution of the elevated velocities.

Discussion

Mature bypass grafts that have previously thrombosed are considered disadvantaged in terms of patency. Graft surveillance with Duplex imaging should be employed on a regular basis to prevent this problem. Chronic warfarin anticoagulation may have a role in improving patency in these situations. Graft replacement versus salvage remains a controversial issue, particularly when autogenous conduit is limited.

Suggested Readings

Avino AJ, Bandyk DF, Gonsalves AJ, et al. Surgical and endovascular intervention for infrainguinal vein graft stenosis. *J Vasc Surg.* 1999;29:60-70.

Berkowitz HD, Kee JC. Occluded infrainguinal grafts: when to choose lytic therapy versus a new bypass graft. *Am J Surg.* 1995;170:136-139.

Nochman GB, Walsh DB, Fillinger MF, et al. Thrombolysis of occluded infrainguinal vein grafts: predictors of outcome. *J Vasc Surg.* 1997;25:512-521.

Sarac TP, Huber TS, Back MR, et al. Warfarin improves the outcome of infrainguinal vein bypass grafting at high risk for failure. *J Vasc Surg.* 1998;28:446-457.

Debabrata Mukherjee, MD, FACC

Presentation

A 63-year-old woman presents for coronary angiography after an abnormal stress test. She undergoes an uncomplicated angioplasty of her right coronary artery. The following morning, she complains of pain at the right groin site. On examination, she has swelling at the access site and a loud continuous murmur.

Ultrasound Scan

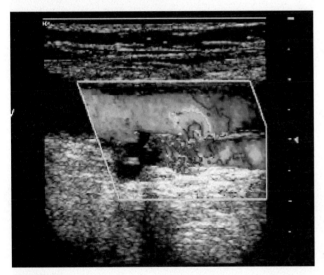

Figure 52-1

Ultrasound Scan Report

Duplex ultrasound scan demonstrates an arteriovenous fistula between the femoral artery and vein with continuous flow noted across the communication.

Differential Diagnosis

Potential groin complications after cardiac catheterization include pseudo-aneurysms, arteriovenous fistulae, hematomas, and arterial thrombosis. Arteriovenous fistulae are abnormal communication between arteries and veins, and need to be differentiated from pseudoaneurysms and simple hematomas. Ultrasound criteria for diagnosis of arteriovenous fistula include (1) colored speckled mass at the level of the groin swelling with turbulent continuous flow in the arteriovenous communication; (2) increased venous flow or arterialization of waveforms proximal to the fistula; and (3) decreased arterial flow distal to the suspected fistula compared to the contralateral side. Pseudoaneurysms typically appear as a perivascular mass with a distinct neck, and color Doppler imaging reveals a classic swirling motion of color inside the mass.

Discussion

Arteriovenous fistulae may occur after penetrating vascular trauma, or may be iatrogenic after vascular access procedures, as in this case. If groin arterial puncture is performed too low, the superficial femoral artery, rather than the common femoral artery, may be punctured. The superficial femoral artery and vein lie directly on top of one another, and a fistula may therefore result. Pain, a bruit, or a thrill may be present over the fistula, and the area may be warm because of increased blood flow. Rarely, high-output cardiac failure can result, particularly with large arteriovenous fistulae. Duplex ultrasound is the diagnostic method of choice.

Diagnosis and Recommendation

The patient has an iatrogenic arteriovenous fistula, and is referred for ultrasound-guided compression repair. The common femoral artery, superficial femoral artery, deep femoral artery, and accompanying veins are identified. A careful search is then performed to identify the communication site of the arteriovenous fistula. Under direct ultrasound monitoring, the tract of the arteriovenous fistula originating from the right superficial femoral artery is manually compressed with the transducer, which interrupts flow into the lesion without compromising flow through the underlying or adjacent normal vasculature. Ideally, only the tract of the arteriovenous fistula should be compressed to prevent interruption of flow in the native artery. Palpation of the dorsalis pedis or posterior tibial pulse is also performed to ensure patency and adequacy of flow through the native vessels.

Discussion

Ultrasound-guided compression repair (UGCR) is the preferred approach to diagnosis and repair in most patients with vascular injuries after cardiac catheterization. The procedure is safe and technically straightforward if performed by an appropriately trained individual, and is associated with minimal patient discomfort. The likelihood of success is highest in patients who are not on anticoagulants at the time of the compression. Even in those patients who are given anticoagulants, an attempt at treatment is warranted because success can still be accomplished in 30% of patients. The success rate is approximately 80% in those not receiving anticoagulants. The key to success of UGCR is the identification of the abnormal communication (tract) between the artery and the vein. The safety of the procedure is contingent on selective obliteration of flow through this tract while maintaining flow through the native vessels. However, patients who are admitted with vascular compromise, rapid expansion of a hematoma causing threatened tissue necrosis, imminent rupture, or other emergency complications should be treated emergently with surgery. Compression is typically maintained for 10 to 15 minutes (or 30 minutes in patients who had received anticoagulants), at which time pressure is slowly released, and flow through the tract is reassessed. Compressions are repeated for these same time increments, if necessary, until the tract is successfully obliterated. Patients successfully treated with UGCR should be on bed rest overnight and allowed to ambulate the next day. All patients with successful UGCR should have a follow-up diagnostic color Doppler ultrasound scan 48 to 72 hours after the initial compression procedure. Subsequently, patients with successful UGCR should have a follow-up examination by their cardiologist in 4 to 6 weeks.

Case Continued

Unfortunately, successful obliteration of the arteriovenous fistula could not be achieved in this patient, and she is referred for angiography. (It should be noted that angiography is not essential prior to consideration for surgical repair.)

Angiography Report

Angiography reveals a large arteriovenous fistula originating from the right superficial femoral artery (Fig. 52-2A).

Endovascular Approach

In individuals who have failed UCGR, endovascular therapy may be an option in selected cases. The technique involves insertion of a 5-French sheath and advancing a 5-French multipurpose catheter (MPA2) from the contralateral common femoral artery. Angiography is performed in multiple oblique projections to localize the origin of the communicating arteriovenous fistula tract. If a covered self-expanding stent is planned for implantation, the diagnostic catheter is exchanged for an 8-French Balkin sheath, which is advanced over a 0.35 guidewire. After advancing the stent to the level of the lesion, it is deployed by withdrawing the sheath. Post dilatation of the stent is performed by an appropriate-sized peripheral balloon. Covered Jostents (Jomed Inc., Rancho Cordova, CA) are now available and may be preferable, particularly for arteriovenous fistula with tracts with a narrow base. After the procedure, all patients are imaged by duplex sonography before discharge and at regular intervals, at 1, 3, and 6 months.

Angiography of the Arterial-Venous Fistula

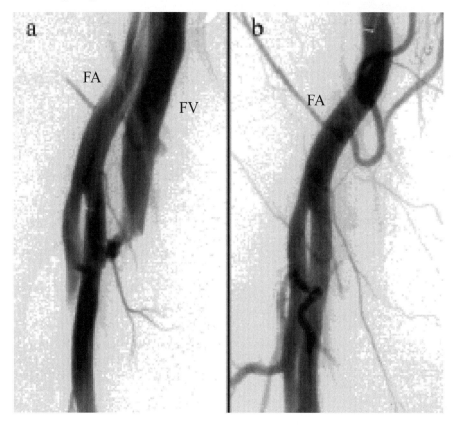

Figure 52-2 (Reproduced with permission from Waigand J, Uhlich F, Gross CM, Thalhammer C, Dietz R. Percutaneous treatment of pseudoaneurysms and arteriovenous fistulas after invasive vascular procedures. *Catheter Cardiovasc Interv.* 1999;47:157-164.) (FA-common femoral artery; FV-common femoral vein.)

Angiography Report

The communicating tract originating from the superficial femoral artery is occluded with a covered stent as shown in Figure 52-2B (12-mm-long Jostent, mounted on a 6.0-mm peripheral balloon).

Discussion

Implantation of covered stents is a feasible and safe option to exclude arteriovenous fistulas in select patients. In patients with lesions at the bifurcation of the common femoral artery, covered stents cannot be used, because this would lead to occlusion of the deep femoral artery. Also, in lesions situated at the level of the common femoral artery, covered stents should not be used because this may preclude the vessel as an entry site for later invasive procedures. When these lesions can be reached selectively with a 3-4-French Tracker catheter, embolization techniques may be the best solution. Typically, embolization coils can be used to occlude all arteriovenous fistulas if a distinct communication tract can be identified. Overall, percutaneous treatment of arteriovenous fistulae appears to be a safe and effective approach with excellent long-term results, and may be an alternative to surgical repair in patients with unsuccessful ultrasound-guided compression repair. In lesions originating from the femoral bifurcation with a broad base, endovascular therapy is not an option.

Surgical Approach

Surgical repair of vascular complications after cardiac catheterization is dependent on the type of vascular complication and the general condition of the patient. Certain technical aspects in the management of vascular complications after catheter injuries deserve consideration. Hemorrhage and hematoma formation can frequently distort normal anatomic relationships in these patients. The risk of additional injury to neurovascular structures can result from overzealous dissection in these circumstances. Similarly, extensive subcutaneous dissection will increase the incidence of local wound complications and should be avoided. Limited vascular control with the use of intraluminal devices, such as balloon catheters, is sometimes preferred. However, in the setting of arteriovenous fistula, the dissection should provide adequate proximal and distal control, as well as for a careful and complete arterial reconstruction.

Prophylactic perioperative antibiotics may reduce the incidence of wound infections/complications. This is particularly important when catheters or sheaths were left in place for long periods of time, or in patients experiencing tissue injury/necrosis because of massive bleeding into surrounding structures. Infection and other wound complications may be reduced further by making an incision through large puncture holes in the skin so that the skin edges can be excised sharply, or by making an incision remote from these large puncture sites to minimize wound contamination from them. Anesthetic technique is an important issue in the management of patients with vascular complications. Local anesthetics, supplemented by short-acting tranquilizers, are usually sufficient for treating acute arterial occlusions. However, local anesthesia may be less satisfactory for the management of large hematomas, pseudoaneurysms, or arteriovenous fistulae where vascular control might necessitate greater dissection. Regardless of the type of injury, local anesthesia incurs the least amount of risk to the patient, but on occasion the operative management of patients will require a general anesthetic. Successful repair typically requires that all 4 limbs of the fistula be controlled. Once control is obtained, the fistula itself should be exposed and directly divided and sutured. The connection itself may be quite small, and can often be repaired with several sutures. Larger defects may require a patch angioplasty or interposition graft. The long-term prognosis after direct repair is excellent.

Discussion

Three different therapeutic strategies are currently available for the management of groin arteriovenous fistulae after cardiac catheterization. These include ultrasound-guided compression repair, endovascular approach using covered stents or embolization coils, and surgical repair. Ultrasound-guided compression repair should be considered as first-line therapy in most patients, and has a very high degree of success in patients not on anticoagulation. Endovascular repair may be considered in selected cases, and preliminary studies report excellent technical success with good long-term results. Surgical repair should be considered in patients with evidence of tissue ischemia, rapidly expanding hematoma with threatened skin necrosis, imminent rupture, and for arteriovenous fistula arising from the common femoral artery bifurcation with a broad base.

Suggested Readings

Feld R, Patton GM, Carabasi RA, Alexander A, Merton D, Needleman L. Treatment of iatrogenic femoral artery injuries with ultrasound-guided compression. *J Vasc Surg.* 1992;16:832-840.

Kelm M, Perings SM, Jax T, et al. Incidence and clinical outcome of iatrogenic femoral arteriovenous fistulas: implications for risk stratification and treatment. *J Am Coll Cardiol.* 2002;40:291-297.

Messina LM, Brothers TE, Wakefield TW, et al. Clinical characteristics and surgical management of vascular complications in patients undergoing cardiac catheterization: interventional versus diagnostic procedures. *J Vasc Surg.* 1991;13:593-600.

Mukherjee D, Roffi M, Bajzer C, Yadav JS. Endovascular treatment of carotid artery aneurysms with covered stents. *Circulation.* 2001;104:2995-2996.

Perings SM, Kelm M, Jax T, Strauer BE. A prospective study on incidence and risk factors of arteriovenous fistulae following transfemoral cardiac catheterization. *Int J Cardiol.* 2003;88:223-228.

Waigand J, Uhlich F, Gross CM, Thalhammer C, Dietz R. Percutaneous treatment of pseudoaneurysms and arteriovenous fistulas after invasive vascular procedures. *Catheter Cardiovasc Interv.* 1999;47:157-164.

Peter K. Henke, MD

Presentation

A 57-year-old man who had an acute myocardial infarction 6 weeks ago, and was treated with a percutaneous intervention, presents to the emergency department with right lower extremity pain and numbness for 5 hours. The patient also feels lightheaded and nauseated, but is without chest pain. The patient notes having difficulty moving his right leg. No history of trauma is elicited. Past medical history includes tobacco use and hypertension, but no diabetes or hyperlipidemia. His discharge medications included an aspirin, a beta-blocker, an angiotensin-converting enzyme (ACE) inhibitor, and a diuretic.

On examination, his pulse is 140 beats per minute and irregular, and his blood pressure is 100/60 mm Hg. His abdomen is soft and he has palpable femoral and pedal pulses in his left leg, but no femoral or pedal pulses in his right leg. The right leg is cool and mottled, with decreased sensation and decreased motor function. Laboratory evaluation reveals creatinine, hematocrit, and leukocyte count and coagulation parameters within normal limits.

Diagnostic Considerations

This patient has potential life- and limb-threatening problems with evidence of a new cardiac event (dysrhythmia), as well as acute limb ischemia (ALI). It is common for patients with ALI to have multiple acute medical problems that must be treated appropriately, and saving life before limb is the overriding priority. First and foremost is evaluation and stabilization of his cardiac issues. An electrocardiogram suggests atrial fibrillation, but no ST segment elevation or depression. The patient also denies any chest pain and a rapid troponin I level is within normal limits. Thus, it is unlikely he has suffered a recurrent major myocardial infarction.

The patient should be started on full-dose intravenous heparin (100 to 150 U/kg bolus and 1000 U/hr), both to decrease the risk of cardiac emboli from atrial fibrillation (which may also be the etiology of his lower extremity ischemia) and to treat potential cardiac ischemia. An aspirin is given orally, as well. The patient's heart rate is controlled with an IV calcium channel blocker, and he converts to a sinus rhythm. The cardiac issues now seem to be stabilized.

The most likely etiology of ALI in this case is a cardiac embolism, and is the most common site of origin in general. Diagnostic tests, such as duplex and/or arteriography, may be considered, but minimizing delay in treatment for ALI is essential, because he has evidence of Society for Vascular Surgery (SVS) grade IIB limb ischemia. The patient needs revascularization within 1 to 2 hours (total ischemic time ≤6 hours), or he may suffer permanent muscle and nerve damage, rendering a nonsalvageable limb. Arteriography with thrombolysis is an option, but given the patient's classic history for an arterial thromboembolism (an antecedent cardiac event and normal vascular examination on his contralateral asymptomatic leg), this step may delay reperfusion that could be achieved more readily with surgery. The physical examination is very helpful to localize the site of occlusion in the setting of ALI. Lack of a femoral pulse on the affected, but not contralateral, limb suggests that he would be a good candidate for open thromboembolectomy at the level of the common or femoral artery via an inguinal exposure (Figure 53-1).

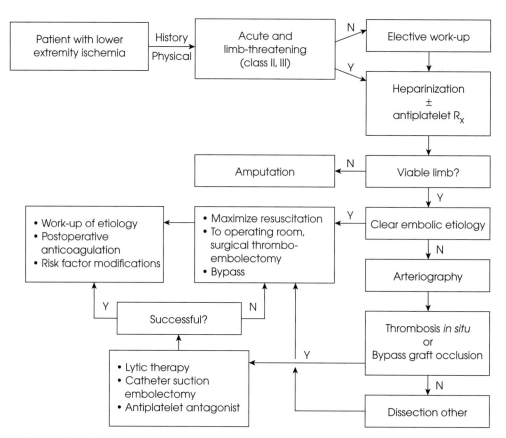

Figure 53-1 Diagnostic and treatment algorithm for acute limb ischemia.

Therapy

The patient is taken to the operating room. His abdomen and both lower extremities are prepped and draped to allow an alternative arterial inflow vessel (eg, axillary artery, contralateral femoral) if the ipsilateral iliac artery cannot be successfully embolectomized. An open thromboembolectomy under local anesthesia with intravenous (IV) sedation is performed, given his recent myocardial infarction. The technique of catheter embolectomy is well established, and a sizable thrombus is extracted from the iliac artery (Figure 53-2).

Further Treatment and Discussion

It is important to continue the heparin throughout the case. In this patient, no significant thrombus is present below the femoral artery. Better equipment in well-outfitted operating rooms includes over-the-wire embolectomy catheters, suction embolectomy catheters, and high-resolution C-arm fluoroscopy that

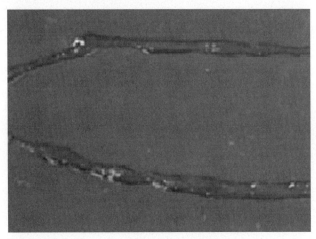

Figure 53-2 Iliac artery thrombus after removal.

allows endovascular and open techniques concurrently. This scenario will likely be the standard of care in the next 5 years.

When the etiology of ALI is not as clear by history and physical, arteriography with thrombolysis is the best option. Indeed, major trials comparing thrombolytic therapy with surgery for ALI included mostly patients with prior failed bypasses or thrombosis *in situ* with up to 14 days of symptoms, and not SVS grade IIB ischemic patients. Thrombolytic therapy may also be less cost effective than open embolectomy because of repeated arteriography and the need for intensive care unit monitoring. Proper case selection is essential, because failed lysis confers a significantly increased risk of limb loss and death. Because this patient has critical late ischemia, surgical embolectomy is the means to most rapidly restore limb blood flow, as compared with thrombolysis, which may take several hours before restoring adequate blood flow. Thrombolytic agents may also cause a systemic fibrinolytic state, and may release thrombus from the atrium or ventricle, causing a stroke or other complications. Thus, an echocardiogram should be obtained prior to beginning thrombolysis if the suspected source of the embolus is intracardiac. Adjunctive pharmacologic agents, such as direct Ib/IIIa platelet inhibitors, also seem to hasten thrombolysis without significantly increasing bleeding risk.

A four-compartment fasciotomy should be considered at this late stage, but there is no good evidence that fasciotomies improve limb salvage. Indeed, fasciotomies have been associated with an increased risk of limb loss, but probably represent a surrogate marker for severe late limb ischemia. Thus, it is still the author's practice to perform fasciotomies in the setting of ALI with neurologic findings.

Follow-up

Postoperatively, the patient should be maintained on heparin and then systematically receive coumadin for at least 3 months. Since he converted to sinus rhythm and the thromboembolism was very likely associated with a cardiac source, no need for longer-term anticoagulation is necessary beyond antiplatelet therapy unless at higher long-term risk. Routine follow-up with history and physical examination is needed, but no specific imaging protocol is required for the affected and contralateral limb. Standard risk factor modification therapies should be pursued. The most common cause of death in patients with ALI is medical comorbidities, reflecting their generalized ill condition.

Selected Readings

Drescher P, Crain MR, Rilling WS. Initial experience with the combination of reteplase and abciximab for thrombolytic therapy in peripheral arterial occlusive disease: a pilot study. *JVIR.* 2002;13:37-43.

Eliason JL, Wainess RM, Proctor MP, et al. A national and single institutional experience in the contemporary treatment of acute lower extremity ischemia. *Ann Surg.* 2003;238:382-390.

Ouriel K, Veith FJ, Sarahara AA. A comparison of recombinant urokinase with vascular surgery as initial treatment for acute arterial occlusion of the legs. *N Engl J Med.* 1998;338:1105-1111.

Palfreyman SJ, Booth A, Michaels JA. A systematic review of intra-arterial thrombolytic therapy for lower limb ischemia. *Eur J Vasc Endovasc Surg.* 2000;19:143-157.

Panetta T, Thompson JE, Talkington CM, Garrett WV, Smith BL. Arterial embolectomy: a 34-year experience with 400 cases. *Surg Clin North Am.* 1986;66:339-352.

Rutherford RB, Baker JD, Ernst C, et al. Recommended standards for reports dealing with lower ischemia: revised version. *J Vasc Surg.* 1997;26:517-538

David K. W. Chew, MBBS, FRSCEd, FACS

Presentation

A 65-year-old man who is a chronic smoker with insulin-dependent diabetes mellitus, hypertension, and hyperlipidemia presents to the emergency department with an ulcer in his left forefoot for 3 weeks. He denies any history of trauma and has minimal pain associated with the ulcer. On examination, he is febrile to 101.5°F; heart rate is 100 beats per minute; and blood pressure is 150/90 mm Hg. His left foot is erythematous and there is an ulcer on the plantar aspect of the forefoot (Figure 54-1). The ulcer penetrates down to the metatarsal head, and there is purulent drainage and adjacent soft tissue swelling. The dorsalis pedis (DP) and posterior tibial (PT) pulses are nonpalpable and have a monophasic signal on Doppler interrogation. His leukocyte count is elevated to 15,000/mm^3. Radiograph of his forefoot does not reveal any gas in the soft tissues or osteomyelitis.

Differential Diagnosis

Patients with diabetes mellitus may develop foot ulceration due to peripheral neuropathy, arterial insufficiency, or other causes. With peripheral neuropathy, loss of sensation and proprioception in the feet result in the development of pressure ulcers over weight-bearing points. Typically, these are on the plantar surface over the metatarsal heads, because the metatarsophalangeal joints are usually hyperextended and subluxated as a result of intrinsic muscular imbalance. As ulcers develop within callosities, they often have a hypertrophic rim and penetrate down to bone (malperforans ulcers). There is usually minimal pain associated with the ulcers.

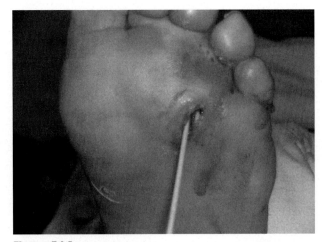

Figure 54-1

Arterial insufficiency related to diabetes mellitus, together with hypertension, hyperlipidemia, and smoking are major risk factors for atherosclerotic occlusive disease. Critical blockage of the tibial and pedal vessels may result in ulceration and gangrene. The ulcers are typically located in the most distal aspect of the extremity (ie, digits) and have a chronic "punched out" appearance. Other stigmata of arterial insufficiency are usually present, such as loss of hair, skin atrophy, dependent rubor, and absent or weak pulses. Pain may not be a significant feature if neuropathy is severe. Other causes of ulceration include trauma, infection (eg, chronic osteomyelitis), and venous stasis ulcers.

Diagnosis and Recommendation

In this patient, the etiology of his ulcer is primarily due to peripheral neuropathy. However, arterial insufficiency, as evidenced by monophasic signals in the dorsalis pedis (DP) and posterior tibial (PT) arteries, may contribute to poor wound healing and has a direct influence on the outcome of treatment of the ulcer. Furthermore, the ulcer has become secondarily infected, resulting in a limb- and life-threatening situation.

Discussion

The principles of treatment of infected diabetic foot ulcers are: (1) infection control using broad-spectrum antibiotics and operative debridement/drainage; (2) arterial reconstruction if necessary, using angioplasty/stent or infrainguinal bypass; and (3) wound management consisting of local wound care, topical growth factors (eg, Regranex), vacuum sponge, skin-grafting, and secondary closure.

Diabetic foot infection can spread rapidly through avascular planes, such as the tendon sheaths in the deep spaces of the foot, resulting in systemic sepsis, limb loss, and death. Intravenous antibiotics should be started immediately after cultures are taken from blood and deep soft tissues. Because the organisms are usually polymicrobial, initial antibiotic coverage is broad-spectrum (eg, clindamycin and levofloxacin). This can be narrowed down as soon as culture and sensitivity results are available.

Surgical Approach

Early operative debridement and drainage is performed. All necrotic soft tissue and exposed bone (which, by definition, is infected) are excised, and adequate drainage of deep infected spaces is ensured. Mechanical pulsatile lavage may further reduce the bacterial load in the remaining soft tissue bed. The amount of bleeding in the wound is indicative of the degree of any underlying arterial insufficiency. Try to preserve as much healthy skin and soft tissue as possible, to facilitate wound closure at a later stage when the infection is under control. The wound is left open, packed daily with normal saline wet-to-dry dressings, and the patient maintained on bed rest with elevation of the leg.

Recommendation

Noninvasive arterial studies are performed to determine the severity of the arterial insufficiency and predict the ability of the wound to heal without vascular reconstruction. These studies include segmental pressures, ankle/brachial index (ABI), and pulse-volume recordings (PVR). Because patients with diabetes tend to have calcified vessels, which are noncompressible, the segmental pressures and ABI may be artificially elevated. In these cases, the transmetatarsal PVR or transcutaneous oxygen tension (PaO$_2$) are useful predictors of healing potential.

▦ Segmental Pressures and PVR

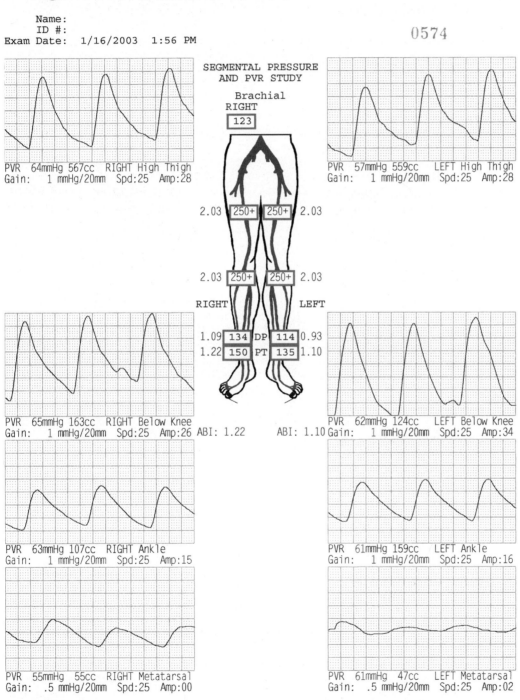

Name:
ID #:
Exam Date: 1/16/2003   1:56 PM   0574

SEGMENTAL PRESSURE
AND PVR STUDY

Brachial
RIGHT
123

PVR 64mmHg 567cc RIGHT High Thigh
Gain: 1 mmHg/20mm Spd:25 Amp:28

PVR 57mmHg 559cc LEFT High Thigh
Gain: 1 mmHg/20mm Spd:25 Amp:28

2.03 250+   250+ 2.03

2.03 250+   250+ 2.03

RIGHT   LEFT

1.09 134 DP 114 0.93
1.22 150 PT 135 1.10

PVR 65mmHg 163cc RIGHT Below Knee
Gain: 1 mmHg/20mm Spd:25 Amp:26 ABI: 1.22

ABI: 1.10 PVR 62mmHg 124cc LEFT Below Knee
Gain: 1 mmHg/20mm Spd:25 Amp:34

PVR 63mmHg 107cc RIGHT Ankle
Gain: 1 mmHg/20mm Spd:25 Amp:15

PVR 61mmHg 159cc LEFT Ankle
Gain: 1 mmHg/20mm Spd:25 Amp:16

PVR 55mmHg 55cc RIGHT Metatarsal
Gain: .5 mmHg/20mm Spd:25 Amp:00

PVR 61mmHg 47cc LEFT Metatarsal
Gain: .5 mmHg/20mm Spd:25 Amp:02

Figure 54-2

Segmental Pressures and PVR Report

The noninvasive arterial studies in this patient show noncompressible distal vessels and artificially elevated ankle pressures. However, the PVR waveforms at the transmetatarsal level are flat.

Recommendation

Given the large size of the wound, revascularization of the lower extremity to facilitate wound healing is indicated. Definition of the arterial anatomy of the lower extremity, using digital subtraction contrast angiography, is performed for operative planning.

Contrast Angiogram of Left Leg

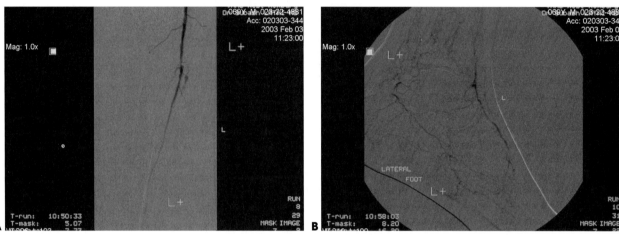

Figure 54-3

Contrast Angiogram Report

Angiogram shows patent popliteal artery to below the knee (Fig. 54-3A) with severe tibial occlusive disease with reconstitution of the dorsalis pedis artery in the foot (Fig. 54-3B).

Surgical Approach

Based on the angiogram, the patient requires a below-knee popliteal to DP artery bypass using ipsilateral greater saphenous vein (GSV). A medial longitudinal incision is made below the knee and the popliteal artery is dissected out. The DP artery is dissected out via a short longitudinal incision on the dorsum of the foot. Using a series of skipped incisions, the GSV is harvested from the groin downward. It is placed in a nonreversed orientation by lysing the valves using the modified Mill's valvulotome. Control of the DP artery is best obtained using a sterile tourniquet. The graft is tunneled subcutaneously. A completion angiogram and duplex scan of the graft are performed to assess the technical adequacy of the bypass procedure.

Control of the infection in the foot is verified (via confirmation of normal temperature, leukocyte count, and absence of necrosis in the wound) before secondary closure of the wound is considered. It is determined that further debridement of the wound or placement of a vacuum sponge is required to facilitate granulation and wound contraction. With improved blood supply and control of the infection, most wounds will eventually heal.

Case Continued

The patient is educated on foot care. Special orthotics and footwear are issued to prevent a recurrence of his neuropathic ulceration.

Suggested Readings

Akbari CM, Macsata R, Smith BM, Sidawy AN. Overview of the diabetic foot. *Semin Vasc Surg.* 2003;16:3-11.

Gibbons GW. Lower extremity bypass in patients with diabetic foot ulcers. *Surg Clin North Am.* 2003;83:659-669.

Jeffcoate WJ, Harding KG. Diabetic foot ulcers. *Lancet.* 2003;361:1545-1551.

Seabrook GR, Towne JB. Management of foot lesions in the diabetic patient. In: Rutherford RB, ed. Vascular Surgery. Vol 1. 5th ed. Philadelphia: WB Saunders; 2000:1093-1101.

Watkins PJ. The diabetic foot. *BMJ.* 2003;326: 977-979.

case 55

Thomas W. Wakefield, MD, and Hemal G. Gada, BA

Presentation

A 59-year-old woman with a history of a patent foramen ovale fell and dislocated her patella. She saw an orthopaedic surgeon, who recommended bed rest and nonweightbearing. One month later, she presented to an outside institution with right-sided facial droop, right-sided hemiplegia, aphasia, and hypoxemia. A computed tomography (CT) scan of the head was unremarkable, and a spiral chest CT scan revealed bilateral pulmonary emboli (PE). At this point, the patient is transferred to your hospital.

On admission, the patient is afebrile with no respiratory distress. Vital signs reveal a regular pulse of 87 beats per minute; pulse oximetry is 91% on 4 liters of oxygen and 100% on 100% oxygen by facemask. On physical examination, a systolic ejection murmur is appreciated, along with ecchymosis of the left patella extending down to the shin without erythema or tenderness. Neurologic examination is significant for right-sided hemianopsia, facial droop, aphasia, and upper and lower extremity weakness.

Differential Diagnosis

Paradoxical embolism causing stroke; simultaneous deep venous thrombosis (DVT)/PE and cerebrovascular accident from an ischemic etiology. An arterial source for cerebral emboli must also be considered.

Diagnostic Tests and Results

Lower extremity duplex scan reveals evidence of an acute DVT of the left leg involving the left posterior tibial, peroneal, and anterior tibial veins. Due to her DVT and patent foramen ovale, it is felt that she likely has developed a paradoxical embolus. Thus, a Greenfield filter is placed. The day after admission, a noncontrast head CT demonstrates mass effect consistent with a left cerebral nonhemorrhagic infarct. Three days after admission, the patient complains of increased right-sided weakness. She undergoes carotid duplex imaging.

◼ Carotid Duplex Scan

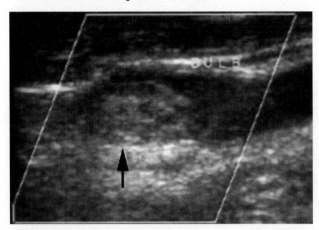

Figure 55-1 Echogenic embolus (*arrow*) just below left carotid bulb. Reproduced with permission from Gada H, Jafer M, Graziano K, Wakefield T. Carotid embolectomy in the treatment of a paradoxical embolus. *Ann Vasc Surg.* 2003;17:457-461.

Duplex Scan Report

A heterogeneous embolus (*arrow*) in the left common carotid artery creating a 60% to 80% diameter stenosis with instability is found (Fig. 55-1). The distal end of the embolus is imaged.

◼ Surgical Approach

The diagnosis of paradoxical embolus to the carotid artery is made. The patient is taken to the operating room for embolectomy, because the embolus appears to be unstable with the potential to cause further cerebrovascular injury. After systemic heparin administration, the carotid artery is opened, revealing a large embolus at the carotid bifurcation. This embolus is removed, but because adequate retrograde flow is not obtained, a 3 Fogarty catheter is carefully passed, extracting a tail of thrombus (6 cm long; Fig. 55-2). A number 12 shunt is rapidly placed, and flow is documented using Doppler. The arteriotomy is closed with a Dacron patch, and minimal atherosclerotic disease is found. A completion intraoperative duplex scan reveals excellent flow throughout the carotid and no debris. The patient is awakened on the table and taken to the recovery room, where she remains stable. Her neurologic examination remains unchanged.

Case Continued

Six days following carotid embolectomy, the patient undergoes percutaneous closure of her patent foramen ovale (PFO). The PFO is sized with a sizing balloon, and an Amplatzer atrial septal occluder device is delivered using fluoroscopic guidance.

    After PFO closure, hemodynamic data indicates no significant shunt by oximetry. The patient is placed on long-term anticoagulation with warfarin for her lower extremity DVT. Six weeks later, a duplex scan of the left carotid artery is performed. The scan reveals no abnormalities (Fig. 55-3). The patient is well at discharge with a stable neurologic exam.

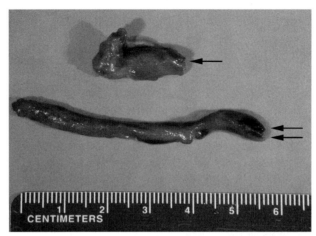

Figure 55-2 Operative specimen revealing embolus. *Arrow* demonstrates echogenic embolus and correlates to the preoperative duplex image (see Fig. 55-1A). *Double arrow* points to thrombus tail. (Reproduced with permission from Gada H, Jafer M, Graziano K, Wakefield T. Carotid embolectomy in the treatment of a paradoxical embolus. *Ann Vasc Surg.* 2003;17:457-461.)

Discussion

Paradoxical embolus (PDE) refers to embolism into the arterial circulation via a shunt. A patent foramen ovale is the major predisposing factor for PDE and is found in 9% to 35% of the population. PDE is infrequent (occurs in only 2% of arterial emboli), although its true incidence may be underestimated. The National Institute of Neurological Disorders and Stroke Data Bank has estimated that approximately 40% of strokes are without identifiable cause and approximately one quarter of these strokes occur in patients with PFO. Thus, a PDE may be involved more often in the pathophysiology of unexplained cerebrovascular accidents than is generally appreciated. The diagnosis of PDE requires: (1) DVT or PE, (2) abnormal communication between the systemic arterial and venous circulations, (3) evidence for arterial embolism, and (4) a gradient favoring right-to-left shunting. PDE should be suspected when large amounts of thromboembolic material are removed during embolectomy, especially if the material

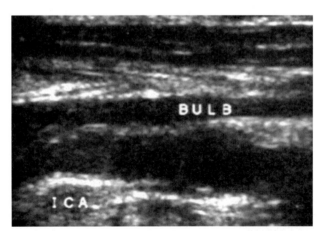

Figure 55-3 Post-procedure duplex scan reveals no abnormalities. (Reproduced with permission from Gada H, Jafer M, Graziano K, Wakefield T. Carotid embolectomy in the treatment of a paradoxical embolus. *Ann Vasc Surg.* 2003;17(4):457-461.)

is well formed and rubbery. On occasion, even indentations caused by venous valves may be noted on the surface of the embolic material.

The patient presented in this case had the important features facilitating a work-up of PDE to the carotid artery circulation. She had an embolizing DVT of the lower extremity causing PE, the etiology of which likely extended back to her patellar injury and the month of bed rest before the ischemic event. The patient also had a PFO documented by transesophageal echocardiography (TEE), the gold standard for PFO detection. Echocardiography (either transthoracic or transesophageal) should be done routinely when patients demonstrate well-formed chronic thrombus during embolectomy. TEE is performed when patients are found to have both peripheral arterial embolism and a negative transthoracic echocardiogram. The right-to-left flow through the PFO was likely facilitated by pulmonary hypertension secondary to the patient's PEs. This progression likely led to the embolus in her left common carotid artery and the ensuing cerebrovascular event.

The treatment of PDE involves immediate anticoagulation once an arterial embolism has been diagnosed. For patients with increased risk of bleeding, other strategies, such as the use of an IVC filter, should be considered. However, the efficacy of such filters in the prevention of small embolic events affecting the intracranial circulation remains controversial. Because most patients presenting with PDE have a PFO, definitive treatment entails direct closure, either by percutaneous transcatheter or surgical means. Success with percutaneous transcatheter closure of a PFO, as an alternative to surgical closure and/or extended anticoagulation, as treatment of PDE has been reported.

Thrombolytic therapy is largely undefined for PDE, but has been shown to have utility in treating ischemic cerebrovascular infarcts. Surgical treatment of carotid embolism caused by PDE is rare. Only three reported cases (including the present case) of surgical management have been described (Table 55-1).

Table 55-1. Carotid Embolectomy as Treatment of Paradoxical Embolus

Author	Age	Sex	Presentation	Location of Obstruction	Type of Surgery	Outcome	Follow-up Treatment
Turnbull et al (1998)	54 y.o.	M	Embolic stroke, pulmonary embolism, patent foramen ovale	Innominate artery	Combined carotid bifurcation and brachial embolectomy	Good	Long-term anticoagulation
McKinney et al. (2001)	67 y.o.	M	Embolic stroke, patent foramen ovale, pulmonary hypertension	Right carotid bifurcation	Carotid embolectomy	Good	Long-term anticoagulation
Gada et al. (2003)	59 y.o.	F	Embolic stroke, pulmonary embolism, patent foramen ovale	Left common carotid artery	Carotid embolectomy	Good	Long-term anticoagulation with percutaneous transcatheter closure of PFO

Modified from Gada H, Jafer M, Graziano K, Wakefield T. Carotid embolectomy in the treatment of a paradoxical embolus. *Ann Vasc Surg.* 2003;17:457-461.

The major risk of carotid embolectomy is further ischemia caused by either embolization or ischemic territory reperfusion. In this case, the benefits outweighed the risks of intraoperative and postoperative stroke extension, because the patient still had movement in her right lower extremity, as well as improving aphasia. If she had evidence of a massive stroke or was unconscious, embolectomy would not have been recommended.

SUGGESTED READINGS

Biller J, Johnson MR, Adams HP Jr, et al. Further observations on cerebral or retinal ischemia in patients with right-left intracardiac shunts. *Arch Neurol.* 1987;44:740-743.

de Belder MA, Tourikis L, Leech G, et al. Risk of patent foramen ovale for thromboembolic events in all age groups. *Am J Cardiol.* 1992;69:1316-1320.

Fisher DC, Fisher EA, Budd JH, et al. The incidence of patent foramen ovale in 1000 consecutive patients: a contrast transesophageal echocardiography study. *Chest.* 1995;107: 1504-1509.

Gada HG, Jafer M, Graziano K, Wakefield T. Carotid embolectomy in the treatment of a paradoxical embolus. *Ann Vasc Surg.* 2003; 17:457-461.

Leonard CF, Neville E, Hall RJ. Paradoxical embolism: a review of cases diagnosed during life. *Eur Heart J.* 1982;3:362-370.

Loscalzo J. Paradoxical embolism: clinical presentation, diagnostic strategies, and thera-peutic options. *Am Heart J.* 1986;112:141-145.

Martin F, Sanchez PL, Doherty E, et al. Percutaneous transcatheter closure of patent foramen ovale in patients with paradoxical embolism. *Circulation.* 2002;106:1121-1126.

McKinney WB, O'Hara W, Sreeram K, et al. The successful surgical treatment of a paradoxical embolus to the carotid bifurcation. *J Vasc Surg.* 2001;33:880-882.

Sacco R, Ellenberg JH, Mohr JP, et al. Infarcts of undetermined cause: the NINCDS Stroke Data Bank. *Ann Neurol.* 1989;25:382-390.

Speechly-Dick ME, Middleton SJ, Foale RA. Impending paradoxical embolism: a rare but important diagnosis. *Br Heart J.* 1991;65: 163-165.

Turnbull RG, Tsang VT, Teal PA, et al. Successful innominate thromboembolectomy of a paradoxic embolus. *J Vasc Surg.* 1998;28: 742-745.

David J Meier, MD, and Sanjay Rajagopalan, MD

Presentation

A 74-year-old woman presents with symptoms of right lower extremity rest pain and multiple areas of ulceration that have persisted for the last 6 weeks. The pain is a constant pressure ache in the right foot, and is particularly intolerable at night in the recumbent position. Over the last 2 weeks, the areas of ulceration have enlarged. Her comorbidities include type II diabetes mellitus for 15 years, coronary artery disease for which she underwent a coronary artery bypass graft (CABG) in 1995, peripheral arterial disease (PAD), hyperlipidemia, and hypertension. She had a right above-the-knee polytetrafluoroethylene (PTFE) femoropopliteal bypass graft 10 years ago. Her medications include aspirin, cilostazol, lisinopril (Prinivil), hydrochlorothiazide, and simvastatin. She has a long-standing smoking (50-pack year) history.

She is afebrile with normal blood pressures in both upper extremities. Examination of the lower extremities reveals mild pitting edema bilaterally, and chronic trophic changes in both lower extremities with absence of hair. The lower extremities on the right side appear pale below the level of the middle third of the calf, with severe dependent rubor. The femoral pulse on the right was not felt, but the left femoral pulse was 3+. The posterior tibial and dorsalis pedis pulses are not felt bilaterally. Multiple small ulcerations are noted on the plantar aspect of the right foot. Two bullae are noted in the dorsal aspect of the foot (Fig. 56-1).

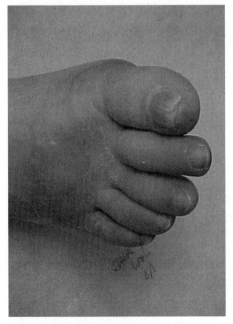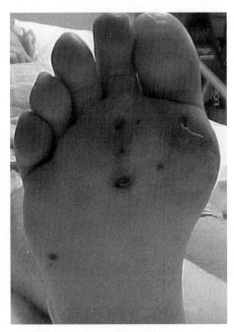

Figure 56-1 Right lower extremity on presentation.

Differential Diagnosis

The differential diagnosis of subacute lower extremity rest pain in conjunction with ulcerations includes lower extremity ischemic syndromes (secondary to progression of native arterial disease, thromboembolism or atheroembolism, occlusion of bypass graft, or a combination of these factors), neuropathic etiologies, infection, and venous gangrene. The presence of pain rules out a predominantly neuropathic cause for the ischemic ulcerations. Venous gangrene usually occurs in the setting of extensive lower extremity deep venous thrombosis (DVT). Infection is always a possibility, and should be considered an etiology by itself or in combination with other etiologies. Infections are often polymicrobial (especially in patients with diabetes) and may be suspected with the onset of rubor and tenderness in a wound. In this elderly patient with classic risk factors for PAD, including known chronic exertional claudication, progression to critical leg ischemia (CLI) may be expected. Furthermore, this patient has several risk factors strongly associated with CLI, including age, smoking, and diabetes. There seems to be a significant interaction between smoking and diabetes in CLI, such that patients with this combination are at highest risk.

Diagnostic Tests and Results

A complete noninvasive arterial evaluation of both lower extremities was obtained. The patient's TBIs were 0.2 in the right lower extremity and 0.4 in the left. This patient's segmental pressures and ankle/brachial index (ABI) were unreliable due to vessel incompressibility. Duplex evaluation revealed an occluded femoropopliteal graft and no named vessels below the level of the knee on the right side. The left lower extremity revealed a patent peroneal artery at the level of the ankle. Laboratory evaluation revealed normal complete blood cell (CBC) count and differential.

Discussion

CLI is characterized by persistent rest pain with or without ongoing tissue loss. The primary amputation rate for patients presenting with CLI is approximately 25%, with subsequent amputation rates of more than 25% at the end of 6 months. In patients with CLI considered unsuitable for reconstructive surgery, up to 46% of limbs are lost at 1 year. Most amputations occur in patients older than 70 years. Patients with diabetes are 10 times more likely to need an amputation than their nondiabetic counterparts, and do so at a younger age. Smoking is a powerful risk factor for the progression to CLI, and interacts synergistically with diabetes. The vast majority of patients with CLI have multilevel, multisegment disease involving both inflow and outflow vessels. More than 85% of patients presenting with CLI in contemporary series have viable treatment options in the form of surgical or percutaneous revascularization options. The procedure(s) chosen should strike a balance between maximizing durability and minimizing risk. It is not uncommon to choose a percutaneous approach alone in view of the substantive risk that surgical bypass may pose. Extremely high-risk patients, particularly if they are nonambulatory, may be best treated with primary amputation even in the presence of revascularizable options. To assess potential revascularization options, an angiogram of the aorta, iliacs and both lower extremities is obtained.

Lower-Extremity Arteriogram

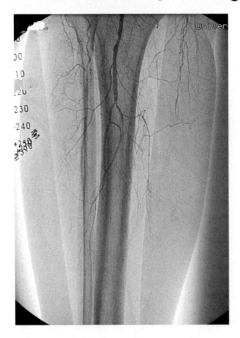

Figure 56-2

Arteriogram Report

Minimal luminal irregularities are noted in the right common iliac, external iliac, and common femoral arteries. An occluded superficial femoral and femoropopliteal graft are seen. The popliteal artery is reconstituted distally by collaterals, and the anterior tibial artery is occluded proximally. The tibial peroneal trunk was severely diseased, with the posterior tibial artery and peroneal arteries occluded proximally (Fig. 56-2). The left lower extremity revealed patent common iliac, external iliac, and common femoral arteries. The superior femoral artery was occluded in the adductor canal and reconstituted below the level of the knee. Single vessel runoff via a patent peroneal artery at the level of the ankle was seen. A duplex evaluation of extremity veins revealed no available conduits in the lower extremity and small-caliber upper extremity cephalic and basilic veins (less than 3 mm in diameter).

Diagnosis

This patient's noninvasive and imaging studies indicate that she has chronic critical limb ischemia (CLI). Given her rest pain with a nonhealing foot ulcer, she has grade III, category 5 peripheral atherosclerotic occlusive disease (PAD).

Approach to Management

The patient with CLI is challenging. A multidisciplinary approach involving a team of individuals proficient in various aspects of vascular disease is most effective.

Case Continued

Despite institution of antibiotics and wound care, the patient's rest pain continued. Potential revascularization options were considered, including femoropopliteal bypass to the below-knee popliteal segment with a synthetic graft; however, these options were felt to be high risk because of the lack of adequate autogenous conduit and the need for a prosthetic bypass for below the knee in the setting of poor distal tibial vessels. A below-knee amputation was recommended. The patient agreed, and she had an unremarkable postoperative course.

Medical Management in CLI

The main tenets of medical management in a patient with nonreconstructible disease include control of infection, management of pain, and adherence to approaches proven to reduce cardiovascular morbidity and mortality, such as the use of aspirin, statins, and angiotensin-converting enzyme (ACE) inhibitors. Prostaglandin formulations have been tested extensively in CLI. In general, the results have been modest at best, with temporary improvement in rest pain and ulcer healing. Prostaglandin formulations are not available in the United States for the treatment of CLI. Drugs such as cilostazol and pentoxifylline have no proven benefit in CLI. A recent meta-analysis of spinal cord stimulation therapy has demonstrated minor benefits that once again are only temporary, because they do not modify the underlying disease state.

Emerging Treatment Options

Vasculogenesis and angiogenesis (referred to as angiogenesis in this chapter) with cell- or growth-factor-based approaches hold considerable promise, because they could potentially address the primary abnormality in CLI: a lack of tissue perfusion. The bone marrow appears to play an important role in the process of angiogenesis, both through the contribution of endothelial precursor cells (EPCs) and through bone marrow-derived hematopoietic precursors. These cells are thought to play a role not only by providing the basic building blocks for a nascent vasculature, but also through the provision of the requisite growth factor and cytokine milieu essential for initiation, sustenance, and stabilization of a vascular network. Contemporary approaches to induce arteriogenesis have evolved, from delivery of single growth factor proteins, such as vascular endothelial growth factor (VEGF) and fibroblast growth factor (FGF) isoforms, to approaches that involve simultaneous delivery of multiple growth factors or the use of gene transfer approaches (both plasmid based and adenoviral platforms) to ensure high local expression of growth factors. However, proof that such approaches indeed result in meaningful improvements in lower extremity perfusion that translates into therapeutic outcomes has been elusive. Emerging evidence in animal models suggest that strategies targeting proximal pathways, such as transcription factors, dual- or multi-gene delivery platforms that deliver a cocktail of factors locally in a sustained and sequential pattern, may confer the requisite set of signals needed to sustain and maintain a more robust vascular network.

Suggested Readings

Anonymous. Second European Consensus Document on Chronic Critical Limb Ischemia. *Circulation*. 1991;84(1V):1-25.

Asahara T, Masuda H, Takahashi T, et al. Bone marrow origin of endothelial progenitor cells responsible for postnatal vasculogenesis in physiological and pathological neovascularization. *Circ Res*. 1999;85:221-228.

Carmeliet P. Angiogenesis in health and disease. *Nat Med*. 2003;9:653-660.

Dormandy JA, Rutherford RB. Management of peripheral arterial disease (PAD). TASC Working Group. *J Vasc Surg*. 2000;31:S198 [Treatment of Critical Limb Ischemia].

Ischemia CCL. Management of peripheral arterial disease. Transatlantic Inter-Society Consensus (TASC). *J Vasc Surg*. 2000;31:S168-280.

Lepantalo M, Matzke S. Outcome of unreconstructed chronic critical leg ischaemia. *Eur J Vasc Endovasc Surg*. 1996;11:153-157.

Rutherford RB, Baker JD, Ernst C, et al. Recommended standards for reports dealing with lower extremity ischemia: revised version. *J Vasc Surg*. 1997;26:517-538.

Ubbink DT, Vermeulen H. Spinal cord stimulation for non-reconstructible chronic critical leg ischaemia. *Cochrane Database Syst Rev*. 2003:CD004001.

case 57

John Pfeifer, MD

Presentation

A 50-year-old woman is referred to you with a history of bilateral varicose veins, first noted 15 years ago after a 100-pound weight loss. She was treated once with injection sclerotherapy, with moderate improvement. Three years ago, the left leg developed a dramatic increase in edema from knee to foot. The edema is painful. After prolonged standing, the ankle doubles in size and the skin becomes bluish in color, with many engorged small surface veins. The left calf swells to the point where it stretches her slacks. The right leg continues to manifest mild edema with minimal discomfort. Physical examination reveals normal arterial pulsations at the femoral, popliteal, and pedal locations. The right leg has slight edema, but the left has significantly more edema, with cyanosis of the entire leg, from the knee down to the foot. Small surface veins in the ankle and foot are distended.

Differential Diagnosis

Diffuse bilateral lower extremity edema may be systemic (renal, cardiac, hepatic, drug induced, endocrine), venous, or lymphatic. Unilateral edema may be secondary to compression of the left iliac vein by the iliac artery, but this edema tends to occur from the proximal thigh distally. In this patient, the edema is clearly from the knee to the foot. Compression of the popliteal vein by a synovial cyst (Baker's cyst) must be considered. Intraoperative trauma, such as that seen with caval ligation or direct venous injury, can also be ruled out in this patient. Similarly, with no history of surgery to the leg itself, injury to or ligation of proximal lymphatics is not a factor. Without the above-mentioned factors, Nicolaides has pointed out that "the most frequent diagnostic problem is to decide whether the origin of the edema is venous or lymphatic." Because of the associated cyanosis and distention of veins, lymphatic disease is unlikely. Thus, venous disease becomes the most likely consideration. With a 3-year history of edema, venous thrombosis seems less likely, and abnormal venous reflux must be presumed as the primary lesion.

Diagnostic Tests and Results

The photoplethysmogram (PPG) is a study that gives general information about the venous status of the limb. If the venous refill time is abnormally shortened, it usually suggests significant venous reflux in the involved extremity. The diagnostic method of choice in this patient is a color duplex scan, using a low-penetration (7.5-MHz) probe. This permits accurate assessment of the saphenofemoral and saphenopopliteal junction, as well as specifically identifies other incompetent perforating veins.

█ **Duplex Scan**

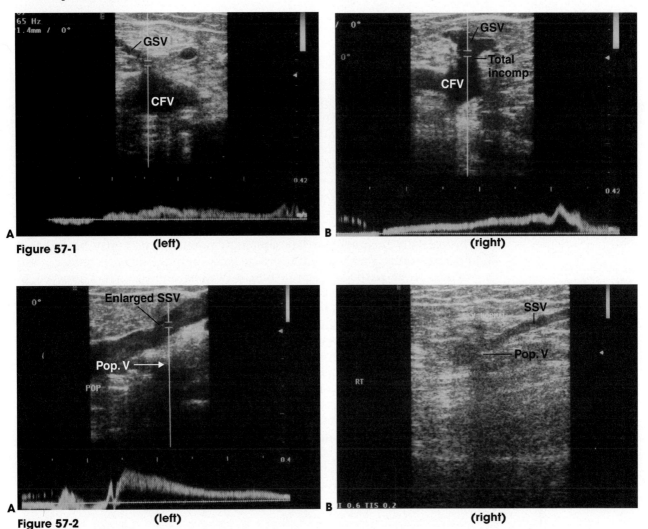

Figure 57-1   (left)   (right)

Figure 57-2   (left)   (right)

Duplex Scan Report

There is partial incompetence of the left saphenofemoral junction (Fig. 57-1A) and total incompetence of the right saphenofemoral junction (Fig. 57-1B). The left saphenopopliteal junction demonstrates complete incompetence, with dramatic enlargement of the short saphenous vein (SSV) (Fig. 57-2A). The right saphenopopliteal junction is normal, with normal diameter seen in the short saphenous vein (SSV) (Fig. 57-2B).

Recommendations

Ligate and divide the left great saphenous vein at saphenofemoral junction (supine position) and excise the distal varicose veins. Then, ligate and divide the left lesser saphenous vein at the saphenopopliteal junction (prone position). Lastly, ligate and divide the right great saphenous vein at the saphenofemoral junction.

◾ Surgical Approach

The principal cause of damaging reflux in this patient is the completely incompetent lesser saphenous vein in the left lower extremity. This is surgically corrected with the patient in the prone position. One day preoperatively, a repeat ultrasound is necessary, because the point of entry of the lesser saphenous vein to the popliteal vein is variable. The technologist identifies the exact level of the union of the lesser saphenous vein with the popliteal vein, and marks the posterior popliteal (or thigh) skin with an indelible marker. The operative incision will be made at this site. On the day of surgery, with the patient in the prone position, a short 2- to 3-inch incision is made at the marked level. The junction of the saphenous vein with the popliteal vein is identified, and the lesser saphenous vein is ligated and divided, flush with the popliteal vein. The remaining ligated distal lesser saphenous vein is left in place. Despite the enlargement of the vein due to reflux, it will usually return to normal size within 6 to 12 months.

The partially incompetent left saphenofemoral junction may be watched and operated on at a later date if it proceeds to complete incompetence. In our experience, these partially incompetent junctions almost always proceed to complete incompetence. Therefore, we would recommend ligation and division of the saphenofemoral junction in the supine position during the same operation as the left saphenopopliteal junction.

On a separate day, the incompetent right saphenofemoral junction should be ligated and divided, with the patient in the supine position. The completely incompetent right saphenofemoral junction should be treated by ligation and division of the great saphenous vein at the saphenofemoral junction, with excision of any large distal varicose veins through small (one-quarter to one-half inch) incisions. In most cases, we do not utilize the stripping operation; we prefer to carry out the procedure described above. Also, a thorough search for significant incompetent perforator veins in the ultrasound suite will reveal those of significant size (larger than 3.5 to 4 mm), and these perforators are ligated at the time of surgery. They frequently are found in deep to large surface varicose veins.

Discussion

The deep compartment of the leg is a high-pressure chamber due to the pumping action of the calf muscle during walking and exercise. The superficial compartment of the leg acts as a low-pressure chamber. Browse et al. have pointed out that if incompetent perforating veins (including the saphenofemoral and saphenopopliteal junctions) render the superficial compartment "hypertensive," venous pathology will develop, including edema, varicose veins, induration, cellulitis, and ulceration. These studies demonstrate almost complete incompetence of the left saphenofemoral junction and complete (grade IV) incompetence of the left saphenopopliteal junction with gross dilatation of the short saphenous vein. This dramatic degree of reflux from both junctions has resulted in overload of the left superficial venous system below the knee and resultant clinical findings. The case described is a classic example of a high-pressure superficial compartment, with edema, cyanosis, distention of skin venules, and varicose veins. The incompetent saphenopopliteal junction has resulted in a dramatic increase in pressure in the lesser (short) saphenous vein, with subsequent enlargement of the vein. Because the enlarging lesser (short) saphenous vein is confined by the overlying fascia, the symptoms are more severe. The increase in flow through this large incompetent vein has created a leg with venous hypertension with all of the described symptoms. Interruption of the high-pressure channels will reduce the venous pressure to normal.

Case Continued

The patient has an unremarkable postsurgical course. She goes home the same day as the surgery, and begins to wear 30- to 40-mm Hg compression hose within 2 weeks.

Suggested Readings

Belcaro G, Nicolaides AN, Stansby G. *The Venous Clinic*. London: Imperial College Press; 1998.

Browse NL, Burnand KG, Irvine AT, Wilson NM. *Diseases of the Veins*. 2nd ed. London: Edward Arnold/Oxford University Press; 1999.

Johnson HD, Pflug J. *The Swollen Leg*. Philadelphia: JB Lippincott Company; 1975.

Kinmoth JB. *The Lymphatics*. London: Edward Arnold; 1982.

Tibbs DJ, Sabistan DC, Davies MG, Mortimer PS, Scurr JH. *Varicose Veins, Venous Disorders, and Lymphatic Problems in the Lower Limbs*. London: Oxford University Press; 1997.

case 58

Jennifer S. Engle, MD, FACS, RVT

Presentation

A 47-year-old man with no significant past medical history presents to your office complaining of left leg pain and swelling with prolonged standing. Results of the physical examination are normal, except for large, bulging varicose veins (Fig. 58-1) and edema of the left lower extremity.

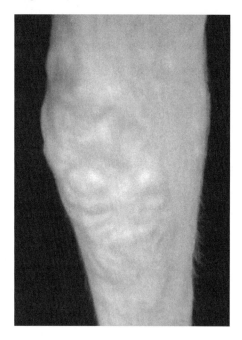

Figure 58-1

Differential Diagnosis

Leg edema can be caused by a pathophysiological process limited to the leg or by a systemic process. Systemic processes responsible for lower extremity edema, which is generally bilateral, include organ failure (heart, liver, kidney); certain medications; and paralysis and muscle atrophy resulting in prolonged periods of extremity dependency. Lymphedema can cause unilateral or bilateral leg swelling.

Swelling may be the result of varicose veins alone or may be attributable to deep venous pathology that can coexist with varicose veins. Thrombosis and congenital anomalies can cause deep venous obstruction and deep venous insufficiency; both of these latter conditions can be associated with unilateral or bilateral edema, with or without varicose veins. The symptoms of deep venous pathology are identical to those associated with varicose veins caused by superficial venous insufficiency, but the treatment of these entities is different.

Discussion

The edema that results from organ failure, paralysis, muscle atrophy, prolonged extremity dependency, or medications can generally be ruled out by a thorough history and physical examination.

Unlike the "pitting" edema associated with venous insufficiency, which begins in the ankles and calves, the "non-pitting" edema of lymphedema begins in the dorsum of the foot, usually involves the toes, and progresses proximally with time. The skin of a lymphedematous limb is characterized by a peau d'orange appearance and papillomas. The skin associated with superficial venous insufficiency and varicose veins can show no changes at all, or can display lipodermatosclerosis and stasis pigmentation changes in the gaiter region. Both varicose veins and lymphedema can result in skin ulceration, but this occurs in the setting of the characteristics described above for each condition.

Varicose veins can result from superficial venous insufficiency, or insufficiency that occurs as a result of deep venous thrombosis or congenital anomalies. The former condition results in primary varicose veins and the latter in secondary varicose veins. The pathophysiology of varicose veins is multifaceted. Failure of the calf muscle pump, failure of the valves within the superficial or deep veins, and deep or superficial venous obstruction can all cause varicose veins. The risk factors for primary varicose veins include a family history of varicose veins, female gender, multiple pregnancies, increased height and weight, and occupations that require standing. The symptoms include pain and swelling with prolonged standing or sitting, which is relieved with leg elevation. Patients may also complain of burning and itching over the varicosities, cramping of the calves at night, lower extremity eczema, and leg ulcers. Venous photoplethysmography is a diagnostic test that measures the venous refill time after foot flexion activates the calf muscle pump to promote venous emptying. A refill time of less than 20 seconds indicates venous insufficiency. Deep venous insufficiency is present when obliterating the superficial venous system with a tourniquet and repeating the test still yields a reduced refill time. Superficial venous insufficiency alone is present when the refill time normalizes with the application of a tourniquet. Venous duplex ultrasonography is capable of detecting both deep and superficial venous thrombosis or insufficiency. It also uses Doppler to measure the duration of valve closure (longer than 0.5 seconds is abnormal).

Recommendation

Venous photoplethysmography and venous duplex ultrasound.

Venous Photoplethysmography

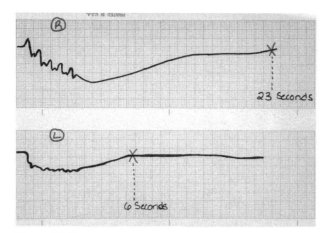

Figure 58-2

Venous Photoplethysmography Report

Without tourniquet: right leg, 23 seconds; left leg, 6 seconds (Fig. 58-2).

With tourniquet: right leg, 30 seconds; left leg, 25 seconds.

Superficial venous insufficiency is noted in the left lower extremity. No evidence of deep venous insufficiency is noted in either lower extremity.

Venous Duplex Ultrasound

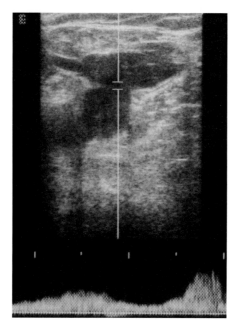

Figure 58-3

Venous Duplex Ultrasound Report

The left greater saphenous vein displays saphenofemoral reflux (duration longer than 0.5 second). No significant reflux is noted in the right lower extremity. No reflux or obstruction is noted in the deep venous system.

Diagnosis and Recommendation

The venous duplex ultrasound shows the etiology of the patient's varicose veins to be saphenofemoral reflux in the left lower extremity. The first line of treatment is leg elevation, exercise, protection of the skin barrier, and compression therapy. Had the venous photoplethysmography and ultrasound showed significant deep venous insufficiency alone or in conjunction with superficial venous insufficiency, the nonoperative management noted above would be the recommended treatment. In this patient, who has superficial venous insufficiency alone, surgical intervention is indicated if he remains symptomatic, develops a complication, or has cosmetic concerns.

Surgical Approach

In the past, either vein stripping or simple varicose vein excisions were the only procedures performed for this problem. With the advent of modern ultrasound and the ability to identify accurately the source of reflux (saphenofemoral, saphenopopliteal, or incompetent perforating veins), outpatient surgical procedures can now be designed to address the specific areas of reflux and subsequently excise the varicose veins without removing normal superficial veins.

In a patient such as this one with saphenofemoral reflux, high ligation of the greater saphenous vein is indicated. This is done through an oblique incision placed slightly above the groin crease between the femoral arterial pulsation and adductor tendon. All five named proximal branches of the greater saphenous should be ligated and divided. Lastly, the greater saphenous vein is ligated and divided just distal to the saphenofemoral junction. Large calf varicosities are subsequently removed through small incisions placed in Langer's lines to minimize the appearance of postoperative scarring. A bulky compression dressing is placed. The patient is discharged home after a brief period in recovery, and returns to the office in 72 hours for dressing and suture removal.

The patient is informed that for the first postoperative week, short intervals of leg elevation are mandatory and high-impact exercise is to be avoided for 1 month. Compression stockings should be worn daily for 1 month and as frequently as possible thereafter, which can reduce the incidence of recurrences. Complications include bleeding; infection; recurrence of varicose veins; injury to the deep vein, artery, nerves, and lymphatics; deep vein thrombosis; pulmonary embolism; and the risks associated with anesthesia.

Discussion

There are acceptable alternatives to the procedures described above. Saphenofemoral reflux can also be treated with a high ligation of the greater saphenous vein, stripping the thigh portion of the greater saphenous vein, and removing the distal calf varicosities. Stripping of the calf portion of the greater saphenous vein is discouraged because of the high incidence of concomitant saphenous nerve injury. Two newer procedures are currently being investigated to treat saphenofemoral reflux. Both employ percutaneous catheters introduced into the greater saphenous at the level of the knee and guided to the saphenofemoral junction via ultrasound. At this point, either radiofrequency or laser energy is dispersed, resulting in contracture of the thigh portion of the greater saphenous vein. Distal varicosities are then removed, as in the previously detailed procedure.

Lesser saphenous varicosities are treated in a similar manner, by ligating and dividing all the proximal branches and then ligating and dividing the lesser saphenous vein at the level of fascial penetration, just distal to the saphenopopliteal junction. Incompetent perforating veins should also be ligated and divided at the fascial level. Preoperatively, the lesser saphenous vein and incompetent perforating veins should be located using ultrasound, and their location marked.

Suggested Readings

Bergan JJ. Excision of varicose veins. In: *Current Therapy in Vascular Surgery*. 4th ed. St. Louis: Mosby; 2001:838-840.

Bergan JJ. Surgical management of primary and recurrent varicose veins. In: *Handbook of Venous Disorders*. 2nd ed. London: Arnold; 2001:289-302.

Scurr JH, Tibbs DJ. Clinical patterns of venous disorder: incompetence in superficial veins: simple or primary varicose veins. In: *Varicose Veins, Venous Disorders, and Lymphatic Problems in the Lower Limbs*. Oxford: Oxford University Press; 1997:47-101.

Weiss RA, Feied CF, Weiss MA. Venous physiology and pathophysiology. In: *Vein Diagnosis and Treatment: A Comprehensive Approach*. New York: McGraw-Hill; 2001:23-30.

case 59

Peter H. Lin, MD, Ruth L. Bush, MD, and Alan B. Lumsden, MD

Presentation

A 53-year-old man presents to the emergency department with a 2-day history of left lower leg swelling. He underwent an 8-hour transatlantic flight 4 days earlier. He complains of significant swelling of the left calf and thigh, which are warm to touch. He also describes severe lower leg pain, which worsens with ambulation. He has no significant past medical history and is not taking any medication. He also denies any trauma to his lower extremity. Physical examination reveals marked swelling of the right lower extremity involving the calf and the thigh, which are tender to touch (Fig. 59-1). Although the calf is soft to touch, it becomes painful with both passive and active dorsiflexion of the foot. The right lower leg is unremarkable in its appearance and upon examination.

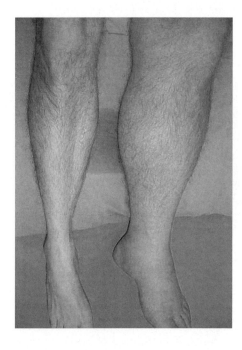

Figure 59-1 Marked left lower swelling.

Venous Duplex Ultrasound

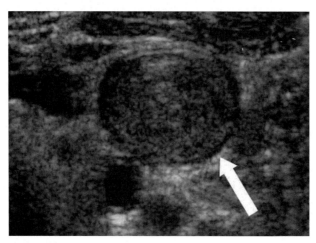

Figure 59-2

Ultrasound Report

Large echolucent density in the left common femoral vein is noncompressible, consistent with acute deep venous thrombosis (DVT). There is a complete venous occlusion with venous thrombus extending proximally to the external and common iliac veins, as well as distally to the superficial femoral and popliteal veins. Doppler signals show absence of normal phasic flow, consistent with venous occlusion.

Differential Diagnosis

The diagnosis for the lower left leg swelling in this patient is DVT, as evidenced by the physical examination and the duplex ultrasound scan. Common risk factors of DVT include age, obesity, hypercoagulable disorders, immobility, pregnancy, oral contraceptive medication, malignancy, ileofemoral venous compression due to abdominal mass, malignancy, May-Thurner syndrome, chronic indwelling catheter in the femoral vein, and leg trauma.

Discussion

The classic presentation of a lower extremity DVT are calf swelling and tenderness, elevated temperature, and a positive Homans' sign (calf pain on dorsiflexion of the foot). The etiology of DVT in this patient is likely related to his immobility during a prolonged flight. The marked swelling of his lower leg suggests an extensive thrombosis of his left lower extremity venous system. In an extreme scenario, phlegmasia cerulea dolens, as evidenced by the painful blue appearance of the leg, can occur due to massive thrombosis involving the iliac veins and extending into the most distal venules in the leg. Phlegmasia cerulea dolens is a condition usually associated with an underlying intraabdominal malignancy, such as pancreatic cancer.

Clinical diagnosis of DVT is unreliable because only 50% of patients with evidence of DVT on venography have any clinical sign. Moreover, the majority of patients suffering fatal pulmonary embolism have no clinical features of venous thrombosis prior to sudden cardiovascular collapse.

Venous duplex ultrasound is the primary imaging technique used to detect DVT. Spectral Doppler can detect the presence of thrombus by determining normal or abnormal flow in the vessels. Normal Doppler will be unidirectional and spontaneous with the respiratory phase. Flow should cease with Valsalva maneuver, and demonstrate augmentation by distal compression. The Doppler will appear abnormal when there is substantial occlusion of the vein. Flow augmentation and Valsalva will be diminished or absent. The most reliable method for detecting thrombus is compression. Compressions are done in gray scale in a transverse plane. Thrombus can only be ruled out when vessel walls completely collapse. Partial thrombosis may be present if the entire vein does not collapse.

Recommendation

Because of the marked leg swelling and constant pain, treatment to remove the DVT and restore the ileofemoral venous flow is indicated. Treatment options for eliminating DVT include surgical thrombectomy, catheter-directed thrombolysis, and percutaneous mechanical thrombectomy.

Discussion

Surgical thrombectomy: Surgical thrombectomy with distal arteriovenous fistula creation for acute DVT is mainly of historical interest only because of its associated operative morbidity, primarily related to blood loss and rethrombosis. However, surgical thrombectomy may still be used in the clinical setting of venous gangrene with impending limb loss. The best reported results are from a 1999 study by Juhan et al. in which they reported an improvement in long-term results following surgical venous thrombectomy for acute iliofemoral DVT. In a review of 77 patients, principally young trauma victims, valvular competency was preserved at 5 years in 80%, while 90% of limbs had either mild symptoms of chronic venous insufficiency or no symptoms at all. Additionally, Meissner et al. reported results of venous thrombectomy with arteriovenous fistula in 30 patients. In all but 3 patients, patency of the iliofemoral segment was maintained 12 months after clot extraction. Most series, however, have demonstrated only average results for this all but abandoned technique.

Catheter-directed thrombolysis: The delivery of a thrombolytic agent directly into an existing venous thrombosis has overtaken systemic thrombolysis due in part to more complete clot lysis combined with a lower rate of bleeding complications. By using one of many commercially available multiple side hole infusion catheters for lytic agent delivery, high drug concentrations can be concentrated at the location of the thrombus. Catheter-directed thrombolysis has been advocated because of its theoretical advantage of complete and rapid clot dissolution. Multiple studies have documented the efficacy of several lytic agents in the treatment of acute DVT, with total infusion times needed for thrombus removal ranging from hours to days. Meissner et al. evaluated an association between time to lysis and the development of venous reflux in patients using serial duplex scans following a DVT episode. With the exception of the posterior tibial vein, early lysis and rapid venous recanalization appears to protect valve integrity in the lower extremity. Although thrombolytic therapy for DVT has excellent outcomes with thrombus clearance, and thus, perhaps, may lower the incidence of post-phlebitic syndrome by preserving valvular function, the complication profile of the treatment secondary to the lytic agent and the infusion times may be limitations for widespread use.

Percutaneous mechanical thrombectomy (PMT): Relief of clot burden by directly extracting thrombus surgically or via lytic dissolution should hypothetically decrease the risk of pulmonary embolus, and also that of post-phlebitic syndrome resulting in manifestations of chronic venous insufficiency. Primarily because of the bleeding risks of catheter-directed thrombolysis, PMT has emerged as an advantageous option for the treatment of acute DVT. One PMT system that has been shown to be effective in the removal of acute DVT is the AngioJet (Possis Medical Inc., Minneapolis, MN) percutaneous mechanical thrombectomy system. The principle of this device is based on the Venturi effect. The AngioJet system creates rapidly flowing saline jets that are directed backward from the tip of the device to outflow channels in a coaxial fashion. This generates a vacuum force, which draws the thrombus into the catheter. A major advantage of this percutaneous treatment modality is that the thrombectomy catheter can be delivered through a small-bore introducer sheath, which reduces access site trauma and avoids operative exposure required with the conventional Fogarty thromboembolectomy. A clinical study conducted by Kasirajan et al., which evaluated the efficacy of the AngioJet system, has demonstrated that such a mechanical thrombectomy system is effective in thrombus removal, venous patency restoration and maintenance, and symptom relief. The AngioJet rheolytic thrombectomy system is designed to produce an area of extremely low pressure at the catheter tip by controlled high-velocity saline jets. Through this mechanism, thrombus surrounding the catheter tip is macerated and rapidly evacuated via an effluent lumen into a collection chamber. In this study, only four (23.5%) patients achieved greater than 90% thrombus clearance with PMT alone. Adjunctive thrombolytic agents were used in 9 of 17 patients, those who had a lesser amount of clot extracted with the use of the PMT catheter. Often, the thrombolytic catheter was left in place and the average duration of lytic therapy was 20.2 hours. Clinical symptomatic improvement was seen in 82% of patients over a follow-up time of 11 months.

Approach

Treatment approach in this patient includes mechanical thrombectomy using the AngioJet system via the left popliteal vein approach.

Venogram

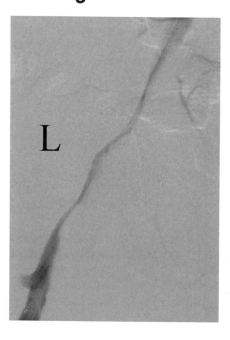

Figure 59-3

Venogram Report

Venogram, performed via the left popliteal vein in the prone position, reveals a complete thrombosis of the superficial femoral vein and extensive DVT in the left ileofemoral venous system.

Surgical Approach

The patient is placed in the prone position. The left popliteal fossa is prepped and draped sterilely. Under ultrasound guidance, the left popliteal vein is percutaneously cannulated using a Micropuncture needle (Boston Scientific, Natick, MA). A 6 French introducer sheath (Boston Scientific) is placed over a guide wire into the popliteal vein. Following the placement of a guide wire through the ileofemoral DVT, an AngioJet thrombectomy catheter is delivered over the guide wire into the venous thrombus. Serial thrombectomy is performed by activating the AngioJet system, which percutaneously removes the thrombus from the superficial femoral vein and the ileofemoral venous system.

Completion Venogram

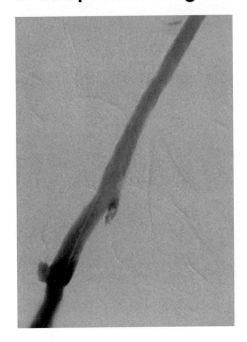

Figure 59-4

Venogram Report

Completion venogram demonstrates complete resolution of the DVT in the entire superficial femoral vein and ileofemoral venous system (Fig. 59-4).

Recommendation

The patient is given systemic heparin bolus (100 U/kg), started in an IV heparin drip, and oral coumadin anticoagulation is begun 3 days later. Repeat venous duplex ultrasound is performed on the following day.

Venous Duplex Ultrasound

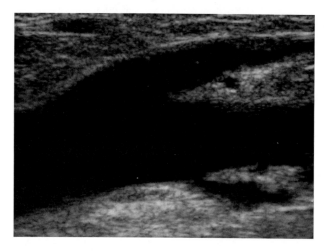

Figure 59-5

Ultrasound Results

Longitudinal image demonstrates a complete resolution of the left femoral and iliac vein without evidence of DVT.

Case Continued

At the time of discharge 4 days later, the patient's left leg swelling has completely subsided without any pain (Fig. 59-6). He remains free of symptoms and has no recurrence of DVT at 1-year follow-up.

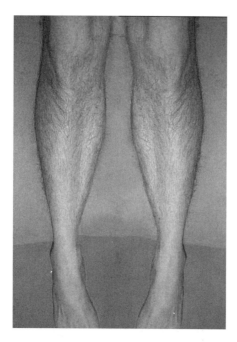

Figure 59-6 At the time of discharge, the patient's left leg has returned to normal without pain or swelling.

Selected Readings

Juhan C, Alimi Y, Di Mauro P, Hartung O. Surgical venous thrombectomy. *Cardiovasc Surg.* 1999;7:586-590.

Kasirajan K, Gray B, Ouriel K. Percutaneous AngioJet thrombectomy in the management of extensive deep venous thrombosis. *J Vasc Interv Radiol.* 2001;12:179-185.

Meissner MH. Thrombolytic therapy for acute deep vein thrombosis and the venous registry. *Rev Cardiovasc Med.* 2002;3(suppl 2): S53-S60.

Meissner MH, Caps MT, Zierler BK, Bergelin RO, Manzo RA, Strandness DE Jr. Deep venous thrombosis and superficial venous reflux. *J Vasc Surg.* 2000;32:48-56.

Meissner AJ, Huszcza S. Surgical strategy for management of deep venous thrombosis of the lower extremities. *World J Surg.* 1996;20: 1149-1155.

Joseph D. Raffetto, MD, FACS

Presentation

A 30-year-old man is referred to the vascular clinic with a nonhealing left leg ulcer of 3 months' duration. He is otherwise healthy. The patient complains of leg and ankle swelling with "weeping" yellow fluid from the ulcer bed. The patient states that at the age of 28 years he fractured his left leg in a car accident, and required open repair with internal fixation. One week after surgery, he developed a blood clot in his left leg that was treated with anticoagulation. On examination, the location of the ulcer is superior to the medial malleolus, and is 3-cm in diameter with a mixed granulating fibrin base. The surrounding skin is dark brown and has a "woody" texture. There is leg and ankle edema, with decreased mobility at the ankle joint and no calf tenderness.

Differential Diagnosis

The differential diagnosis for a leg ulcer includes chronic venous insufficiency, arterial insufficiency, diabetes, vasculitis, cryoglobulinemia, trauma, infection, malignancy, and decubitus. In African-American patients, one must consider sickle cell disease as a cause of perimalleolar ulcers. Bilateral lower extremity arterial pulses are normal. A venous duplex and APG are ordered.

■ Venous Duplex Ultrasound

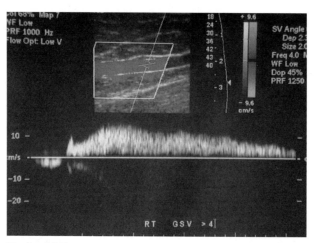

Figure 60-1

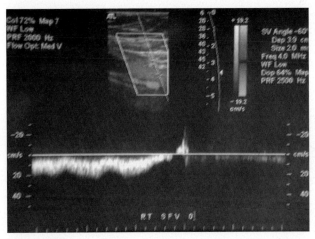

Figure 60-2

Duplex Ultrasound Report

Duplex ultrasound (DUS) demonstrates severe reflux (incompetent valves) of the entire left long saphenous vein (greater saphenous vein), common femoral vein, and popliteal vein, with two incompetent perforator veins in the leg. There is no deep venous thrombosis. When the valve is incompetent, there is severe (greater than 4 seconds) reflux following compression of the leg, with a long segment of flow reversal (long segment of venous spectra). Figure 60-1 demonstrates a normal superficial femoral vein. Note the absence of reflux following compression of the leg when the valve is competent, and with no flow reversal (long area void of venous spectra) (Fig. 60-2).

Case Continued

Air plethysmography (APG) demonstrates a venous filling index (a measure to evaluate the severity of the reflux) of 6 mL/s (normal is less than 2 mL/s) and an ejection fraction (a measure to determine the calf muscle pump function) of 35% (normal is greater than 60%). The history of leg trauma complicated by a venous thrombosis and the clinical examination is suggestive of a venous ulcer.

Diagnosis and Recommendation

The diagnosis is chronic venous insufficiency with venous ulcer. Unlikely diagnoses include arterial insufficiency due to lack of further ischemic signs (gangrene, loss of hair, shiny taut skin-atrophic, loss of muscle mass, dystrophic toenails), abnormal pulses, and older age. Diabetic foot ulcer is classically on the plantar surface at the metatarsal phalangeal joints, interphalangeal joints, or heel and dorsal foot. Vasculitis or cryoglobulinemia would have other systemic manifestations and require further serologic tests and biopsy for confirmation. A rare manifestation of various skin cancers is the presence of leg ulcers, and in the epithelium of chronic ulcers (Marjolin ulcer). Systemic myeloproliferative disorders can present with skin ulceration.

Treatment recommendations include compressive therapy with either bandages (Unna's boot) or garment stockings, or surgery with ligation and stripping of the long saphenous vein with perforator interruption. Indications for surgery are failure of compressive therapy due to poor fit or noncompliance, recurrent venous ulcer despite aggressive medical management, severe reflux in the deep system, and as an adjuvant to medical compression therapy.

Surgical Approach

A standard approach is to exise the long saphenous vein with high ligation at the saphenofemoral junction and endoscopic perforator vein ligation under general anesthesia. Subfascial endoscopic perforator surgical ligation (SEPS) is performed first. The concept is to divide perforators that are present in both the superficial and deep posterior compartment of the leg. The important perforator veins of the leg are the Cockett perforators (I, II, and III) originating from the posterior arch vein, and the proximal paratibial perforators that connect the posterior arch vein and long saphenous vein to the posterior tibial and popliteal veins. The limb is exsanguinated using an esmarque wrap, and a pneumatic tourniquet placed on the proximal thigh is inflated to 250 to 300 mm Hg to obtain a bloodless field. Two skin incisions are required, and are in the midcalf posterior-medial skin 4 cm and 10 cm from the tibia. Two endoscopic ports are placed in the subfascial plane: a 10-mm port housing the camera, and 5-mm working port (to pass scissors, clips, dissecting instruments). A balloon space-maker is inserted to widen the subfascial space (superficial posterior compartment), and carbon dioxide insufflation is maintained at 30 mm Hg to provide visualization. The subfascial space is assessed for perforators from the proximal border of the tibia to the ankle level, and perforators are clipped and divided. The paratibial fascia is opened next to enter the deep posterior compartment, and this allows for division of the Cockett II and III perforators, the proximal paratibial perforators, and Boyd's perforator (at the knee just above the paratibial perforators). The Cockett I perforator is retromalleolar and usually requires a separate direct incision to divide and ligate it.

Once all the perforators are divided, the ports are removed and the remaining carbon dioxide is manually expressed, followed by tourniquet removal. At this stage, a 4-cm incision in the groin, 4 cm lateral to the pubic tubercle, is made to expose the saphenofemoral junction. High ligation of the saphenofemoral junction along with all tributaries is performed, and the long saphenous vein is stripped from the groin to the level just below the knee. All wounds are closed and an elastic bandage is applied from the foot to the thigh.

The patient is given instructions to maintain leg elevation for 1 to 2 days, remove the bandages on day 2 to check the wounds, and reapply an elastic wrap to minimize leg swelling. Usually, patients are able to ambulate 4 to 6 hours following surgery. The patient should be instructed that there may be bruising along the medial thigh and leg from the stripping, and occasionally there may be an associated hematoma. After surgery, patients usually return to work in 1 to 2 weeks. Compression stockings are recommended for 3 to 4 weeks following surgery, and should be worn during extensive periods of standing or sitting.

Discussion

Chronic venous insufficiency (CVI) is estimated to affect between 0.5% and 3% of the adult population. CVI affects women 3 times more than men. However, venous ulcers are more commonly seen in males and the elderly. CVI results from persistent venous hypertension that can be measured by ambulatory venous pressure (measured from the dorsal foot vein). Normal baseline venous pressure on standing is 80 to 90 mm Hg. In normal functioning veins, when ambulating the venous pressure in the leg decreases to less than 40 mm Hg. An ambulatory venous pressure greater than 40 mm Hg is considered abnormal and suggestive of CVI. The venous recovery time, defined as the time required for return to a baseline venous pressure during standing, is normally between 17 and 20 seconds. Patients with CVI have venous recovery times that are significantly lower.

The etiology of CVI can be from a primary cause (unknown etiology) resulting in venous reflux (incompetent valves), or from a secondary known cause such as occurs with venous thrombosis with obstruction with or without concomitant valvular reflux, and leg trauma that results in poor calf muscle pump function. In rare cases, CVI can be from a congenital cause, as in patients with Klippel-Trenaunay syndrome (venous malformation including varicosities, limb hypertrophy, and capillary dermal hemangioma—the port wine stain).

A significant cause of CVI is the postphlebitic syndrome (or postthrombotic syndrome) that occurs as a late complication of an acute deep venous thrombosis (DVT). The postthrombotic syndrome can affect 29% to 79% of post-DVT patients; however, interestingly, about 38% of patients who have had a venous thrombosis have no valvular incompetence and usually have complete and early resolution of thrombus. Following venous thrombosis, veins undergo partial or complete recanalization, or remain thrombosed with collateral flow. The resulting vein segments that have recanalized or remain thrombosed may have damaged or nonfunctioning valves, leading to chronic venous hypertension. It is important to note that incompetent valves alone, venous thrombosis alone, or a combination of both can result in the same clinical manifestations in patients with CVI.

Patients with CVI can have the following lower extremity presentations: varicose veins associated with pain, leg edema, venous claudication (leg swelling with heaviness and leg cramps), skin hyperpigmentation and fibrosis affecting the dermis and subcutaneous fat (lipodermatosclerosis), decreased ankle mobility, and leg ulceration. Patients with CVI, especially with skin changes of lipodermatosclerosis are at risk for delayed wound healing from repetitive trauma to the limb. Patients with long-standing CVI may also have lymphedema, representing a combined disease process. Initial attention to the venous abnormalities with proper treatment for resolution of the lymphedema may be required.

The evaluation of patients with CVI begins with a complete history and physical examination. One should determine if deep or superficial venous thrombosis is present. The use of anticoagulants and prior venous surgery should be documented. Examination of the extremities requires assessment of arterial pulses, tissue evaluation for ulceration and skin color changes, toenail hypertrophy, edema, and varicosities. Confirmatory tests using DUS to evaluate for venous thrombosis, anatomic pattern, and reflux (defined as valve closure time of greater than 0.5 seconds), and APG should be performed. Patients with cellulitis and ulcer bed infections should be treated with 1 to 2 weeks of antibiotics, with frequent dressing changes.

Therapeutic considerations for CVI include compression therapy with elastic compressive stockings, paste gauze boots, layered bandaging, or adjustable layered compression garments. Surgery should be considered in patients who have persistent discomfort, refractory venous ulcers, inability to comply with compression therapy, and as an adjuvant to compressive stocking treatment. In general, patients with venous ulcers require 3 to 6 months before complete healing is achieved. Recurrent ulceration is frequent if compression therapy is not maintained.

Suggested Readings

Chrisopoulos DG, Nicolaides AN, Szendro G, Irvine AT, Bull ML, Eastcott HHG. Air-plethysmography and the effect of elastic compression on venous hemodynamics of the leg. *J Vasc Surg.* 1987;5:148-159.

Gloviczki P, Bergan JJ, Rhodes JM, Canton LG, Harmsen S, Ilstrup DM. Mid-term results of endoscopic perforator vein interruption for chronic venous insufficiency: lessons learned from the North American subfascial endoscopic perforator surgery registry. The North American Study Group. *J Vasc Surg.* 1999;29:489-502.

Johnson BF, Manzo RA, Bergelin RO, Strandness DE. Relationship between changes in the deep venous system and the development of the postthrombotic syndrome after an acute episode of lower limb deep vein thrombosis: a one- to six-year follow-up. *J Vasc Surg.* 1995; 21:307-313.

Kahn SR, Solymoss S, Lamping DL, Abenhaim L. Long-term outcomes after deep vein thrombosis: postphlebitic syndrome and quality of life. *J Gen Intern Med.* 2000;15: 425-429.

Meissner MH, Manzo RA, Bergelin RO, Strandness DE. Deep venous insufficiency: the relationship between lysis and subsequent reflux. *J Vasc Surg.* 1993:18:596-605.

Scott TE, LaMorte WW, Gorin DR, Menzoian JO. Risk factors for chronic venous insufficiency: a dual case-control study. *J Vasc Surg.* 1995;22:622-628.

van Bemmelen PS, Bedford BS, Beach K, Strandness DE. Quantitative segmental evaluation of venous valvular reflux with duplex ultrasound scanning. *J Vasc Surg.* 1989;10:425-431.

Thomas W. Wakefield, MD, and Jonathan L. Eliason, MD

Presentation

A 46-year-old man with a 20-year history of severe chronic venous insufficiency (CVI) that he attributes to two leg fractures presents to you with a healed right medial malleolar ulcer for Unna boot therapy. He has no history of deep venous thrombosis (DVT) and has never been on anticoagulants. He presents with a significant history of swelling in his right lower extremity, which worsens with standing. The patient is a sheet metal worker and is on his feet for significant lengths of time. On physical examination, the patient is found to have classic changes of stasis dermatitis and statis pigmentation in the right lower extremity. He has no obvious phlebitis, although he has significant varicose veins. His varices are located from just above the knee and extend down to the area of his medial ankle. On presentation, the patient brings a venogram that suggests that he has no evidence of current or previous DVT and that his deep venous system is open and intact.

Differential Diagnosis

The differential diagnosis for a patient with ulcers involves venous, arterial, neuropathic, or mixed etiology. Venous ulcers are typically located in the medial and lateral malleolar area and associated with stasis dermatitis and stasis pigmentation. Arterial ulcers are typically located on the distal extremity with associated signs and symptoms of peripheral vascular occlusive disease, including thickened toenails, loss of hair, and pallor, along with severe pain. Neuropathic ulcers are typically located over pressure points such as the first and fifth metatarsal heads of the foot and over the heel. They are often painless, deep, and indolent and associated with a significant surrounding callus. This patient's history and presentation are classic for a venous etiology to his ulceration. A photoplethysmograph, venous duplex scan, air phlethysmograph, and venogram are ordered.

Photoplethysmography Study

INDICATIONS: Unexplained LE edema.
HISTORY:
Previous studies for comparison: No
This patient presents with a history of right LE DVT and venous ulcerations, r/o deep venous insufficiency.

VENOUS REFLUX (PPG):
   Refilling time after Dorsal Plantar Fle

  RIGHT TOURNIQUET:
     None: 9 sec
     Ankle: 18 sec

  LEFT TOURNIQUET:
     None: 26 sec

FINAL IMPRESSION: The right LE PPG shows evidence of deep venous insufficiency. The left LE PPG is within normal limits.

Figure 61-1

Photoplethysmography Study Report

Photoplethysmography (PPG; Fig. 61-1) reveals that the patient has right lower extremity deep venous insufficiency, while the left leg is within normal limits (greater than 26 seconds).

▮ **Venous Duplex Scan**

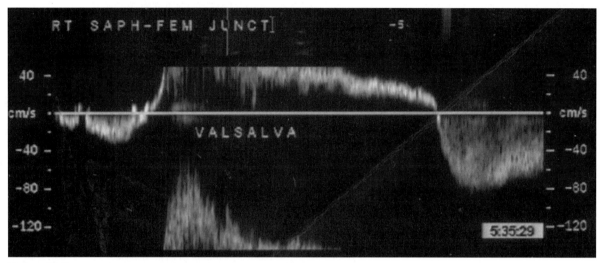

Figure 61-2

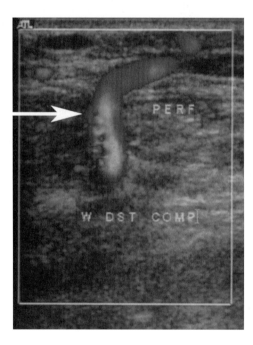

Figure 61-3

Venous Duplex Scan Report

No evidence of DVT is seen in the right lower extremity, but the greater saphenous vein appears varicosed. The saphenofemoral junction is imaged with and without Valsalva maneuvers and shows evidence of venous reflux (Fig 61-2). An incompetent perforator in the distal calf involving the posterior tibial vein is noted (*arrow,* Fig. 61-3). This perforator is marked and measured at 0.51 cm.

▉ Air Plethysmography

	ACI MEDICAL INC. APG-1000C/CP PATIENT REPORT					Normal Values
	Name: Date: Time:	RIGHT LEG stocking		LEFT LEG stocking		
REFLUX	Venous Volume (VV) ml	135.9				
ml/sec - - -	Venous Filling Index VFI	9.905				<2 ml/sec
ml/sec - - -	VFI with superficial occ	8.548				<3.5 ml/s
CALF MUSCLE PUMP FUNCTION	Ejection Volume (EV) ml	117.9				
	Ejection Fraction (EF)%	86.77				> 40%

Figure 61-4

Air Plethysmography Report

Air plethysmography (APG) reveals that the patient has significant venous reflux with venous filling index (VFI) at 9.9 mL/s; with superficial occlusion, the VFI actually improves to 8.6 mL/s (Fig. 61-4). The patient has a normal ejection volume and ejection fraction of 87%.

▉ Ascending and Descending Venography

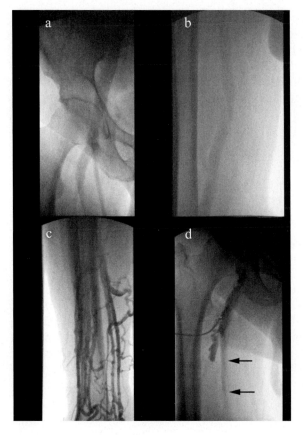

Figure 61-5

Ascending and Descending Venography Report

The ascending venogram reveals widely patent calf and thigh veins. Descending venogram with valsalva demonstrates lack of valves at the superficial femoral vein and reflux of contrast down both the superficial femoral (*arrows*) and profunda femoris veins (Fig. 61-5).

Diagnosis and Recommendation

The patient's diagnosis is superficial and deep venous insufficiency as the cause of his venous ulceration. The recommendation includes saphenofemoral disconnection, inversion stripping of the greater saphenous vein to just above the knee, stab-avulsion phlebectomy of the varicosities, and finally interruption and ligation of the incompetent calf perforator underneath the area of his stasis ulcer.

The patient has reflux at the groin in both the superficial (from APG) and deep (from venogram) venous systems. His reflux improves with superficial occlusion, suggesting that removal of the superficial system would be helpful. Because of the reflux at the level of the groin, disconnection at the saphenofemoral junction of the saphenous vein from the deep venous system is recommended. The patient also has an incompetent perforator documented by venous duplex imaging, which will be ligated at the time of superficial venous excision. Finally, as the patient has a widely patent deep venous system, it is felt appropriate to proceed with the removal of the superficial venous varicosities.

Surgical Approach

The patient's veins are marked in the preoperative holding area and the calf perforator is located by duplex ultrasound imaging. The patient is then taken to the operating room. The operation begins by making a small incision in the right groin. The saphenofemoral junction is disconnected and a section of the saphenous vein removed after 5 proximal branches have been ligated and divided. Then, using a stripper, the saphenous vein is stripped with an inversion technique down to just above the knee. Small incisions are then made with a number 11 blade and stab-avulsion phlebectomies performed to remove the entire previously marked vein. Finally, a small incision is made posterior to the location of an incompetent perforator that had been marked and is ligated and divided.

Discussion

Chronic venous insufficiency is a condition in which lower extremity venous hypertension occurs due to abnormalities of the venous wall and venous valves. This can occur in the setting of previous DVT or secondary to primary venous valvular dysfunction. CVI is quite common and its prevalence increases with age. The overall incidence of venous stasis syndrome is 76 in 100,000 patient years. The incidence of venous ulceration is much less common, but still significant with an incidence of 18 in 100,000 patient years. The economic impact thereforer is significant, with an estimated 200 million 1990 dollars per year spent on their treatment in the United States alone. This figure is likely much higher today.

The pathophysiology of CVI is primarily the result of venous valvular dysfunction. With valvular insufficiency, the resulting standing column of blood leads to venous hypertension. This in turn leads to capillary dysfunction and tissue injury. Elevated venous pressures can occur due to either venous reflux from valvular incompetence of either the superficial, deep, or perforator veins and less commonly venous obstruction from DVT or venous compression syndromes, such as iliac vein compression.

Clinical characteristics of CVI include symptoms related to reflux and obstruction. From reflux, patients present with edema, aching, fatigue, night cramps, and associated stasis dermatitis and stasis pigmentation. If these changes proceed unabated, they can lead to ulceration. Patients with obstruction have pain with ambulation, significant thigh and leg swelling, and a poor response or no response to a program of CVI management.

The diagnosis of CVI involves both noninvasive and invasive testing. Noninvasive tests include PPG, APG, and venous duplex ultrasound imaging. Invasive tests include venography. Treatment of CVI involves the wearing of surgical support stockings, intermittent leg elevation, and a good exercise program such as walking, bicycling, or swimming. Adequate compression remains the foundation for healing. The most common methods for applying wound treatment and wound compression include multiple layer compression bandages or the Unna boot, and occlusive dressings underneath ace wrapping. If compression and wound coverings are utilized, patients require intermittent leg elevation until their edema is lessened to allow for the placement of appropriately fitted surgical support stockings. The combination of wound covering and compression allows for most venous ulcers to heal over time.

Meticulous local wound care and careful attention to the skin surrounding the ulcer are also paramount to allow ulcer healing. Topical wound care agents are available, but many are costly and efficacy beyond standard compression along with wound covering has been difficult to demonstrate. For large venous ulcers expected to show low rates of healing, cultured human skin equivalent (Apligraf, Ortho-McNeil Pharmaceuticals) or split thickness skin grafting may be considered.

In addition to good wound care, a mainstay of treatment is to correct points of reflux and, if necessary, open up areas of obstruction. For the correction of reflux, procedures available include superficial venous vein resection such as performed in this patient, with or without perforator ligation using either the open or the endoscopic technique (SEPS), and procedures that restore valvular competency, such as valvuloplasty, vein segment transposition, or vein valve transplantation. For patients who have chronic venous obstruction, bypasses such as a femorofemoral venous crossover bypass for an iliac vein obstruction or a saphenopoplital bypass for a femoral vein obstruction are available. One of the procedures that has gained favor recently and has shown tremendous promise is venoplasty and stenting for patients who have iliac vein compression syndrome, the so-called May-Thurner syndrome.

Suggested Readings

Burnand KG. The physiology and hemodynamics of chronic venous insufficiency of the lower limbs. In: Glovkczki P, Yao JST, eds. *Handbook of Venous Disorders*. 3rd ed. New York: Arnold, 2001:49-57.

Christopoulos DG, Nicolaides AN, Szendro G, Irvine AT, Bull ML, Eastcott HH. Air plethysmography and the effect of elastic compression on venous hemodynamics of the leg. *J Vasc Surg*. 1987; 5:148-159.

Gloviczki P, Bergan JJ, Rhodes JM, Canton LG, Harmsen S, Ilstrup DM, The North American Study Group. Mid-term results of endoscopic perforator vein interruption for chronic venous insufficiency: lessons learned from the North American Subfascial Endoscopic Perforator Surgery registry. *J Vasc Surg*. 1999;29:489-502.

Heit JA, Rooke TW, Silverstein MD, et al. Trends in the incidence of venous stasis syndrome and venous ulcer: a 25-year population-based study. *J Vas Surg*. 2001;33:1022-1027.

Hurst DR, Forauer AR, Bloom JR, Greenfield LJ, Wakefield TW, Williams DM. Diagnosis and endovascular treatment of iliocaval compression syndrome. *J Vasc Surg*. 2001;34:106-113.

Iafrati MD, Pare GJ, O'Donnell TF, Estes J. Is the nihilistic approach to surgical reduction of superficial and perforator vein incompetence for venous ulcer justified? *J Vasc Surg*. 2002;36:1167-1174.

Masuda EM, Kistner RL. Long-term results of venous valve reconstruction: a four- to twenty-one-year follow-up. *J Vas Surg*. 1994; 19:391-403.

Pappas PJ, You R, Rameshwar P, et al. Dermal tissue fibrosis in patients with chronic venous insufficiency is associated with increased transforming growth factor β_1 gene expression and protein production. *J Vasc Surg*. 1999;30:1129-1145.

Rohrer MJ, Claytor RB, Garnette CS, et al. Platelet-monocyte aggregates in patients with chronic venous insufficiency remain elevated following correction of reflux. *Cardiovasc Surg*. 2002;10:464-469.

Rutherford RB, Padberg FT Jr, Comerota AJ, Kistner RL, Meissner MH, Moneta GL. Venous severity scoring: an adjunct to venous outcome assessment. *J Vasc Surg*. 2000;31: 1307-1312.

Zajkowski PJ, Proctor MC, Wakefield TW, Bloom J, Blessing B, Greenfield LJ. Compression stockings and venous function. *Arch Surg*. 2002;137:1064-1068.

Jonathan D. Gates, MD

Presentation

A 19-year-old male presents to your emergency department (ED) with multiple gunshot wounds (GSW) to the right and left flanks and the left thigh. He is hemodynamically unstable at the scene, where he is resuscitated with 500 mL of saline. When he arrives in the ED, his airway is intact, blood pressure is now stable, and he has a single GSW in each flank, with moderate tenderness in the right flank and anterior abdomen without obvious peritonitis. Gross hematuria is noted in the Foley catheter. He has a single GSW in the left thigh with an appropriate exit wound in the posterior thigh, with intact distal pulses. He is unable to move his lower extremities and has markedly decreased sensation in both legs. He is sent for a computed tomography (CT) scan of the abdomen and pelvis.

Abdominal/Pelvic CT Scan

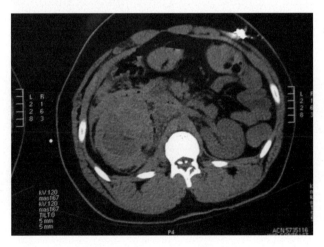

Figure 62-1

CT Scan Report

Abdominal/pelvic CT scan shows injury to the right kidney with hematoma around the kidney (Fig. 62-1) and an intact left kidney. There is a fracture of the L1 lumbar spine with bone fragments in the canal without epidural hematoma. There is no free fluid in the abdomen.

Surgical Approach

The patient is taken to the operating room immediately following his scan. Laparotomy reveals a retroperitoneal right colon injury, and a stable right retroperitoneal perinephric hematoma. The patient undergoes right ileocolectomy with primary anastomosis, and intraoperative urologic consultation results in nonoperative therapy to the right kidney injury.

An intraoperative intravenous pyelogram demonstrated a normal functioning left kidney and delayed function of the right kidney. Given the inherent hypercoagulability from the recent trauma, laparotomy, and new onset of paraplegia from the spinal GSW, this patient is at high risk for deep venous thrombosis (DVT). Selection of appropriate prophylaxis against venous thromboembolic events is warranted.

Discussion

New onset paraplegia in the trauma patient represents a high-risk category for the development of DVT. The penetrating wound to the kidney and the surrounding retroperitoneal hematoma confers a risk of bleeding should the patient be placed on prophylactic pharmacologic anticoagulation. Subcutaneous unfractionated heparin for DVT prophylaxis is inferior to low-molecular-weight heparin (LMWH) in most trauma scenarios. Most practitioners would not acutely anticoagulate a patient in whom there is a diagnosis of a nonsurgically treated solid organ injury. Over time, the risk of bleeding from the injured solid organ in the presence of anticoagulation diminishes.

The retrievable inferior vena cava (IVC) filter may be the solution to this dilemma, but is not yet approved in the United States.* The IVC filters have been shown to reduce the incidence of pulmonary embolism (PE) in the short term, but long term (2 years), there seems to be an associated increase in symptomatic DVT in those patients with a filter in place. There is also a small (4% to 6%) but real risk of IVC occlusion in the presence of an IVC filter. Some practitioners now place their patients on Coumadin in the presence of a permanent IVC filter. Lifelong administration of Coumadin also carries a risk of life-threatening hemorrhage, and might impose restrictions on the activities of an otherwise healthy young person. Hence, there appears to be a downside to having a long-term IVC filter in place.

This patient's risk of DVT/PE is highest within the first 6 weeks following his injury and the risk of anticoagulation is highest within the first 4 weeks. The retrievable IVC filter would remain in place during the period when the DVT/PE risk is highest, and it is known that an IVC filter is most effective. Over time, as that risk diminishes and the patient becomes more mobile, the filter could be removed and more appropriate prophylactic anticoagulation achieved thereafter, when it has become safe to do so. However, defining this period must be made on a case-by-case basis.

Recommendation

A Gunther-Tulip retrievable IVC filter (Fig. 62-2) is placed percutaneously. Administration of Lovenox, 40 mg daily, is started after 10 days and used for DVT prophylaxis.

Case Continued

A urine leak develops, and a right nephrostomy tube is placed to control the urine from the right kidney. Neurosurgical evaluation of the lumbar spine fracture indicates that no operative intervention is needed.

Four weeks postoperatively, the patient is improving and is moved from bed to chair in a clamshell brace. An attempt is made in interventional radiology to remove the IVC filter, but the cavagram demonstrates partial filling of the filter

---

*Since April 2003, these filters have been placed with good success at the author's institution.

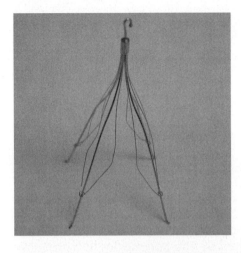

Figure 62-2 Gunther-Tulip temporary filter prior to insertion.

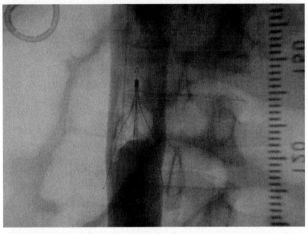

Figure 62-3 Inferior cavagram demonstrating the IVC filter with partial occlusion by thrombus.

with clot (Fig. 62-3). Therefore, the filter is left in place and the patient is fully heparinized with subcutaneous LMWH twice a day until a therapeutic international normalized ratio is achieved with oral anticoagulation. The temporary filter now remains in place as a permanent device. Because this patient is young and should recover from his traumatic injuries, lifelong follow-up with abdominal ultrasound and examination should be done.

Suggested Readings

Cahn MD, Rohrer MJ, Martella MB, Cutler BS. Long-term follow-up of Greenfield inferior vena cava filter placement in children. *J Vasc Surg*. November 2001;34:820-825.

Decousas H, Leizorovics A, Parent F, et al. A clinical trial of vena caval filters in the prevention of pulmonary embolism in patients with proximal deep-vein thrombosis. *N Engl J Med*. 1998;338:409-415.

Magnant JG, Walsh DB, Juravsky LI, Cronenwett JL. Current use of inferior vena cava filters. *Vasc Surg*. November 1992;16:701-706.

Rousseau H, Perreault P, Otal P, et al. The 6-F nitinol TrapEase inferior vena cava filter: results of a prospective multicenter trial. *J Vasc Interv Radiol*. March 2001;12:299-304.

Schutzer R, Ascher E, Hingorani A, Jacob T, Kallakuri S. Preliminary results of the new 6F TrapEase inferior vena caval filter. *Ann Vasc Surg*. 2003;1:103-106.

Spain DA, Richardson JD, Polk HC Jr, Bergamini TM, Wilson MA, Miller FB. Venous thromboembolism in the high-risk trauma patient: do risks justify aggressive screening and prophylaxis? *J Trauma*. March 1997;42: 463-467; discussion 467-469.

Yazu T, Fujioka H, Nakamura M, et al. Long-term results of inferior vena cava filters: experiences in a Japanese population. *Intern Med*. September 2000;39:707-714.

Joseph D. Raffetto, MD, FACS

Presentation

A 21-year-old man is involved in an altercation resulting in a single gunshot wound to the abdomen. He is conscious at the scene, and is brought in by the emergency medical service. En route, he becomes lethargic with increasing abdominal distension, and is rapidly intubated by the paramedics. On arrival in the emergency department, the patient's heart rate is 140 beats per minute, blood pressure is 80 systolic and 40 diastolic, and he is ventilated at a rate of 30 breaths per minute. The patient was resuscitated with 2 L of normal saline and started on O-negative blood through two large bore intravenous (IV) lines. Rapid assessment revealed clear breath sounds bilaterally, normal heart sounds, a firm distended abdomen with a single entrance wound in the right upper quadrant, and no other injuries noted.

Differential Diagnosis

A patient presenting with an acute penetrating injury to the abdomen must be suspected of having an injury to a solid organ (liver, spleen), hollow viscera (small bowel, colon, bile duct), or major vascular structure (vena cava, aorta, mesenteric vessels). Abdominal distension in the presence of a penetrating injury is concerning for intraabdominal hemorrhage. Patients presenting in shock with or without abdominal distension following penetrating trauma, as well as blunt trauma, should be suspected of having a significant vascular injury and warrant prompt surgical treatment. In this case, the patient has a single gunshot wound to the abdomen and presents with shock and abdominal distension, making the likelihood of a vascular injury very high. However, patients with penetrating and blunt injuries to the abdomen can also have other reasons for shock, including cardiac tamponade; pneumothorax; hemothorax; transected thoracic aorta; tracheal disruption; and massive pulmonary (air) embolism. Although less likely in the differential for the case presented, patients may present with major abdominal vascular trauma and concomitant chest trauma, especially in penetrating wounds that cross the chest, mediastinum, and abdomen from multiple projectiles (bullets, knives).

Diagnostic Tests and Results

Rapid resuscitation and recognition of imminent life-threatening injuries from penetrating injuries is paramount in patients presenting in shock. Therefore, patients in extremis are immediately assessed and brought to the operating room for surgical exploration, avoiding unnecessary tests and delays that may jeopardize survival. Occasionally, patients who lose their vital signs at arrival require an immediate thoracotomy in the resuscitation room to reestablish cardiocirculatory integrity prior to definitive surgical repair. However, the outcomes for these patients are usually dismal.

In patients who sustain penetrating or blunt injuries who are hemodynamically stable, but potentially have intraabdominal injuries, several diagnostic tests are useful. In patients with penetrating trauma who are completely asymptomatic, diagnostic laparoscopy is very useful before performing a full laparotomy to visualize directly the intraperitoneal organs. The potential pitfall of laparoscopy is the difficulty in assessing the retroperitoneal structures, and a missed injury, depth of organ injury, and lower sensitivity for hollow viscus injury. Computed tomography (CT) with intravenous contrast is useful in demonstrating large vascular structures, solid organs, and intraperitoneal/retroperitoneal fluid. CT angiography is very useful in evaluating arterial injuries of the trunk, neck, and extremities, usually avoids delays in mobilizing the angiography team, and is less invasive. Diagnostic peritoneal lavage (DPL), which requires placement of an intraperitoneal catheter under local anesthesia, is useful in rapidly assessing patients with blunt abdominal trauma for gross bleeding (10 mL of blood aspirated) and for occult injuries by evaluating the effluent after instilling 1 L of normal saline in the abdominal cavity and determining the presence of greater than 500 WBC, 100,000 RBC, elevated amylase or bilirubin, and particulate enteric matter (food fibers, stool). Although DPL is rapidly performed, it is limited by the lack of specificity to which organ is injured; moreover, the ability of DPL to detect very small amounts of blood in the peritoneal cavity makes it difficult to ascertain significant injuries (mesenteric tear) versus insignificant injuries (abdominal wall peritoneal tear). With rapid CT (spiral, helical) scanners, the initial evaluation of abdominal trauma is now commonly by CT, essentially replacing DPL. Ultrasonography is a rapid noninvasive test to determine the presence of fluid (blood in penetrating or blunt trauma) in the abdominal cavity with sensitivities of 80% to 95%. The major drawback is a low specificity and this method's dependence on the operator/interpreter. The test of choice for vascular injuries is angiography. Angiography has exceptional sensitivity and specificity (greater than 95%), and although an invasive diagnostic tool, it has the advantage of providing therapeutic options by endovascular techniques in the treatment of pelvic arterial trauma, arteriovenous fistulas, and pseudoaneurysms.

Diagnosis and Recommendation

In the case presented, the type of injury (penetrating), clinical presentation, and hemodynamic compromise are strongly suggestive for a diagnosis of acute intraabdominal vascular injury. The patient needs emergent operative intervention without any further tests.

Approach

In evaluating abdominal vascular injuries, it is important to subdivide the major vascular structures into vascular regions by the location of the hematoma or hemorrhage. The patient's abdomen, chest, and thighs are prepped and draped. Principles of vascular injuries require proximal and distal control, debridement of devitalized tissue, and coverage of suture lines and grafts with viable tissue, peritoneum, retroperitoneum, or omentum. Vascular injuries can be repaired primarily by end-to-end reanastomosis, by interposition grafting (vein, Dacron, or polytetrafluoroethylene), or by patch angioplasty.

Supramesocolic

A midline supramesocolic vascular injury is best approached laterally unless the site of hemorrhage can be easily visualized in the lesser sac. If hemorrhage is rapid, an aortic compression device or manual hand compression may be used to occlude the aorta at the diaphragmatic hiatus prior to clamping. If the supramesocolic injury is close to the abdominal aortic hiatus, the left chest is made available for possible thoracic aortic clamping through a left anterolateral thoracotomy. Injuries to the supramesocolic area include suprarenal aorta, celiac axis, proximal superior mesenteric artery, or renal artery. The left colon, left kidney, spleen, tail of the pancreas, and gastric fundus are mobilized past the midline by a combination of sharp and blunt dissection. Once the aorta is exposed, an aortic clamp is used to occlude it. Dissection then proceeds distally so that the actual bleeding site in the aorta or one of the visceral branches is exposed and distal vascular control obtained.

Inframesocolic

The inframesocolic injury is best approached directly in the midline just below the mesocolon, just as one would approach an infrarenal abdominal aortic aneurysm transperitoneally. Injuries to the inframesocolic region are associated with the infrarenal aorta or inferior vena cava or inferior mesenteric artery.

Inferior Vena Cava and Branches

The infrahepatic inferior vena cava and both renal veins may be exposed by mobilizing the right colon and hepatic flexure past the midline and performing a Kocher maneuver. The retrohepatic vena cava is exposed by dividing the triangular and anterior and posterior coronary ligaments of the hepatic lobe and mobilizing this lobe to the midline. Vascular control of the infrarenal vena cava can usually be obtained by applying sponge sticks or vascular clamps both proximally and distally around the perforations. With injuries at the level of the renal veins, both renal veins should be controlled with vessel loops, and the vena cava should be controlled at the infrarenal level and suprarenal infrahepatic level as it passes beneath the liver.

Retrohepatic Vena Cava

The rare injuries to the retrohepatic vena cava can be approached in several ways. Adequate liver mobilization is required for proper visualization and vessel control. The coronary ligaments and triangular ligaments are incised, being careful with the medial coronary ligament due to the proximity of the hepatic veins. In the hemodynamically stable patient, simultaneous cross clamping of the portal triad, suprahepatic (intraabdominal) vena cava, and suprarenal vena cava (below the liver) may occasionally slow bleeding enough to allow for the placement of sutures. If this maneuver fails, or if the patient is unstable, a sternotomy incision is added to the celiotomy incision and an atriocaval shunt is placed. Umbilical tape tourniquets around the vena cava are pulled tight on the shunt, thus excluding the area of injury and allowing direct repair.

Pararenal

Injuries to the lateral pararenal region include the renal artery, renal vein, or kidney. Vascular control is obtained at the midline as in the exposure for inframesocolic injuries. Control of the right renal vein requires mobilization of the C-loop of duodenum and exposure of the vena cava at the junction with the renal veins.

Lateral Pelvic

Injuries to the iliac arteries and veins present with lateral pelvic hemorrhage or hematomas. Proximal vascular control is obtained by exposing the infrarenal abdominal aorta and vena cava (inframesocolic exposure) in the midline. Distal control is obtained by dividing the peritoneum over the external iliac vessels proximal to the inguinal ligament as the vessels exit the pelvis. Full exposure of the right iliac vessels usually necessitates mobilization of the cecum and right colon. On the left, the sigmoid colon must be mobilized for complete exposure. The confluence of the common iliac veins is difficult to expose and may necessitate temporary transection of the right common iliac artery with mobilization to the left of midline, and following repair of the venous injury, a primary end-to-end reanastomosis of the artery.

Portal

Injury to the portal triad may involve the portal vein, hepatic artery, and bile duct. Control is obtained at the hepatoduodenal ligament by looping the structures posterior and anterior on the ligament (Pringle maneuver). Finger control of the bleeding is performed, and the vascular structures are dissected carefully to avoid inadvertent injury to the bile duct. Distal vessel control is then obtained on the hepatic artery and portal vein.

Case Continued and Surgical Approach

The patient was taken emergently to the operating room where a celiotomy was performed. On exploration, 2 L of blood were identified. Exploration of the abdomen demonstrated a right colonic perforation, a left lobe liver injury, small bowel perforation, and a large central retroperitoneal hematoma with ongoing venous and arterial bleeding. The patient became hypotensive and the diaphragmatic hiatus was rapidly identified, the left lobe of the liver attachments (coronary and triangular ligaments) divided, and the crus fibers divided with exposure of the supraceliac aorta for clamping and control. Sponge stick control on the vena cava was utilized for tamponade. A right-to-left medial visceral rotation (right colon and duodenum) was performed, exposing the infrarenal vena cava and aorta. The transverse mesocolon and small bowel was eviscerated. The patient's blood pressure had stabilized and the aortic clamp was placed infrarenal and above the bifurcation. The inferior vena cava demonstrated a 2-cm tangential anterior medial tear that extended into the adjacent aorta with a 1-cm tear. The vein was repaired by lateral venorrhaphy using 5-0 polypropylene sutures. The aortic wall was inspected and débrided, leaving a defect approximately 2 cm long. The aorta was repaired by placing an interposition polytetrafluoroethylene tube graft and was anastomosed end to end. Following repair of the vascular injuries, the colonic perforation and the small bowel perforations underwent resection with plans for delayed reanastomosis. The liver injury required debridement and ligation of intrahepatic vessels and omental packing. The abdomen was irrigated and a tongue of omentum placed over the aortic repair, and the retroperitoneum closed. The patient remained stable over the next 24 hours, and was brought back for a second-look operation. There was no further hemorrhage and the bowel was viable. The small bowel and colon were reattached in continuity and the abdominal fascia was closed, leaving the skin and subcutaneous fat open. The patient did well. He resumed oral nutrition 8 days following the injury, and on examination, had a normal lower extremity pulse. He was discharged to a rehabilitation facility 26 days later.

Discussion

In civilian trauma, major intraabdominal vascular injuries from blunt trauma occur in 5% to 10% of cases, and penetrating stab wounds in 10.3% of cases; gunshot wounds have the highest incidence at nearly 25% of reported cases. Abdominal gunshot wounds are responsible for 70% to 78% of abdominal vascular injuries. All intraabdominal hematomas, including supramesocolic, inframeso-colic, perirenal, pelvic, portal, and mesenteric, are opened in penetrating trauma. The aorta, inferior vena cava, and external iliac artery and vein are most commonly injured. Overall mortality rate is 45%, but injuries to the abdominal aorta, hepatic veins, retrohepatic inferior vena cava, and portal vein increases the mortality rate between 70% and 90%. Data from the American College of Surgeons National Trauma Data Bank Report of 2002 demonstrates a change in pattern of trauma in the United States (www.facs.org/trauma.ntdb). Penetrating injuries occur predominantly in males, with a peak frequency in the ages between 18 and 21 years and a second peak at ages 36 and 37years, and 11% of the injuries are due to violence from gunshots, shotguns, stabs, and fights. Blunt injuries are caused by accidents involving deceleration of motor vehicles, falls, altercations with direct blows, and contact sports. It is noteworthy that patients presenting with abdominal vascular injuries commonly have concomitant injuries to solid organs and hollow viscus, ranging from 40% to as high as 75%, as seen in pancreatic or duodenal injuries, due to the proximity of the vena cava and aorta.

Basic principles of trauma with priority to the airway, breathing, and circulation are mandatory. Patients with abdominal trauma are resuscitated, and determination of hemodynamic stability is performed rapidly. Examination is performed to identify associated injuries to the head, neck, chest, back, and extremities. Unstable patients with penetrating abdominal trauma, or patients with blunt trauma with a positive ultrasound (presence of blood) or DPL, require emergent surgical exploration. Hemodynamically stable patients with either penetrating or blunt abdominal trauma should undergo further diagnostic testing to define possible vascular or solid organ injuries.

Stab wounds or small-caliber gunshot wounds of the abdominal aorta can be repaired directly. If excessive narrowing is present, a patch aortoplasty utilizing prosthetic graft is used to maintain luminal diameter and blood flow. When the aorta suffers extensive destruction, as can occur in seatbelt-associated blunt abdominal aortic trauma, an appropriately sized prosthetic interposition graft is inserted. Extensive experience with aortic prosthesis in the face of enteric or fecal contamination from penetrating wounds has clearly demonstrated efficacy and safety. However, it is important to note that suture lines and graft should be covered by peritoneum or omentum. Mortality from aortic injury approaches 60%.

Iliac artery injuries should be repaired because ligation carries amputation rates in excess of 50%. The iliac artery can be repaired primarily or using a saphenous vein or prosthetic graft. When extensive fecal contamination is present, repair of the iliac artery is dangerous due to a high rate of pelvic sepsis and possible anastomotic disruption. In this circumstance, the iliac artery is ligated and a femoral-to-femoral bypass with prosthetic graft is performed to reestablish blood flow. Iliac vein injury should be repaired, if possible, by lateral venorrhaphy. However, if the vein has extensive destruction, it should be ligated. The patient's legs should be wrapped with elastic bandages and elevated. Survival from iliac vessel injuries varies with associated injuries, and ranges from 60% to 80% for iliac artery, and 70% to 90% for iliac vein.

Injuries to the celiac artery can be managed by repair or ligation. Unless a small injury is present at the origin of the celiac axis, this vessel is ligated because there is essentially no morbidity in young trauma patients due to a generous collateral circulation via the superior mesenteric artery. Injury to the common hepatic artery is rare, and can often be ligated due to the collateral flow from the gastroduodenal artery. Portal vein injuries are difficult to manage because of their posterior location and retropancreatic portion, as well as significant associated injuries to the pancreas, vena cava, duodenum, liver, and kidney. Attempts at repair should be made, because ligation could lead to compromised midgut, and if associated with hepatic artery ligation could cause liver ischemia and necrosis. The mortality of portal vein injury is 40% to 60% due to associated injuries.

Extensive injury requiring ligation of the superior mesenteric artery at its origin or distal to the midcolic artery or inferior pancreaticoduodenal artery can lead to ischemia of the entire midgut. Due to the vicinity of the pancreas and commonly associated pancreatic and duodenal injuries, and the potential for pancreatic leaks near the arterial repair, such wounds present a challenge for revascularization. Retrograde bypass grafting with saphenous vein or prosthetic from the distal infrarenal abdominal aorta to the superior mesenteric artery is usually necessary to avoid anastomotic dehiscence and ischemic intestine.

When life-threatening hemorrhage necessitates ligation of a renal artery, a nephrectomy should be performed. On rare occasions in stable patients with penetrating renal artery injury, bypass grafting from the infrarenal abdominal aorta to the distal renal artery may be justified. When renal artery thrombosis secondary to an intimal contusion from blunt trauma is recognized soon after it occurs, resection of the renal artery with an end-to-end anastomosis is preferred. As soon as the abdomen is entered, the affected kidney is packed in ice and flushed with cold Collins solution. If the warm ischemia time is longer than 6 hours, nephrectomy is recommended. A recent multicenter study determined that blunt renal injuries had a worse renal salvage than penetrating trauma, and that renal injuries requiring arterial reconstruction versus only renal vein injury also had a poor prognosis. The study concluded that immediate nephrectomy of the injured kidney should be performed in patients with blunt renal vascular injuries, who also sustained significant parenchymal disruption, in the presence of a functioning contralateral kidney.

Vena cava injuries, especially in the retrohepatic region, can present a formidable challenge to repair, and are usually associated with high mortality. Patients requiring an atriocaval shunt for a retrohepatic caval injury have mortality rates between 50% and 90%. The vena cava is repaired, preferably in a transverse fashion, using a running suture of 4-0 or 5-0 polypropylene. Primary venorrhaphy has been demonstrated to be effective, especially for anterior cava perforations, and have low thrombosis and embolic complication rates. Extensive infrarenal injuries to the vena cava can be ligated. The patient's lower extremities are wrapped with elastic bandages, or placed in compression stockings, and the extremities are elevated for the first 1 to 2 weeks after operation. Extensive suprarenal vena cava injuries below the liver should be treated by patch venoplasty or the insertion of an externally supported polytetrafluoroethylene conduit of appropriate size. The right renal vein and left renal vein near the left kidney are repaired by lateral venorrhaphy, and the left renal vein at the midline may be ligated. Overall survival from inferior vena cava injury is between 48% and 65%. Survival is based on severity of patient presentation, anatomic location of the vena cava injury, and associated aortic injury.

Suggested Readings

Accola KD, Feliciano DV, Mattox KL, et al. Management of injuries to the suprarenal aorta. *Am J Surg.* 1987;154:613-618.

Davis TP, Feliciano DV, Rozycki GS, et al. Results with abdominal vascular trauma in the modern era. *Am Surg.* 2001;67:565-571.

Jackson MR, Olson DW, Beckett WC, Olsen SB, Robertson FM. Abdominal vascular trauma: a review of 106 injuries. *Am Surg.* 1992; 58:622-626.

Knudson MM, Harrison PB, Hoyt DB, et al. Outcome after major renovascular injuries: a Western trauma association multicenter report. *J Trauma.* 2000;49:1116-1122.

Kuehne J, Frankhouse J, Modrall G, et al. Determinants of survival after inferior vena cava trauma. *Am Surg.* 1999;65:976-981.

Tyburski JG, Wilson RF, Dente C, Steffes C, Carlin AM. Factors affecting mortality rates in patients with abdominal vascular injuries. *J Trauma.* 2001;50:1020-1026.

Wendy L. Wahl, MD

Presentation

A 40-year-old woman is transferred to you from an outside hospital emergency department after a motorcycle crash in which she was thrown from the vehicle. She arrives 5 hours after the time of the initial injury. The outside hospital sent all studies performed, including computed tomography (CT) scans of the head, chest, and abdomen, and plain radiographs of the extremities. She was transferred for care of her mangled left upper extremity. Her identified injuries are her left upper extremity fractures, rib fractures, and an associated pulmonary contusion. She arrives hemodynamically stable and intubated. Her left upper extremity examination reveals bony deformity of the distal humerus and proximal forearm, with no pulses by palpation or Doppler signal at the antecubital fossa or wrist. There are open traumatic amputations of the left fourth and fifth fingers. She has a pulse by Doppler in the proximal upper arm above the site of her fracture. There are skin lacerations over the mid forearm and mid upper arm with no associated pulsatile bleeding.

■ Left Upper Extremity X-Ray

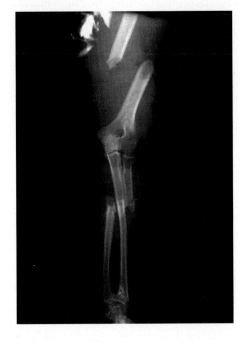

Figure 64-1

X-Ray Report

Displaced fracture of the left distal humerus with displaced proximal ulna and radius fractures (Fig. 64-1).

Her left hand is mottled with firmness of the forearm. Her motor examination is limited by pain, but she appears to have gross motor function in the remaining fingers and can flex and extend at the wrist.

Approach

The patient has documented evidence of a blunt vascular injury to her upper extremity, either secondary to contusion from a direct crush mechanism or from laceration and/or intimal injury from the bony injury or shear. An arteriogram will help in determining the level and extent of injury. If the patient presented immediately after injury, an arteriogram done in Radiology may be appropriate. Because she has had no pulsatile blood flow to her hand and forearm for almost 6 hours, the risk of irreversible ischemia is increased. The most expeditious evaluation for this patient would be an on-table arteriogram done in the operating room prior to vascular repair. The patient's clinical examination is also worrisome for compartment syndrome, which can also be addressed in an expedited manner in the operating room.

Recommendation

On-table arteriogram of the upper extremity in the operating room with exploration of the brachial and axillary arteries. Ideally, the orthopedic injuries should be stabilized to prevent further movement and injury of the vessels. However, in this patient, stabilizing the orthopedic injuries would increase the duration of ischemia and potentially lead to irreversible injury. Vascular repair prior to fracture stabilization is recommended in this instance.

Case Continued

At the time of arterial exploration, a crush injury to the distal brachial artery is identified. Above the level of the injury, a 23-gauge butterfly needle is placed in the brachial artery, and an arteriogram is performed.

Arteriogram

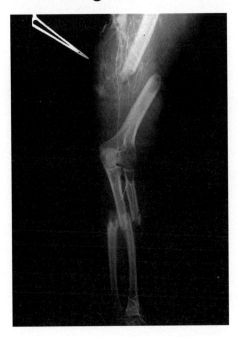

Figure 64-2

Arteriogram Report

A small brachial artery with single-vessel runoff to the hand via a diminutive radial artery is visualized (Fig. 64-2).

Recommendation

There is no filling of the ulnar artery, with poor filling of the radial artery. A thrombectomy to remove thrombus in the vessels should be performed. Further inspection of the affected area should also be done to evaluate for a contused segment.

Surgical Approach

The brachial artery should be exposed over the area of injury. In this case, there is an area of contusion of the brachial artery measuring 4 to 5 cm in length. An arteriotomy is made with a No. 11 blade. A No. 3 Fogarty embolectomy catheter is passed proximally with restoration of pulsatile flow. The catheter is passed distally with removal of thrombus from the radial and ulna arteries, but flow is still suboptimal with poor Doppler waveforms at the wrist.

Diagnosis and Recommendation

The brachial vessel may have extensive intimal injury at the level of contusion, or there may be more distal thrombus present. There is also the possibility of arterial spasm, Injection of intra-arterial papaverine may improve this. In this patient, it is more likely that the poor arterial flow is from the long segment of vascular injury, and this area should be resected. The decision to perform a primary vascular anastomosis or to use vein conduit depends on the length of the defect and the ability to create an anastomosis that will not be under tension. In this case, at least 5 cm of artery is damaged, and replacement with saphenous vein is recommended.

Surgical Approach

A bypass with reversed saphenous vein is created between the debrided ends of the brachial artery. Restoration of brachial artery flow is continued with much improved Doppler signals at the wrist. Next, the fractures are stabilized under direct vision, with no obvious kinking or redundancy of the arterial graft.

Case Continued

The forearm is noticeably tense after restoration of arterial inflow. The patient is more than 6 hours from the time of her initial injury.

Diagnosis and Recommendation

Compartment syndrome of the forearm is likely and can be readily measured using a needle connected to a pressure transducer. (Please see Case 71 for further details.) The three compartments of the forearm include the dorsal and volar compartments and the mobile wad. The dorsal compartment contains the extensors of the fingers and wrist. The volar compartment contains the flexors and pronators of the forearm and wrist, as well as the median and ulnar nerves and the radial and ulnar arteries. The mobile wad does not need to be separately decompressed because of its close association to the dorsal compartment.

Surgical Approach

The dorsal compartment of the forearm should be released via a straight incision. The volar compartment should be opened through a "lazy-S"-shaped incision to avoid later skin contracture.

Case Continued

The dorsal and volar compartments are opened with extensive bulging of the muscle. All muscles appear viable, with bleeding when cut and contraction when stimulated. Orthopedic fixation is completed. The patient is returned to the ICU with dressings to her open fasciotomy sites. She returns to the operating room 5 days later for closure of her fasciotomy sites.

Discussion

The most common cause of compartment syndrome in the forearm is elbow dislocation, but coexistent arterial injury is not uncommon. Factors that predispose to arterial injury in the forearm are open elbow dislocations, absence of a radial pulse before reduction of the elbow, and other systemic injuries at the time of elbow dislocation. The timing of repair of the vascular injury can be debated, but in general, if there is prolonged ischemia, the vascular repair should precede orthopedic stabilization. A temporary carotid shunt can be used to bypass the injured segment and provide arterial flow during the orthopedic repair. A member of the vascular team should be present to ensure that the vascular repair is not jeopardized during the above reduction and that the bypass lies properly in the wound after reduction.

Suggested Readings

Endean ED, Veldenx HC, Schwarcz TH, Hyde GL. Recognition of arterial injury in elbow dislocation. *J Vasc Surg.* 1992;16:402-406.

Flynn LM, Kazmers A. Blunt arterial injuries of the shoulder and elbow. In: Ernst CB, Stanley JC, eds. *Current Therapy in Vascular Surgery.* 4th ed. St. Louis: Mosby, 2001: 598-602.

Velhamos GC, Toutousaz KG. Vascular trauma and compartment syndromes. *Surg Clin North Am.* 2002;82:125-141.

Timothy A. Schaub, MD, and Gilbert R. Upchurch, Jr., MD

Presentation

A 24-year-old, unrestrained, male driver with no significant past medical or surgical history presents to the emergency department via ambulance 30 minutes after a head-on car-versus-tree collision. An airbag was deployed. He complains of severe pain in his left lower extremity. After a complete primary and secondary survey, he is alert and oriented, has several minor facial lacerations, and a notable deformity of the left knee. There is no exposed bone or active external bleeding from the left lower extremity. Peripheral pulses on the right lower extremity are all palpable. The left lower extremity has a palpable femoral pulse; however, weak popliteal, dorsalis pedis, and posterior tibial Doppler signals are found. The left foot and toes are cool to touch. Motor function appears to be intact in the legs bilaterally, with decreased sensation on the left. Ankle/brachial index (ABI) of the right lower extremity is 1.0; the left lower extremity is 0.3. Diagnosis of dislocation of the left knee based on clinical data and presentation made. The left knee is reduced in the emergency department. The ABIs remain unchanged after reduction.

Differential Diagnosis

Diminished pulses in the left foot in this setting could be due to direct compression of the popliteal artery, damage to the artery, or arterial spasm. In this patient, given the high likelihood of a dislocated knee joint and decreased pulses, any one, or a combination of the above three etiologies, is possible. The knee was reduced in the emergency department in hopes of returning normal vascular supply, but was not successful. The reduction removes direct compression from the differential.

Discussion

Posterior knee dislocation, defined as loss of the tibiofemoral articulation, is an uncommon but potentially devastating injury. It usually occurs during motor vehicle accidents, industrial accidents, or following sports injuries. Because the popliteal artery is relatively fixed in position in the popliteal fossa, a large force is required to cause dislocation and can result in avulsion, shearing, intimal injury, or traction on the popliteal artery. While the knee is dislocated, mechanical compression of the artery may also diminish or obliterate the pulses distally. This lack of inflow can lead to thrombosis of the vessels forming the tibial trifurcation (anterior tibial, posterior tibial, and peroneal arteries).

Failure to identify a popliteal injury after a blunt trauma can result in major morbidity and lower extremity amputation. The incidence of injury to the popliteal artery for "low-velocity" injuries is approximately 5% and is as high as 45% for "high-velocity" trauma. Importantly, in patients with a significant popliteal injury, as many as 10% have been reported to have palpable pulses. Sixty percent of vascular injuries involving an extremity have a concomitant peripheral nerve injury. The six indices of acute loss of arterial flow (pulselessness, pain, paralysis, pallor, paresthesias, and poikilothermia) are critical signs in this type of trauma. A full neurovascular assessment of the extremity, including ABIs, should be performed, when feasible.

Recommendation

Following sedation and reduction of the knee, repeat ABIs if pulses are present (as performed above). Perform angiography and heparinization if ABIs are less than 0.9 or if pulses remain diminished, and if there are no contraindications secondary to other traumatic injuries. If no pulses are present after reduction, heparinize and take emergently to operating room. If ABIs are normal after reduction, observe pulses closely; perform knee repair by orthopedic surgery.

Discussion

Traditionally, arteriography was used in any patient with a suspected injury to the popliteal artery regardless of physical examination findings. The only exception was if no pulses could be found, at which point the patient would be taken directly to the operating room. Recently, selective arteriography has been proposed as an alternative to mandatory arteriography based on several limited series due to the expense, time commitment, pain, and associated risks of arteriography. Patients with a normal neurovascular examination who have a blunt knee dislocation can be closely observed, with studies showing a 100% negative predictive value for prediction of a popliteal artery injury after knee dislocation. Another study recommended differentiating patients by presence of "abnormal pulses" based on a meta-analysis of seven articles. Individuals may construe "abnormal" differently, and determining "abnormal" requires a great deal of experience. It is important to note that as many as 10% of patients with a significant popliteal injury have been reported to have palpable pulses.

Based on the available data, if the ABI is less than 0.9, arteriographic evaluation is indicated. If the ABI is greater than 0.9, the patient should be closely observed and the knee repaired as necessary. If no pulse is present, administer heparin and take the patient directly to the operating room for on-table arteriography and revascularization.

Case Continued

The patient undergoes angiography of the left lower extremity. An arteriogram is performed using a transfemoral approach. During angiography, pain in the left lower extremity increases significantly, and the patient now has decreased plantarflexion and dorsiflexion (paralysis). The foot appears pale, and is cool to the touch (poikilothermic).

◼ Angiogram

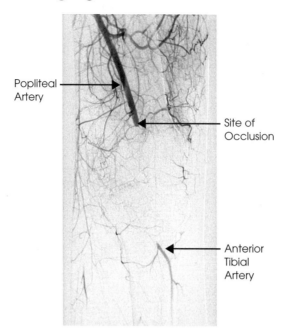

Popliteal
Artery

Site of
Occlusion

Anterior
Tibial
Artery

Figure 65-1

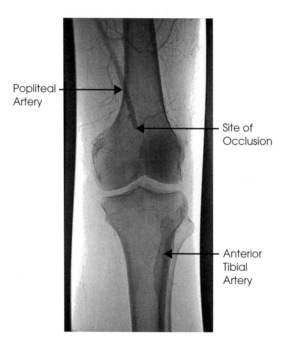

Popliteal
Artery

Site of
Occlusion

Anterior
Tibial
Artery

Figure 65-2

Angiogram Report

Traumatic occlusion of the left popliteal artery with reconstitution separately of anterior and posterior tibial arteries near their respective origins.

Diagnosis and Recommendation

An arterial injury of the left popliteal artery with occlusion of the popliteal artery and reconstitution of branches distal to occlusion via collaterals is present. Vascular repair of the popliteal artery should be performed by means of an above-knee popliteal artery to below-knee popliteal artery bypass, using the contralateral reversed autologous saphenous vein. If further complicated by compartment syndrome, four-compartment calf fasciotomy of the left lower extremity can be performed. It is recommended that the consent for operation include the small, but significant, chance that amputation may need to be performed, above or below the knee, with the associated risks during this operation, if revascularization is not feasible.

Surgical Approach

Both the right and left legs should be prepped and draped. Greater saphenous vein is harvested from the leg contralateral to the injury. Using a medial approach, an incision is made above and below the left knee, with the incision above the knee extending well up into the medial thigh. The distal incision should be able to connect with a medial incision of a fasciotomy, if necessary. The distal incision may be necessary for removal of clot from the popliteal trifurcation. Careful thrombectomy of the distal arteries may be beneficial to remove fresh clot and promote arterial patency.

The popliteal artery is identified at its origin as the superficial femoral artery passes through the adductor hiatus above the knee. The artery is again identified below the knee as it passes deep to the medial head of the gastrocnemius muscle. The proximal anastomosis to the above-knee popliteal artery is performed. The vein is placed anatomically between the incision sites. It is important to remember to completely extend the leg prior to performing the distal anastomosis to ensure that the vein will not be under tension or kink. The distal anastomosis is then performed to the below-knee popliteal artery. A postoperative angiogram or ultrasound scan is performed to ensure adequate revascularization and repair. Distal pulses are assessed and marked.

Case Continued

The greater saphenous vein from the right leg is harvested and the proximal end marked. Next, a four-compartment fasciotomy is performed on the distal left lower extremity. The muscle appears healthy and contracts with touch of Bovie. Using a medial approach with the patient in supine position, exploration of the popliteal artery above and below the popliteal fossa is performed. The area of damage is found just above the popliteal fossa as noted on the arteriogram. The popliteal vein is undamaged and patent. An arteriotomy of the popliteal artery is performed, and an intimal tear is noted in the lumen. A Fogarty catheter is passed distally and fresh clot is removed. An above-knee popliteal artery to below-knee popliteal artery bypass is performed with end-to-side anastomoses using reversed saphenous vein. Signals are found in both the posterior tibial and anterior tibial arteries following bypass. An on-table arteriogram is performed, and a patent proximal and distal anastomosis site as well as posterior and anterior tibial arteries are noted. The peroneal artery was not well visualized. The patient is extubated and sent to the recovery room in stable condition. Postoperatively, the patient has palpable dorsalis pedis and posterior tibial pulses bilaterally.

Discussion

Autologous saphenous vein, usually the greater saphenous, is preferred over polytetrafluoroethylene (PTFE) grafts in infrageniculate bypasses, because long-term patency in vein grafts is superior to PTFE. However, no studies have been performed to compare PTFE and vein grafts in patients undergoing bypass grafts solely for revascularization after trauma.

Advances in the treatment of traumatic arterial injuries, as seen in this patient, have decreased the rate of required amputations. One of the first published studies on popliteal artery injuries was from World War II, when ligation was the standard of care for popliteal artery injury. The associated amputation rate was 73%. During the Korean War, the reported rate dropped to 32% with popliteal repair, with similar results during the Vietnam Conflict. Today, the rate is quoted as less than 15%. It is important to note the amputation rate rises to 85% when operation is delayed more than 8 hours following injury.

Up to 50% of knee dislocations that occur in the field are reduced either spontaneously or by emergency personnel prior to arrival in the emergency department. This emphasizes the importance of the history and physical examination during resuscitation. When a patient has had bilateral popliteal artery injuries, a posterior approach with some success has been described.

Case Continued

On postoperative day 7, the patient was discharged to home. His wounds were healing well. At 2-week follow-up, he was progressing well with physical therapy. ABIs were 1.0 bilaterally. The graft had no evidence of stenosis on follow-up duplex imaging. On physical examination, he had palpable distal pulses bilaterally and normal dorsiflexion and plantarflexion. The fasciotomy sites were closed the following week.

Suggested Readings

Baker WH, Kahn SS. Arterial injuries. In: *Textbook of Surgery: The Biological Basis of Modern Surgical Practice*. 15th ed. Philadelphia: WB Saunders; 1997:1711-1722.

Barnes CJ, Pietrobon R, Higgins LD. Does the pulse examination in patients with traumatic knee dislocation predict a surgical arterial injury? A meta-analysis. *J Trauma*. 2002;53:1109-1114.

Gable DR, Allen JW, Richardson JD. Blunt popliteal artery injury: is physical examination alone enough for evaluation? *J Trauma*. 1997; 43:541-544.

Miranda FE, Dennis JW, Veldenz HC, et al. Confirmation of the safety and accuracy of physical examination in the evaluation of knee dislocation for injury of the popliteal artery: a prospective study. *J Trauma*. 2002;52:247-252.

Moursi MM. Blunt arterial injuries to the knee. In: Ernst CB, Stanley JC, eds. *Current Therapy in Vascular Surgery*. 4th ed. St. Louis: Mosby; 2001:614-618.

Perron AD, Brady WJ, Sing RF. Orthopedic pitfalls in the ED: vascular injury associated with knee dislocation. *Am J Emerg Med*. 2001;19:583-588.

Veith FJ, Gupta SK, Ascer E, et al. Six-year prospective multicenter randomized comparison of autologous saphenous vein and expanded polytetrafluoroethylene grafts in infrainguinal arterial reconstructions. *J Vasc Surg*. 1986;3:104-114.

Matthew J. Eagleton, MD

Presentation

A 25-year-old man presents to the emergency department with complaints of severe pain in his right lower extremity. The patient's past history is significant for intravenous drug abuse (IVDA). Several hours prior to presentation the patient injected methamphetamine into his right femoral vein. He reports that immediately after injection, he developed severe pain in his right leg and foot. On physical examination, the right foot and calf are mottled and swollen. There are palpable femoral and popliteal pulses. Pedal pulses are absent on the right, but Doppler signals are present. Motor and sensory functions are intact. The remainder of the physical examination is normal.

Differential Diagnosis

The differential diagnosis for lower extremity pain and cyanotic discoloration in this 25-year-old with a history of IVDA includes a variety of pathologies. Injection into the femoral vein may have resulted in venous thrombosis, and he has subsequently developed symptoms consistent with phlegmasia cerulea dolens. The patient may also have inadvertently injected methamphetamine into his femoral artery. The intra-arterial injection could have caused distal embolization and occlusion of the lower extremity vessels, or there may be profound vasospasm due to the drug's effect.

Recommendations

Based on the clinical assessment and subsequent differential diagnosis, the patient is immediately anticoagulated with a bolus of heparin (100 units/kg) and begun on a heparin infusion. A duplex ultrasound (US) is ordered to assess for the presence of deep venous thrombosis (DVT). In addition, a right lower extremity arteriogram is requested. Because it is clear that this patient has a significantly ischemic limb and Doppler signals, it was felt that noninvasive vascular surgery laboratory studies were not indicated.

Ultrasound Report

There is no evidence of acute, subacute, or chronic deep venous thrombosis in the femoral or popliteal veins. The tibial veins could not be adequately visualized due to the swelling in the leg; therefore, a thrombus in these vessels cannot be ruled out.

Arteriogram Report

The common femoral, superficial femoral, and popliteal arteries are patent with no luminal irregularities. There is a patent tibioperoneal trunk and anterior tibial artery proximally. The distal peroneal artery, posterior tibial artery, and anterior tibial artery are diminutive with evidence of vasospasm. There is minimal visualization of vessels in the foot, and the digital arteries are not seen.

Diagnosis

Acute limb ischemia due to vasospasm caused by inadvertent intra-arterial drug injection, but distal embolization of the digital arteries cannot be ruled out.

Discussion

The incidence of intra-arterial injections associated with drug abuse is not known. The most common sites of arterial injection include the brachial artery, the superficial femoral artery, and, less commonly, the carotid artery. Numerous mechanisms have been proposed to explain the onset of ischemia following intra-arterial drug injection. These include embolization of inert particles, endothelial damage and vessel thrombosis, vasospasm, and venous thrombosis. After intra-arterial drug injection, drug and particulate matter pass through the arteriolar and capillary system and into the venous system. Vessel obstruction and endothelial damage can therefore occur at any of these sites. Drug crystals can cause digital artery obstruction, as can other materials mixed with the drug. Vasospasm can occur secondary to drug acidity or alkalinity, vascular trauma, and norepinephrine or epinephrine release. The contribution of vasospasm to the ischemic effects of intra-arterial drug injection is controversial.

Patients generally present with severe, persistent pain after intra-arterial drug injection. The physical examination should assess the extent of ischemia and document the degree of motor and sensory function deficits. The affected extremity is typically swollen, and if the hand is affected the finger and wrist will often be flexed in a "claw-like" position. Distal limb pulses are usually normal, which can help to distinguish this from other disease processes. The degree of ischemia at presentation has been shown to directly correlate with outcomes. Arteriography is not always mandated in the evaluation of intra-arterial drug injection. This procedure itself may aggravate the ischemic injury and promote further vasospasm. However, it is useful in determining the extent of injury and monitoring the response to therapy, and should be used in almost all cases with diminished or absent pulses.

Treatment protocols are designed to minimize stasis, thrombosis, and inflammation. Patients are treated with an initial bolus of heparin, usually 10,000 units followed by a continuous infusion. Some have recommended the addition of low-molecular-weight dextran. Tolazoline, a vasodilator, in doses of 25 to 50 mg injected intra-arterially at the time of angiography, have been used to successfully treat the vasospastic response due to intra-arterial drug injections. Other vasodilators that have been used include verapamil and phentolamine.

The use of steroids, delivered either intra-arterially or systemically, is also advocated by some and has been associated with improved outcomes. Narcotics are administered for pain control. This protocol is generally continued for at least 48 hours, and there is complete resolution of symptoms or no further improvement in function. The use of thrombolytic agents is controversial and has not been shown to significantly improve outcomes. Rarely is revascularization indicated or possible. Fasciotomies may be required in selected cases associated with massive edema and the development of compartment syndrome.

Approach

Anticoagulants are administered to the patient prior to the angiogram, and a heparin infusion is continued. At the time of the angiogram, 25 mg tolazoline is injected in the proximal artery, with angiographic improvement in the vasospasm. The patient is continued on combination therapy of heparin, dexamethasone, and morphine for 48 hours.

Case Continued

Patient has complete resolution of his symptoms.

Discussion

The outcome from inadvertent intra-arterial drug injection can be estimated by evaluating the color, capillary refill, temperature, and sensory function of the affected extremity at the time of presentation. Patients with deficits in one to two of these areas have excellent outcomes, while those with three or more defects are likely to develop neurologic dysfunction and have subsequent tissue loss.

Case Continued

The patient is eventually discharged to home. He returns to the emergency department approximately 1 month later with complaints of a painful, tender mass in his right groin. On physical examination, he is tachycardic and febrile, and has a pulsatile, tender mass in the right groin with overlying skin erythema. The remainder of his physical examination is normal.

Differential Diagnosis

The differential diagnosis of a painful, tender groin mass associated with fever in a person with a history of IVDA is vast. In this scenario, however, the leading diagnoses to be ruled out are mycotic aneurysm or a mycotic pseudoaneurysm.

Discussion

Mycotic aneurysms and pseudoaneurysms are the most common complication following intra-arterial drug injection in the population of IVDA patients. A mycotic aneurysm and pseudoaneurysm are caused by embolic or local infectious process. Often, the aneurysm results from repetitive needle trauma to an artery, with subsequent bacterial contamination. Sites frequently associated with the development of mycotic aneurysms include the most common sites for intra-arterial injection: the femoral and brachial arteries. However, septic emboli can result in more remote aneurysms, including involvement of the visceral vessels. Endocarditis is a common finding. Often, drug addicts will inject repeatedly into aneurysms or pseudoaneurysms due to their easy accessibility.

The majority of intra-arterial drug injections involve vessels of the lower extremity. Pseudoaneurysms are the most common arterial injury observed, followed closely by arteriovenous fistula, which may accompany a pseudoaneurysm. In cases of mycotic pseudoaneurysms, patients often present with a painful, pulsatile mass and overlying cellulitis. Occasionally the mass is not palpable due to the edema caused by the infectious process. Patients may be febrile, and there is a high incidence of bacteremia. The predominant infectious bacteria are *Staphylococcus aureus*. Although embolization can occur, distal pulses are usually intact. Duplex US should be obtained because it can provide a great deal of information about the degree of tissue involvement, vessel (artery or vein) from which the aneurysm arises, and presence of an arteriovenous fistula. Arteriography is not necessary if distal pulses are palpable and the US provides sufficient information, but it should be performed if there is any question about distal vessel patency, or if the aneurysm involves the visceral vessels, carotid artery, or pulmonary vasculature.

Recommendation

A complete blood count, cultures, and ultrasound of the right groin are ordered.

Laboratory Results

The patient is found to have a significant leukocytosis.

Duplex Ultrasound Report

There is a pseudoaneurysm measuring 3.5 × 3.0 cm arising from the common femoral artery. The pseudoaneurysm is patent. There is edema in the surround-

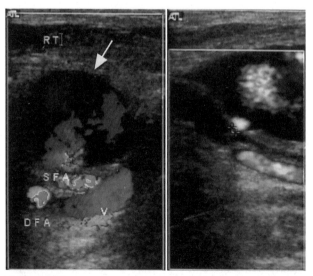

Figure 66-1

ing tissue. The common femoral artery, deep femoral artery, and superficial femoral artery are patent.

Diagnosis

Mycotic pseudoaneurysm of the right common femoral artery.

Recommendations

The presence of a mycotic aneurysm warrants surgical intervention. Prior to surgery, the patient undergoes vein mapping to assess for adequate vein should a bypass be required. Most IVDA patients have no usable superficial vein, because it has been injured from repeated injections. The patient is started on intravenous antibiotics immediately.

Surgical Approach

The patient is brought to the operating room and placed under general anesthesia. The abdomen, both groins, and right lower extremity are prepped into the operative field. An incision is made in the right groin, and circumferential control of the proximal common femoral artery is obtained. Distal control of the deep femoral and superficial femoral artery is obtained. After anticoagulation, the region of the aneurysm is then dissected. The area is grossly infected, and resection of the infected portion of the common femoral artery involved in the pseudoaneurysm is necessary. The common femoral artery is ligated proximally at the level of the inguinal ligament and distally just above its bifurcation. The intervening segment is resected, and infected tissue surrounding the pseudoaneurysm is debrided as well. Samples of tissue are sent to the microbiology laboratory for further evaluation. Closure of the deep tissue with rotation of the proximal sartorius is done to cover the arterial stumps, but the skin is left open and allowed to close secondarily. The patient has monophasic Doppler signals in his feet at the end of the case.

Discussion

Complications from mycotic aneurysms include rupture, thrombosis, and distal embolization. Treatment of mycotic aneurysms and pseudoaneurysms warrants excision of the aneurysm and debridement of all surrounding infected tissue in addition to antibiotic therapy. Any remaining infected tissue can lead to eventual disruption of the ligated artery. The need for subsequent revascularization is controversial. Often these patients have no adequate autologous vein to perform a revascularization procedure, and placement of a prosthetic graft, even if via an extra-anatomic route, places the patient at risk for developing a graft infection. The use of contralateral superficial femoral-popliteal vein has been described if immediate revascularization is necessary and no superficial vein is available. Generally, revascularization is reserved for patients with profound ischemia. If the infected aneurysm involves the common femoral artery and ligation can occur above the level of its bifurcation, fewer than 50% of patients will have severe ischemic symptoms, and less than one-third require early revascularization to prevent amputation. Almost all patients who undergo ligation of the common femoral artery complain of some degree of claudication. Postoperative hemorrhage, graft infections (if a bypass is performed), and amputation are common complications. Amputation rates vary from as low as 10% to as high as 33% in some series. If revascularization can be delayed after infection has cleared, grafts can be placed in a more normal anatomic location.

Suggested Readings

Cooper JC, Griffiths AB, Jones RB, et al. Accidental intra-arterial injection in drug addicts. *Eur J Vasc Surg.* 1992;6:430-433.

Padberg F, Hobson R, Lee B, et al. Femoral pseudoaneurysms from drugs of abuse: ligation or reconstruction? *J Vasc Surg.* 1992; 15:642-648.

Silverman SH, Turner WW. Intraarterial drug abuse: new treatment options. *J Vasc Surg.* 1991;14:111-116.

Treiman GS. Vascular injury secondary to drug abuse. In: Ernst CB, Stanley JC, eds. *Current Therapy in Vascular Surgery.* 4th ed. St. Louis: Mosby; 2001:618-623.

Treiman GS, Yellin AE, Weaver FA, et al. An effective treatment protocol for intraarterial drug injection. *J Vasc Surg.* 1990;12:456-465.

Valentine RJ, Turner WW. Acute vascular insufficiency due to drug injection. In: Rutherford RB, ed. *Vascular Surgery.* 5th ed. Philadelphia: WB Saunders 2000:846-855.

Yeager RA, Hobson RW, Padberg FT, et al. Vascular complications related to drug abuse. *J Trauma.* 1987;27:305-308.

Mark R. Hemmila, MD

Presentation

A 29-year-old man with no significant past medical history presents to the emergency department 1 hour following an altercation. He has two gunshot wounds in his left anterior thigh from a handgun and a small amount of blood is emanating from these wounds. On physical examination, he has an obvious distal left femur deformity with swelling in the region of the wound and associated long-bone instability. Examination of bilateral lower extremities reveals a cool, mottled left lower extremity with numbness and weakness in the foot. The right femoral, popliteal, dorsalis pedis, and posterior tibial pulses are all easily palpable and normal. The left femoral pulse is 2+ and the left popliteal, dorsalis pedis, and posterior tibial pulses are absent on both palpation and Doppler interrogation.

▩ Left Lower Extremity X-Ray

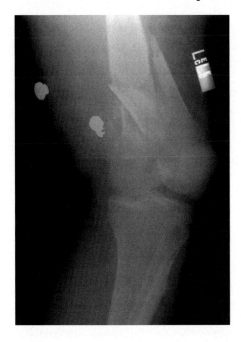

Figure 67-1

X-Ray Report

Severely comminuted supracondylar fracture of distal left femur with possible extension to the articular surface. Soft tissue changes with adjacent foreign bodies consistent with history of gunshot wound.

Differential Diagnosis

Potential injured neurovascular structures in this patient include the superficial femoral artery, popliteal artery, superficial femoral vein, popliteal vein, and sciatic nerve. The neurologic changes can be associated with direct trauma to the peripheral nerves or secondary injury from ischemia.

Case Continued

The patient is taken emergently to the operating room where he undergoes left medial thigh exposure of the popliteal artery, debridement of the damaged arterial tissue, and primary reanastomosis of the popliteal artery. A thromboembolectomy of the popliteal and both tibial arteries is performed. The orthopedic surgeon stabilizes his supracondylar femur fracture by placing a spanning external fixator across the left knee. It is now 7 hours since his injury and 1 hour since his left lower extremity was revascularized.

Diagnosis and Recommendation

This extremity has been ischemic for 6 hours. Arterial circulation has been reestablished, and the patient is currently in the reperfusion period. Concern for compartment syndrome of the left lower leg should be extremely high based on the injury sustained, duration of ischemia, and the preoperative neurologic examination. Three options exist: (1) assume presence of compartment syndrome based on the history of the case and immediately perform four-compartment fasciotomies; (2) measure compartment pressures and proceed with fasciotomy if values greater than 25 to 30 mm Hg are obtained; (3) observe the patient postoperatively for signs and symptoms of compartment syndrome and return to the operating room for fasciotomy if clinically indicated. You choose option 1 as the safest approach for the patient in this case. Option 3 requires an awake, cooperative patient, with the ability to perform hourly neurovascular examinations. To safely pursue option 3, the patient must have no neurologic deficits preoperatively or postoperatively and the ability to return promptly to the operating room should the need for fasciotomy arise.

Discussion: Measurement of Compartment Pressures

Intracompartmental tissue pressure in the extremities can be measured directly using a sterile needle connected to a pressure transducer. A commercial device manufactured by Stryker Instruments (Stryker Corporation, Kalamazoo, MI) is commonly used for this purpose (Fig. 67-2) and uses a needle with a side hole to avoid incorrect readings from tissue occlusion of the needle lumen. To perform a pressure measurement, the skin over the central region of the compartment is swabbed with aseptic solution and anesthetized with local anesthetic. A tiny incision is made in the skin with a No. 11 scalpel blade, and the needle of the pressure transducer is inserted through the opening and advanced until it penetrates the fascia surrounding the compartment to be measured. A small amount (0.5 mL) of saline is injected and the equilibrated pressure measured. It is important to measure all of the individual compartments in the region of interest because the different compartments can have elevated pressures independent of each other. A pressure of less than 10 mm Hg is considered normal. Pressures of

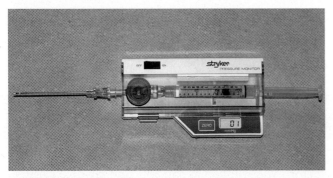

Figure 67-2 Stryker intracompartmental pressure monitor.

10 to 20 mm Hg are considered mildly elevated, but present a low risk for permanent tissue injury. A pressure greater than 30 mm Hg with clinical signs is indicative of compartment syndrome and requires immediate fasciotomy. Pressures between 20 and 30 mm Hg represent a "gray zone" where the concern for compartment syndrome must be entertained, but the choice to perform a fasciotomy is usually correlated with the clinical course and whether or not continued tissue swelling is expected. It must be emphasized that pressure measurements are not a substitute for sound clinical judgment and prudent operative management when compartment syndrome is suspected.

Surgical Approach

Release of pressure in the compartment is performed by longitudinally incising the fascia in one location per compartment in the affected extremity. In general, all compartments of the involved portion of the extremity should undergo fasciotomy. The calf has 4 compartments, the thigh 2, the foot 10, the arm 3, and the forearm 2. Following release of the compartment, the exposed muscle should be assessed clinically for tissue damage and viability. Does it bulge through the fascial incision? Is it beefy red or dusky, purple, gray, black, or brown? Does the muscle contract when stimulated with the electrocautery? All clearly nonviable tissue should be debrided. Equivocal tissue should be reassessed for viability with serial examinations, and the patient returned to the operating room for debridement if marginal tissue progresses to nonviability.

The standard incisions for a 4-compartment lower leg fasciotomy are lateral and medial through the skin of the calf. The lateral incision is placed slightly anterior to the fibula and lateral to the anterior tibial crest. This provides access to the anterior and lateral compartments of the lower leg. Creating a short transverse incision through the leg fascia can aid in locating the intramuscular septum between the two compartments. The superficial peroneal nerve lies posterior to this membrane in the lateral compartment. When longitudinally dividing the fascia of the lateral compartment, care must be taken to avoid dividing or injuring this nerve. The medial incision is created 2 cm posterior to the posterior crest of the tibia, which is midway between the anterior and posterior calf borders. The surgeon should avoid injuring the saphenous nerve and vein. Another transverse incision is made to identify the intramuscular septum between the superficial and deep posterior compartments. Using Metzenbaum scissors, longitudinal fasciotomies are performed to open the two posterior compartments. Generous skin incisions should be made, and usually run at least 15 to 20 cm in length. If any doubt is present about the adequacy of fasciotomy, the incisions in the skin and fascia should be extended until this uncertainty is eliminated.

A four-compartment, two-incision left lower extremity fasciotomy is performed. Extensive bulging of the muscle bellies through the fasciotomy and skin openings occurs. The open skin wound is approximated using staples, elastic vessel loops, and the shoelace technique.

Two days later, the patient is taken to the operating room by orthopedic surgery for removal of his external fixator and open reduction and internal fixation of his left supracondylar femur fracture. The skin incisions of his fasciotomy wounds are closed with a combination of delayed primary closure and split-thickness skin grafting on post-injury day 10.

Discussion

Compartment syndrome develops when tissue expansion in a rigidly confined space generates increased compartmental pressure that exceeds the capillary perfusion pressure of the tissue residing in the closed space. This leads to tissue ischemia, eventual permanent injury, and death to the involved organs. Traditionally, compartment syndrome has been considered a disease of the fascial compartments that enclose muscle and neurovascular structures within the extremities. However, compartment syndrome can occur in other fascial compartments of the body, such as the abdomen. The development of compartment syndrome is usually an unavoidable process associated with trauma or acute vascular occlusion and ischemia. However, permanent damage to the compartmental contents is preventable, and in most circumstances represents a delay in diagnosis or inadequate treatment.

Compartment syndrome should be considered in every patient with an injured extremity or acute vascular compromise. Conditions that are associated with a high incidence of compartment syndrome include fractures, crush injuries, large volume resuscitation, acute arterial compromise, and acute venous occlusion. Less common potential causes of compartment syndrome are a tight dressing or cast, eschar from a circumferential burn, soft tissue swelling from envenomation, and application of military antishock trousers. The initial injury or ischemic event leads to tissue edema and/or hematoma, which result in an increase in the volume of soft tissue within the myofascial compartment. Noncompliance of the fascial envelope leads to a rapid increase in the compartmental pressure, which may exceed the capillary perfusion pressure. This causes further ischemia, added tissue injury, more edema, and increased pressure—a cycle that eventually results in severe and permanent tissue damage.

The five Ps (pain, paresthesias, paralysis, pulselessness, and pallor) are a common mnemonic for signs and symptoms consistent with compartment syndrome. Pain out of proportion to the severity of injury is a sensitive symptom in an awake patient. Stretching of the muscle group involved often exacerbates the pain caused by excessive pressure in the compartment. The appearance of paresthesias can be early and sensory abnormalities are indicators of nerve compression and ischemia. Paralysis is typically a late finding due to prolonged nerve compression or irreversible muscle damage. Pulselessness from compartment syndrome alone is a late event and indicates a delay in diagnosis. Often, pulselessness results from acute occlusion of the artery from emboli, thrombus, or trauma and initiates the tissue ischemia leading to compartment syndrome. Early discovery of pulselessness and paralysis, which are typically late findings in the setting of compartment syndrome, should raise the possibility of neurovascular injury. As pressure builds in the compartment, it causes compression of the capillaries, leading to decreased skin perfusion and localized pallor. Physical examination revealing a tense firm extremity during palpation of the tissue is worrisome and can be easily compared to the contralateral fascial compartment.

Open long-bone fractures with extensive soft tissue injury is an unusual setting in which compartment syndrome can occur. A common pitfall is to assume that the open nature of injury provides complete decompression. This rationale is false and can lead to catastrophic results. Initial treatment should be triggered when suspicion arises for compartment syndrome based on clinical findings. Orthopedic casts or tight dressings are removed; escharotomies are performed in burn patients. If the patient's symptoms do not improve, a decompressive fasciotomy is indicated. In equivocal cases measurement of the compartment pressure as previously described may be helpful. No established benefit has been proven in humans from the administration of pharmacologic agents such as antioxidants or mannitol.

Most of the negative sequelae from compartment syndrome can be avoided by early diagnosis if the clinician has a high index of suspicion and implements appropriate monitoring in patients who are at risk for elevated compartmental pressures as well as correcting the underlying cause (eg, acute limb ischemia). Pain out of proportion to the injury sustained is an important finding in the setting of potential compartment syndrome and should not be ignored. Correlation of the history, physical findings, and pressure measurements will yield the best results when ruling in or out the diagnosis of compartment syndrome. Be wary of overlying dressings, tight casts, and splints in the newly injured patient, and be vigilant in examining these patients for signs and symptoms of compartment syndrome. When performing a fasciotomy and caring for patients with fasciotomies, use sterile technique because infection of the muscle tissue can lead to further tissue loss and morbidity.

Suggested Readings

Bergstein JM. Extremity compartment syndrome. In: Cameron JL, ed. *Current Surgical Therapy*. 7th ed. St. Louis: Mosby; 2001: 1140-1144.

Blaisdell FW. The pathophysiology of skeletal muscle ischemia and the reperfusion syndrome: a review. *Cardiovasc Surg*. 2002;10: 620-630.

Nypaver T. Fasciotomy in vascular trauma and compartment syndrome. In: Ernst CB, Stanley JC, eds. *Current Therapy in Vascular Surgery*. 4th ed. St. Louis: Mosby; 2001: 624-628.

Velmahos GC, Toutouzas KG. Vascular trauma and compartment syndromes. *Surg Clin North Am*. 2002;82:125-141.

case **68**

Mark G. Davies, MD, PhD

Presentation

An 80-year-old woman presents to the emergency department with a 4-hour history of sudden onset of pain in her left leg, below the knee, associated with weakness. The weakness resolved over the next hour. She has no past history of similar events. She has non-insulin-dependent diabetes with statin-controlled hypercholesterolemia. The patient does not give a history of any recent cardiac symptoms. On examination, the patient is noted to be alert and oriented and to favor her left leg. She has an irregular heart rate (150 beats per minute). She is on nasal cannulae with home oxygen. Examination of the peripheral pulses notes intact pulses in the right leg, but only a palpable femoral pulse in the left leg. The leg is cool to touch below the knee. Sensation and motor function are intact. No continuous-wave Doppler signals are identified in the anterior tibial or posterior tibial vessels at the level of the left ankle.

Differential Diagnosis

The differential diagnosis in this case is that of acute lower extremity embolism or *in situ* thrombosis below the level of the common femoral artery (Table 67-1).

Diagnosis

Grade II ischemia.

▧ Approach

The patient is prepared for possible surgical intervention. Her previous electro-cardiogram (ECG) shows normal sinus rhythm. Given her new-onset atrial fibrillation, the patient is begun on a protocol to rule out a myocardial infarction and is rate controlled with intravenous metoprolol.

Table 68-1. Classification of Critical Ischemia

Category	Status	Description	Capillary Refill	Muscle Changes	Sensory Loss	Arterial Doppler	Venous Doppler
I	Viable	No threat	Intact	None	None	+	+
II a	Threatened	Salvageable with intervention	Intact but slow	None	Partial	−	+
II b	Threatened	Salvageable with early intervention	Slow or absent	Diminished	Partial function	−	+
III	Irreversible	Nonsalvageable, amputation required	Absent	No function	Insensate	−	+

Note: +, present; −, absent.

ECG

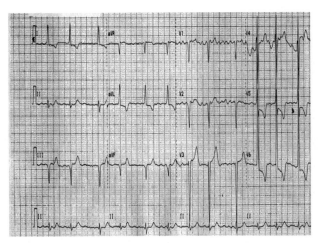

Figure 68-1

ECG and Echo Report

ECG reveals arterial fibullation (Fig. 68-1).

Approach

Heparin (80 IU/kg IV bolus, and 18 IU/kg/h IV continuous infusion) is administered to the patient. Complete blood count and serum chemistry are obtained. These are within normal limits. A duplex ultrasound examination of the left lower extremity is performed in the emergency department, and reveals occlusion of the popliteal artery with no proximal tibial vessel runoff. Her ankle/brachial index is zero. She is sent for lower extremity angiography. The right common femoral artery is cannulated, and a left lower extremity angiogram is performed.

Angiogram

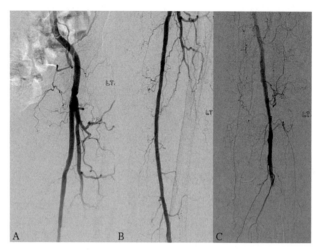

Figure 68-2

Angiogram Report

The angiogram reveals no evidence of inflow disease or superficial femoral artery (SFA) disease (*A* and *B*). There is complete occlusion of the popliteal artery with no distal runoff (*C*)

Diagnosis and Recommendation

The diagnosis is acute lower extremity embolism with no runoff. The options for this patient are surgical embolectomy, with or without intraoperative thrombolysis, or intra-arterial thrombolysis. The patient is considered high risk, but she has intact motor and sensory function, which allows time for a trial of thrombolysis. In the presence of deteriorating motor and sensory function, open surgical intervention of femoral embolectomy and intraoperative arteriography, and possibly intraoperative thrombolysis, would be required. We choose to offer the patient a trial of intra-arterial thrombolysis, because she does not have contraindications to lytic therapy. See Table 68-2.

Surgical Approach

In the angiography suite, a 6F Balkan sheath is placed from the right groin and allowed to lie within the left external iliac artery. A pressurized, heparinized saline infusion is commenced at 60 mL/h through the sheath. A 5F vertebral catheter is advanced into the above-knee popliteal artery over a guide wire. A guide wire is then passed easily through the clot until it lies in the peroneal artery. An infusion catheter is then placed over this wire to lie in the popliteal artery and the tibioperoneal trunk (Fig. 68-3). An infusion wire is directed into

Table 68-2. Contraindications to Thrombolysis

Absolute

 Active internal bleeding
 Recent cerebrovascular accident (< 2 months)
 Intracranial pathology

Relative

 Major:
  Recent (< 10 days) major surgery, obstetric delivery or organ biopsy
  Active peptic ulcer or other gastrointestinal pathology
  Recent major trauma
  Uncontrolled hypertension

 Minor:
  Minor surgery or trauma
  Recent cardiopulmonary resuscitation
  High likelihood of left heart thrombus
  Bacterial endocarditis
  Hemostatic defects

the peroneal artery. A tissue plasminogen activator (tPA) infusion of 1 mg/h (0.5 mg through the infusion catheter and 0.5 mg through the infusion wire) with a peripheral IV infusion of 300 IU/h unfractionated heparin is commenced. See Table 68-3.

Case Continued

The patient is transferred to the surgical intensive care unit (ICU) for monitoring. Clinical findings in the limb improve gradually, with increasing warmth in the calf over time. A Doppler signal is appreciated at the ankle 6 hours after

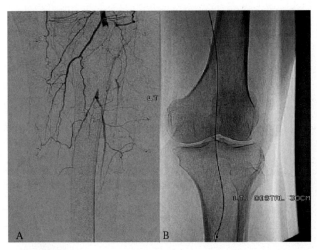

Figure 68-3

Table 68-3. Likelihood of Success for Thrombolysis

FACTOR	HIGH	LOW
Guidewire	Pass	Does not pass
Duration of occlusion	Short (hrs/days)	Long (wks/months)
Location for occlusion	Proximal	Distal
Distal vessel	Visualized	Nonvisualized
Distal doppler signal	Audible	None

commencing the infusion. After 12 hours, the patient is returned to the angiography suite for a follow-up angiogram, which demonstrates marked interval improvement in her angiographic findings. There is more than 80% lysis of the embolus with TIMI (Thrombosis in Myocardial Infarction) grade 3-4 flow and restoration of outflow through the peroneal artery (Fig. 68-4). The patient is returned to the surgical ICU for an additional 12 hours. Follow-up angiograms are performed.

Discussion

Clinical improvement is associated with return of continuous-wave Doppler signals at the foot (anterior and posterior tibial arteries) and an ankle/brachial index of 0.9. Rare but important events to watch for during thrombolytic infusions are the phenomenon of the "storm before the calm" (increasing pain secondary to lysis of clot and distal embolization), acute compartment syndrome (due to rapid skeletal muscle reperfusion in a very ischemic limb), and distant occult bleeding into the brain and retroperitoneum (most often seen with higher doses of tPA and full heparinization). At 24 hours, lysis of the clot, restoration of inline flow, and tibial vessel runoff are evident (Fig. 68-5).

▣ Approach

The angiogram findings, in association with the improvement in the patient's symptoms, allowed the infusion therapy to be stopped. The patient's sheath is

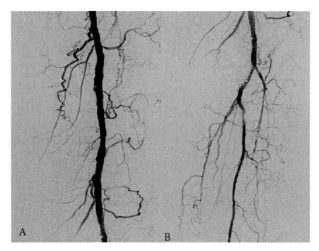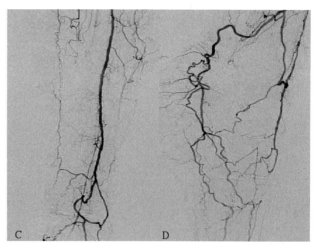

Figure 68-4

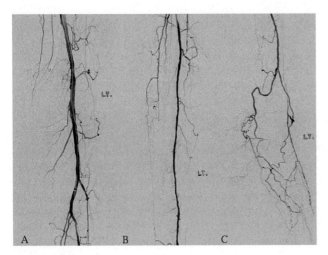

Figure 68-5

removed 4 hours after cessation of the tPA infusion, and hemostasis is achieved by manual pressure. Care must be taken with prolonged tPA infusions, due to the build up of fragment X, which can result in unrecognized abnormal coagulation in a patient. She is fully heparinized with the goal of an activated partial thromboplastin time (aPTT) of 60 to 80 seconds.

Case Continued

The patient is seen by the cardiology consult service, and is fully anticoagulated with warfarin with a target international normalized ratio (INR) of 2 to 3. She will be continued on chronic anticoagulation, because in the presence of her pulmonary disease the likelihood of successful cardioversion is low.

Discussion

Acute Limb Ischemia

Acute limb ischemia caused by embolism is associated with a cardiac origin in more than 75% of patients; 80% of these emboli lodge in the aortoiliac and femoral vessels. The most common etiology for these cardiac embolic events to the lower limb is acute myocardial infarction or new-onset atrial fibrillation. The morbidity and mortality of operations in patients with recent myocardial infarction exceed those for patients who undergo operations for emboli without corresponding myocardial infarction, and have encouraged clinicians to consider therapeutic thrombolysis.

Thrombolysis

Two scenarios exist for the use of thrombolysis in lower-limb arterial occlusion: preoperative thrombolysis and perioperative thrombolysis. The success of treatment is determined by correct patient selection. The Working Party on Thrombolysis was formed to develop a consensus on the use of thrombolytic therapy in peripheral arterial disease. It made 37 recommendations, which encompassed the results of clinical trials and accumulated clinical experience from Europe and North America.

In a recent meta-analysis of the literature, a systemic review of intra-arterial thrombolytic therapy for peripheral vascular disease was undertaken. A total of 32 articles were found, but only 12 were assessed to be of sufficient quality to be included in the analysis. There was a distinct lack of large randomized controlled trials comparing thrombolysis with surgical management. The exceptions were the TOPAS (Thrombosis or Peripheral Arterial Surgery) and STILE (Surgery versus Thrombolysis for Ischemia of the Lower Extremity) trials, although both had methodological flaws. The STILE trial did not achieve the sample size that was originally determined, and the TOPAS trials had a large number of contributing centers (113) compared with the sample size (548). Meta-analysis of the abstracted data sets showed no significant difference between thrombolysis and surgery in terms of major amputation (relative risk [RR] 0.9, 95% confidence interval, 0.6-1.4) and death (RR, 1.2; 0.8-1.9). There was an increased risk of residual ischemia with thrombolysis (RR, 1.8; 1.2-2.5) and hemorrhage (RR 2.9; 1.1-7.9). Patients who were shown to benefit from thrombolysis were those with short duration ischemia (RR reduction, 72%) and occluded grafts (RR reduction, 58%). The conclusions of this meta-analysis were, despite the theoretical advantages of thrombolysis, there was still insufficient evidence to justify its widespread use except in patients with graft occlusions and short duration ischemia.

Suggested Readings

Davies MG, Lee DE, Green RM. Current spectrum of thrombolysis. In: Moore W, Ahn S, eds. *Endovascular Surgery*. 3rd ed. Philadelphia: WB Saunders; 2001:255–274.

Palfreyman SJ, Michaels JA, Booth A. A systematic review of intra-arterial thrombolytic therapy for peripheral vascular occlusions. *Euro J Vasc Endovasc Surg*. 2000;19:143-157.

Working Party on Thrombolysis in the Management of Limb Ischemia. Thrombolysis in the management of lower limb peripheral arterial occlusion: a consensus document. *Am J Cardiol*. 1998;81:207-218.

Peter L. Faries, MD, Joshua Bernheim, MD, Rajeev Dayal, MD,
Scott Hollenbeck, MD, Albeir Mousa, MD, and K. Craig Kent, MD

Presentation

The patient is a 67-year-old woman who presents with intermittent abdominal pain. The pain is vague in nature and typically occurs 20 to 40 minutes after eating. It lasts 1 to 2 hours and resolves spontaneously. It is unclear if fatty food is more likely to generate the symptoms, but antacids do not relieve the pain.

Differential Diagnosis

Intermittent abdominal pain may originate from a wide variety of etiologies. These include symptomatic cholelithiasis, chronic pancreatitis, peptic ulcer disease, inflammatory bowel disease, irritable bowel syndrome, constipation, viral gastrointestinal illness, diverticulitis, abdominal malignancy, renal lithosis, pelvic inflammatory disease, uterine fibroids, or ovarian pathology. Therefore, it is important to characterize the pain with respect to its associated signs and symptoms. In this case, the pain is postprandial. The most common causes are likely to be symptomatic cholelithiasis or chronic cholecystitis. Other sources of intermittent abdominal pain are frequently associated with alterations of bowel habits or other associated symptoms.

Patients with symptomatic chronic mesenteric ischemia will typically have associated weight loss. The age of the patient may also provide some insight to the potential etiology of the abdominal pain. Patients with symptomatic mesenteric occlusive disease frequently are over 50 years old and may exhibit other manifestations of peripheral vascular disease. Radiological imaging studies are essential to evaluate for abdominal malignancy as an alternate source of intermittent abdominal pain associated with weight loss, as well as for mesenteric arterial occlusive disease.

Case Continued

The patient reports an 18-pound weight loss over the preceding 7 months and she appears thin. She has not been trying to lose weight, but has been avoiding food because eating is associated with the onset of pain. She denies any alteration in her bowel habits and denies blood in the stools, or black stools; she denies diarrhea or loose stools, and denies constipation. She had no episodes of abdominal pain prior to 7 months ago, and has no history of peptic ulcer disease. She has a 30-pack-year history of smoking, and discontinued smoking 8 years ago.

On physical examination, she is in no acute distress and has normal vital signs. She has no scleral icterus and no palpable adenopathy. Her abdomen is flat and nondistended, with normal active bowel sounds. She has no palpable abdominal masses, no abdominal tenderness, and no evidence of peritoneal irritation. Rectal examination demonstrates no masses, with stool that appears normal, but is trace positive for occult blood. Bimanual examination reveals no adnexal masses or evidence of uterine abnormalities. Laboratory examination is unremarkable, with normal serum chemistry and liver function profiles and normal amylase and lipase. Urinalysis is negative for red blood cells or evidence of urinary tract infection.

Extensive evaluation is necessary to ensure that no other, more common, causes of abdominal pain are present. Radiological evaluation is performed, including an ultrasound. This demonstrates a normal gallbladder, common bile duct, and liver. There is no evidence of hydronephrosis. An upper endoscopy shows no evidence of peptic ulcer disease. A computed tomography (CT) scan indicates no evidence of intraabdominal pathology with no evidence of malignancy or chronic pancreatitis. Serum markers suggestive of malignancy, including cancer antigen (CA)-125, carcinoembryonic antigen (CEA), and alpha-fetoprotein (AFP), are negative. Colonoscopy reveals only occasional diverticula without evidence of inflammation and no mucosal abnormalities.

Discussion

Without evidence of an alternative source of abdominal pain, evaluation for mesenteric ischemia should proceed. Noninvasive imaging techniques to evaluate the visceral circulation may be employed as the initial screening tests. Duplex ultrasound may be used in highly experienced centers; however, difficulty in obtaining adequate imaging may be encountered when bowel gas is present. Duplex evaluation also tends to be highly operator dependent.

Magnetic resonance arteriography (MRA) using gadolinium-contrast enhancement has become increasingly accurate for the evaluation of the visceral circulation. When appropriate protocols are utilized, MRA can detect the presence of mesenteric arterial occlusive disease. In general, it is necessary to have hemodynamically significant stenoses in at least 2 of the 3 mesenteric vessels (celiac axis, superior and inferior mesenteric arteries); more commonly, occlusion of 2 of the 3 with hemodynamically significant stenosis of the third is necessary to develop chronic mesenteric ischemia.

Occasionally, MRA may have artifactual flow defects, particularly if tortuosity of the vessels is present. To definitively establish the diagnosis of chronic mesenteric ischemia, contrast angiography is preferred. Images may be obtained in multiple projections, with the lateral projection providing the best demonstration of the origin of the visceral vessels. Selective cannulation and injection of the visceral vessels may provide additional anatomic detail. In instances of significant mesenteric occlusive disease, extensive collateral vessel communication is typically present. A prominent marginal artery of Drummond or arc or Riolan is often present to provide additional collateral arterial flow to the intestine. Findings of hemodynamically significant stenoses in at least 2 and more typically all 3 visceral arteries, combined with the appropriate clinical scenario and the absence of an alternative source of abdominal pain, are used to establish the diagnosis of chronic mesenteric ischemia. Intervention is necessary both to alleviate the chronic abdominal pain and to prevent progression to frank bowel infarction. MRA and visceul angiogram is recommended.

▨ MRA and Angiogram

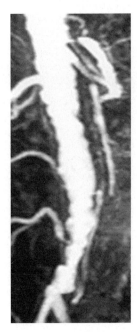

Figure 69-1

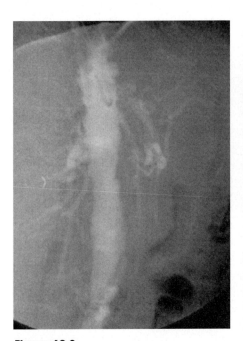
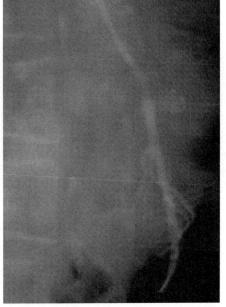

Figure 69-2

MRA and Angiogram Reports

MRA reveals occlusion of the inferior mesenteric artery with high-grade stenoses of the superior mesenteric artery and occlusion of the celiac axis at its origin (Fig. 69-1). These findings are confirmed at contrast arteriography performed via the femoral approach (Fig. 69-2).

Discussion

Intervention for mesenteric occlusive disease may be carried out using either percutaneous transluminal angioplasty (PTA) or direct operative revascularization with bypass or endarterectomy. Percutaneous techniques have been used increasingly in recent years, and can provide revascularization and relief of ischemic symptoms with minimal morbidity. Angioplasty, with or without placement of a stent, has been demonstrated to be successful in a high proportion of patients who have appropriate anatomic criteria. Patients who respond most favorably include those with incomplete occlusion that is short and focal in nature. Long-segment occlusions are considerably more difficult to treat successfully, because dissection in a subintimal plane occurs frequently during attempts at recanalization. Difficulty may be encountered in reestablishing wire position within the mesenteric arterial lumen distally, and compromise of mesenteric branch vessels may be precipitated by more distal dissection in the subintimal plane. In contrast, when PTA is used for focal, nonocclusive stenoses, arterial perfusion may be restored in over 90% of cases.

It is possible to treat multiple mesenteric stenoses using percutaneous techniques at the same setting. The lesions may be tandem within the same vessel, or more commonly may be in distinct vessels. When tandem lesions are present within the same vessel, simultaneous treatment is required to adequately restore mesenteric perfusion. In instances of isolated lesions in distinct arteries, the decision to perform multiple interventions simultaneously may be made after consideration of additional factors. Treatment of multiple lesions is more likely to provide optimal blood flow to the visceral circulation. In addition, compromise of one PTA site by restenosis during follow-up may be less likely to generate recurrent ischemia. Other factors that should be considered when the treatment of multiple vessels is being contemplated include the patient's ability to tolerate further intervention and their overall physiologic condition, as well as the adequacy of the primary PTA with regard to alleviating mesenteric ischemia. Other risk factors may also influence the decision, including the presence of aortic luminal debris that may be the source of embolization during wire and catheter manipulation, and baseline renal insufficiency that may be exacerbated by increased contrast dye loads.

The durability of percutaneous repair is of significant concern, particularly because restenosis at the angioplasty site is likely to result (at a minimum) in return of the chronic mesenteric symptoms, and may precipitate frank acute mesenteric ischemia with resultant bowel necrosis. Published durations of follow-up are shorter for PTA than for direct surgical revascularization. During follow-up that is typically less than 2 years, restenosis has been observed in approximately 10% of patients. Restenosis generally requires repeated angioplasty or an alternative revascularization procedure. The absence of extensive long-term follow-up may limit enthusiasm for use of percutaneous techniques in patients who are considered good candidates for open surgical revascularization. However, in patients with significant comorbid medical illnesses in whom major aortic surgery may be poorly tolerated, mesenteric PTA is likely to provide the best initial approach for restoration of mesenteric blood flow.

Case Continued: Open Surgical Revascularization

In the current patient, attempts at percutaneous intervention are carried out from the femoral approach initially. However, despite the use of multiple hydrophilic angiographic wires of varying diameter and shape, augmented with the use of directional catheters and guide sheaths, the lesion in the superior mesenteric artery (SMA) cannot be crossed with a wire. The brachial artery is then used to provide better in-line access to the origin of the SMA. However, even with direct in-line access via a left brachial artery puncture, wire access across the ostial SMA lesion cannot be obtained. Therefore, open surgical revascularization is required.

Discussion

Several options for surgical revascularization exist. These include transaortic endarterectomy, antegrade bypass to one or two mesenteric arteries or retrograde bypass to one or two mesenteric arteries. Transaortic endarterectomy may be performed with a thoracoabdominal exposure or transabdominally with median visceral rotation. After dissection and mobilization of the central aorta, including division of the medial arcuate ligament, the renal, superior mesenteric, and lumbar arteries, as well as the branches of the celiac axis, are dissected to allow individual control. Once aortic clamping has been performed, a trapdoor incision is used to enter the aortic lumen. An endarterectomy is performed in the deep medial layer with eversion endarterectomy of the visceral branches. Extensive experience with the use of transaortic endarterectomy in the United States is limited to relatively few centers of excellence. The long-term patency results of this repair are excellent at these centers.

Case Continued

Mild aneurysmal dilatation is noted to be present in the suprarenal aorta. Although this does not warrant surgical repair, it may make suprarenal clamping difficult. The common iliac arteries are widely patent bilaterally and free of occlusive disease. Consequently, the decision is made in this instance to proceed with mesenteric revascularization using the common iliac artery as the inflow source vessel. A single bypass graft using an externally supported prosthetic graft is planned. The abdomen is explored through a midline incision. Evaluation for alternative sources of the chronic intermittent abdominal pain and weight loss reveals no intraabdominal pathology. The bowel is noted to be pale, but it is viable. The small intestine is retracted to the right side of the abdomen. The superior mesenteric artery is identified as it emerges from behind the body of the pancreas at the root of the mesentery. A segment of undiseased SMA is dissected free to allow vascular control to be obtained. The common iliac artery is then dissected free from the surrounding structures, with care being taken not to injure the adjacent iliac vein. The bypass graft is laid in a gently curving arc to prevent kinking or collapse when the small intestine is returned to its anatomic position. Externally supported prosthetic graft material may aid in preventing kinking of the graft. The adequacy of the bypass graft may be assessed intraoperatively by Doppler insonation of the mesenteric vessels, palpation for pulsation in the arterial branches in the mesentery, observation of the small intestine for peristalsis, and observation of the appearance of viability in the intestine, liver, and spleen.

Discussion:

The supraceliac aorta provides an excellent source of arterial inflow for mesenteric bypass. In instances where it is used, dissection begins either with a left medial visceral rotation or dissection through the lesser sac to expose the supraceliac aorta. Division of the crura of the diaphragm provides additional exposure. Hemodynamic control to allow the proximal anastomosis to be fashioned frequently requires clamping of the entire diameter of the aorta. The thickness of the supraceliac aorta often prohibits the use of partially occluding vascular clamps in this position. When a bifurcated graft is used for antegrade bypass, the first limb is brought directly onto the hepatic or celiac artery and anastomosed in an end-to-side fashion. The second limb is brought into position adjacent to the superior mesenteric artery. A retropancreatic tunnel is frequently employed to allow passage of the graft limb. The anastomosis is again performed in an end-to-side fashion. The long-term durability of mesenteric bypass is excellent. These procedures are often well tolerated and remain the gold standard for mesenteric revascularization.

Suggested Readings

Cunningham CG, Reilly LM, Rapp JH, et al. Chronic visceral ischemia: three decades of progress. *Ann Surg.* 1991;214:276-288.

Gentile AT, Moneta GL, Taylor LM Jr, et al. Isolated bypass to the superior mesenteric artery for intestinal ischemia. *Arch Surg.* 1994;129:926-932.

Johnston KW, Lindsay TF, Walker PM, et al. Mesenteric arterial bypass grafts: early and late results and suggested approach for chronic and acute mesenteric ischemia. *Surgery.* 1995;118:1-7.

Matsumoto AH, Tegtmeyer CJ, Fitzcharles EJ, et al. Percutaneous transluminal angioplasty of visceral arterial stenoses: Results and long-term clinical follow-up. *J Vasc Intervent Radiol.* 1995;6:165-174.

Stoney RJ, Ehrenfeld WK, Wylie ET. Revascularization methods in chronic visceral ischemia caused by atherosclerosis. *Ann Surg.* 1977;186: 468-476.

Taylor LM, Porter JM. Treatment of chronic mesenteric ischemia. *Semin Vasc Surg.* 1990; 3:186.

Robert D. Brook, MD

Presentation

A 72-year-old man with a significant past medical history for coronary artery disease, systolic dysfunction, congestive heart failure (ejection fraction = 25%), mild chronic renal insufficiency (baseline creatinine = 1.6), and hypertension is admitted to the cardiac care intensive care unit for acute dyspnea and a presumed exacerbation of heart failure. A myocardial infarction is excluded during the first 24 hours by the absence of changes in serial myocardial enzyme measurements and the electrocardiogram. He is treated with nasal oxygen (6 Ls/min), a doubling of the dosage of his angiotensin-converting enzyme inhibitor, continuation of digoxin and low-dose beta blockade therapy, and aggressive diuresis using intravenous furosemide. He responds well to therapy within 24 hours. Prior to transfer to the step-down unit, he develops a low-grade fever (temperature 100.5°F). His blood pressure decreases from his usual levels of 90/60 to 78/40 mm Hg. Slow intravenous hydration is provided and his blood pressure medications are held. Shortly afterward, he develops severe acute abdominal pain and nausea.

On examination, vital signs reveal a blood pressure of 82/48 mm Hg, heart rate of 102 beats per minute, respirations of 24 per minute, and oxygen saturation of 92% on 3 L/min. He appears to be in acute distress with anxiety and severe abdominal pain. His neck, lung, cardiac, venous, and arterial examinations are unchanged. His abdominal examination reveals absent bowel sounds, mild diffuse periumbilical pain with guarding, and no rebound tenderness. His rectal examination reveals normal tone and is trace-positive for occult blood. Abdominal plain films and laboratories are ordered.

■ Test Reports

Normal abdominal plain films without evidence of obstruction, ileus, mass, or lumen perforation.

Complete blood cell (CBC) count showed a modest leukocytosis (white blood cells [WBC] = 11.9). Comprehensive chemistry panel was unchanged from baseline, except for a small increase in lactate dehydrogenase (LDH = 250 IU/L) and reduction in serum bicarbonate (HCO_3 = 19 mEq/L). Blood and urine cultures pending. Urinalysis negative for hematuria or pyuria.

Differential Diagnosis

The differential diagnosis for acute periumbilical abdominal pain, fever, hypotension, and leukocytosis is broad. *Peritonitis*: lumen perforation (eg, ulcer), ruptured diverticuli, or infectious bacterial and nonbacterial organisms. *Gastrointestinal*: pancreatitis, early small bowel obstruction, diverticulitis, early appendicitis, inflammatory bowel disease, gastroenteritis, or *Clostridium difficile* colitis. *Vascular*: aortic dissection, aortic aneurysm leakage, and acute mesenteric ischemia. The latter includes splanchnic arterial thrombosis (usually in the setting of underlying atherosclerotic disease), arterial embolus or dissection, small vessel disease and vasculitis, venous thrombosis, watershed ischemic colitis, and nonocclusive mesenteric ischemia.

Discussion

In a patient with sudden relative hypotension, poor cardiac output, history of atherosclerosis, and severe abdominal pain greater than physical examination findings, mesenteric ischemia should be rapidly considered as the primary diagnosis. The increase in LDH, rectal examination positive for occult blood, and metabolic acidosis are all nonspecific findings that are suggestive of this diagnosis. Due to the high morbidity and mortality rates and emergent nature of this diagnosis, immediate testing should focus on excluding this diagnosis and differentiating between occlusive versus nonocclusive mesenteric ischemia (NOMI) once the initial testing described above has been performed. Hypotension and the use of digoxin increases the risk for NOMI by causing vasoconstriction of the splanchnic vessels. The use of diuretics may increase renal blood flow and further diminish mesenteric perfusion. Any concomitant infection, septicemia, and volume depletion will also contribute to NOMI.

▌ Diagnostic Tests

Abdominal computed tomography, magnetic resonance imaging, or ultrasonography cannot exclude NOMI. To avoid unnecessary delay, an emergent digital-subtraction mesenteric angiography should be the initial test if mesenteric ischemia (particularly NOMI) is considered and no signs of sepsis or peritonitis are present.

▌ Mesenteric Angiography

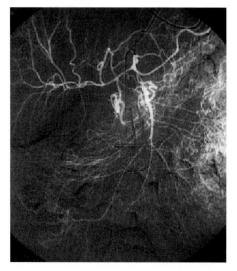

Figure 70-1

Mesenteric Angiography Report

An emergent mesenteric angiogram demonstrates NOMI. Four arteriographic criteria for NOMI have been presented: (1) narrowing at the origins of multiple superior mesenteric branches; (2) alternate arterial dilatation and narrowing; (3) mesenteric arcade spasms and; (4) impaired perfusion of intramural vessels.

Discussion

Acute NOMI is caused by severe and diffuse superior mesenteric artery narrowing due to vasospasm that is triggered by malperfusion secondary to hypotension (heart failure), dehydration (aggressive diuresis with furosemide), and digoxin therapy.

Diagnosis and Recommendation

The diagnosis of acute NOMI is made. In contrast to acute occlusive disease (eg, emboli, thrombosis), surgery is not indicated for early NOMI without mucosal necrosis.

Approach

After angiography displays NOMI, vasodilator therapy should immediately begin. Direct intra-arterial mesentery infusions of papaverine and prostaglandin E_1 have been used with success. Vasospasm is known to persist even after correction or resolution of the inciting events. However, measures should also be taken to reduce the hypotension and to treat any precipitating dehydration or infection, including careful hydration (Swan-Ganz catheter may guide this) and broad-spectrum empirical antibiotics.

Surgical Approach

Control of NOMI with vasodilator therapy should be tried initially. Indications for initial or subsequent laparotomy are failure of intra-arterial vasodilators to restore splanchnic perfusion, an increase in serum markers suggesting bowel necrosis, peritonitis, and persistent symptoms of abdominal pain after 24 to 72 hours.

Case Continued

An initial 20-µg bolus of prostaglandin E_1 was followed by an infusion at 2.5 to 5.0 µg/h. Symptoms of nausea with abdominal pain resolved within 24 hours. LDH and HCO_3 returned to normal. Repeat angiogram demonstrated a significant restoration of splanchnic perfusion (Fig. 70-2). Intravenous glucagon may be used in this setting as a splanchnic vasodilator, though clinical experience is anecdotal.

Discussion

NOMI is a medical emergency with continued high rates of mortality ranging from 50% to 80%. It accounts for 20% to 30% of all syndromes of mesenteric ischemia. Conditions that predispose to the syndrome are previous heart disease and reduced cardiac function, older age, renal impairment, aortic insufficiency, and use of certain medications including diuretics and digoxin. Dehydration, hypotension, shock, and infection precipitate acute malperfusion of the mesentery, which triggers severe microvascular vasoconstriction and spasm. Immediate angiography and direct intra-arterial vasodilator therapy offer the best outcomes.

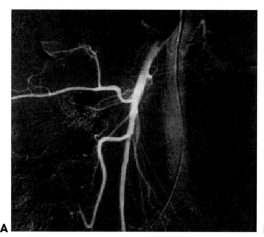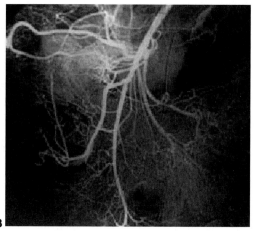

Figure 70-2 A: Severe NOMI at baseline before vasodilator therapy. Extreme mesenteric vasoconstriction is evident. **B:** Post-treatment repeat angiogram demonstrates improved filling of vessels.

Suggested Readings

Bassiouny HS. Nonocclusive mesenteric ischemia. *Surg Clin North Am.* 1997;77:319-325.

Kim AY, Ha HK. Evaluation of suspected mesenteric ischemia: efficacy of radiologic studies. *Radiol Clin North Am.* 2003;41:427-442.

Lock G. Acute mesenteric ischemia: classification, evaluation and therapy. *Acta Gastreoenterol Belgica.* 2002;65:220-225.

Mansour MA. Management of acute mesenteric ischemia. *Arch Surg.* 1999;134:328-330.

Park WM, Gloviczki P, Cherry KJ. Contemporary management of acute mesenteric ischemia: factors associated with survival. *J Vasc Surg.* 2002;35:445-452.

Trompeter M, Brazda T, Remy CT, Vestring T, Reimer P. Nonocclusive mesenteric ischemia: etiology, diagnosis, and interventional therapy. *Eur Radiol.* 2002;12:1179-1187.

Michelle T. Mueller, MD, Mark R. Sarfati, MD, and Larry W. Kraiss, MD

Presentation

A 48-year-old man with a past medical history of gastroesophageal reflux disease but no previous surgeries presents to the emergency department complaining of abdominal pain. He has had intermittent abdominal pain for years, but the symptoms have dramatically worsened over the last 2 weeks. The onset of pain occurs approximately 30 minutes after meals and lasts for hours, and is now associated with nausea and vomiting. The patient denies any weight loss, melena, or hematochezia. A recent upper endoscopy was unremarkable and colonoscopy showed benign polyps.

On physical examination, the patient is noted to be afebrile and hemodynamically stable. The examination reveals the abdomen to be soft and mildly distended with slight tenderness to palpation, but without peritoneal signs. There are no hernias. The white blood cell count is 7,000 and hematocrit 40. The electrolyte levels, liver function tests, amylase, lipase, and lactate levels are normal. To further evaluate the abdominal pain, a computed tomography (CT) scan with oral and intravenous contrast is ordered.

Differential Diagnosis

The differential diagnosis for abdominal pain without peritonitis is extensive. Chronic abdominal pain narrows the differential, yet it remains lengthy. Possible diagnoses in this case include gastroesophageal reflux disease, peptic ulcer disease, biliary colic, chronic cholecystitis, chronic pancreatitis, partial small bowel obstruction, tumor, chronic mesenteric ischemia, and mesenteric venous thrombosis.

CT scanning has become an important part of the evaluation of abdominal pain. Initial diagnostic impressions based solely on clinical findings are changed by the CT scan nearly one third of the time; post-CT scan diagnoses are correct 92% to 95% of the time compared to 50% to 71% of pre-CT scan diagnoses. The addition of intravenous contrast to a CT scan of the abdomen and pelvis aids in the diagnosis of venous thrombosis, aneurysms, bowel ischemia, and bleeding.

■ CT Scan

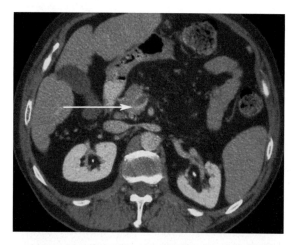

Figure 71-1

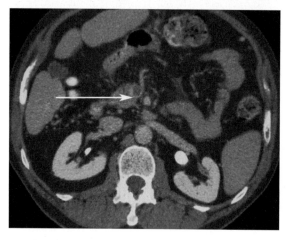

Figure 71-2

CT Scan Report

The CT scan reveals mesenteric venous thrombosis (MVT Fig. 71-1). There is mesenteric stranding and a filling defect in the superior mesenteric vein ringed with contrast (*arrow*) (Fig.71-2).

Discussion

The diagnosis of MVT depends upon visualization of the clot. Abdominal and pelvic CT scans have the greatest accuracy for detecting thrombus in the large mesenteric veins. In addition, associated confirmatory findings are also seen, such as ascites, bowel wall thickening, stranding of the mesentery, pneumatosis, or even portal venous air. Duplex ultrasound, mesenteric angiography with venous phase imaging, and magnetic resonance imaging (MRI) have also been used to diagnose MVT, but with lower accuracy. Abdominal radiographs typically show nonspecific findings consistent with an ileus pattern or generalized edema of the bowel wall.

Recommendation

At this point, the patient has no signs of bowel infarction and no indications for surgical exploration. The patient is admitted to the hospital for fluid resuscitation, immediate anticoagulation with full-dose intravenous heparin, and serial abdominal examinations. A hypercoagulability screen was sent prior to anticoagulation.

Case Continued

The patient's abdominal pain improves, and he tolerates oral intake. He is transitioned to subcutaneous low-molecular-weight heparin and coumadin. Discharge occurs 2 days later. At follow-up approximately 2 weeks later, the patient is clinically well. His hypercoagulability screen revealed no abnormalities for protein C, protein S, or antithrombin III. Mutations in the factor V and prothrombin genes were absent. Lifelong anticoagulation is recommended.

Discussion

MVT is a broad term that includes thrombosis of the inferior mesenteric vein, superior mesenteric vein, splenic vein, or portal vein. MVT is responsible for approximately 2% to 15% of all cases of acute intestinal ischemia. MVT obstructs venous return, which can lead to edema of the bowel wall, distention, and eventual infarction. MVT is difficult to diagnose initially because of the typical insidious onset and subtle early clinical findings. Early symptoms are produced by congestion of the bowel and are visceral in character. Patients often present with signs and symptoms that are nonspecific and vague, including crampy abdominal pain, abdominal distention, nausea, anorexia, malaise, ascites, diarrhea, gastrointestinal bleeding, and pain out of proportion to examination. About half of patients will have leukocytosis; an elevated lactate is unusual. Delays in diagnosis are common and contribute to the reported high morbidity and 15% to 40% mortality.

The traditional separation of MVT into primary or secondary categories is arbitrary. All patients with MVT should be regarded as harboring a hypercoagulable state. The hypercoagulability may be endogenous and related to a defined abnormality in the coagulation system (eg, protein C deficiency, protein S deficiency, antithrombin deficiency, antiphospholipid antibody syndrome, lupus anticoagulant, factor V Leiden, prothrombin gene mutation). Alternatively, the hypercoagulable state producing MVT may result from other processes, such as intra-abdominal inflammation (pancreatitis, diverticular disease, peritonitis, appendicitis), trauma, portal hypertension, intra-abdominal or hematologic malignancy, polycythemia vera, myeloproliferative disorders, splenomegaly, oral contraceptives, cirrhosis, or even severe dehydration.

It is more relevant clinically to categorize MVT on the basis of duration of symptoms as well as whether portal or splenic vein thrombus is present. MVT can present acutely with a more fulminant course lasting only days or as a chronic condition (arbitrarily defined as lasting at least 4 weeks). Acute MVT more often results from small mesenteric vein branch involvement, and is more difficult to diagnose with CT scanning or duplex ultrasound because the larger mesenteric veins may not contain thrombus. These patients have poor venous collateralization and are more likely to have peritoneal signs on examination indicating bowel infarction. Acute MVT is often first recognized intraoperatively. A clear majority of patients with acute MVT will require an operation and probable bowel resection. Acute MVT has been more often associated with a thrombophilic complication than the chronic form.

Patients with chronic MVT often have symptoms lasting weeks, involvement of larger vessels (focal thrombus at the portomesenteric confluence or splenic vein), and are usually diagnosed with a CT scan (or possibly a duplex scan) identifying the large-vessel thrombus as well as collateral circulation. When compared to acute MVT, these patients are more likely to have thrombosis related to a postoperative complication or cirrhosis. These patients rarely need an operation and almost never require a bowel resection. The Mayo Clinic experience suggests that patients with acute MVT fare worse than patients with chronic MVT. Mortality in acute MVT is higher at both 30 days (approximately 30% versus 6%) and 3 years (64% versus 17%).

Surgical Approach

Patients with suspected MVT and an abdominal examination with peritonitis should go to the operating room. Intraoperatively, the surgeon may find bloody ascites, and dusky, thick, and rubbery appearing intestine. All patients should be anticoagulated as soon as possible once the diagnosis of MVT is made, even intraoperatively. If necrotic bowel is identified, resection should be performed. The surgeon must then decide if a second-look laparotomy should be scheduled for 24 to 48 hours to re-evaluate areas of questionable bowel viability. Additional bowel resections at second-look procedures are common.

Very rarely, a large-vessel venous thrombectomy or local thrombolysis may be indicated. However, there are only isolated case reports of success. Mechanical thrombectomy should be reserved for patients who do not respond to other therapies. It is not surprising that such treatment is often futile, because the patients most likely to need surgery are those with small-vessel involvement.

Patients diagnosed with MVT, but without peritonitis, should be admitted to the hospital for fluid resuscitation and anticoagulation. These patients should be closely observed for the development of peritoneal signs, which should then prompt exploratory laparotomy, but there is no benefit to surgery without signs of peritonitis.

Complications associated with MVT include bowel necrosis, portal hypertension, variceal bleeding, and recurrent thrombosis. Indefinite (ie, lifelong) anticoagulation is often recommended because patients so treated have a lower recurrence rate and better survival. However, if the cause of the MVT is clearly identified and temporary, it may be reasonable to discontinue the anticoagulation after 3 to 6 months. Individualized therapy is advised. The patient in this scenario was anticoagulated indefinitely because of the idiopathic nature of his MVT; it is presumed that he has a hypercoagulable state even though it is undefined.

Summary

Mesenteric venous thrombosis is difficult to diagnose secondary to the vague presenting symptoms. The high morbidity and mortality is related to a delay in diagnosis. A high index of suspicion and liberal use of CT scanning in patients with abdominal pain may shorten this delay. It is useful to categorize patients based on duration of symptoms and isolated large mesenteric vein involvement. All patients with MVT should be anticoagulated as soon as possible after the diagnosis is made. Patients should be operated upon selectively, based on clinical findings that suggest bowel infarction. All patients with MVT should be regarded as hypercoagulable. Because of lower rates of recurrent MVT and better survival, indefinite anticoagulation is usually recommended.

Suggested Readings

Clement DJ. Evaluation of the acute abdomen with CT: is image everything? *Am J Gastroenterol.* 1993;88:1282-1283.

Gore RM, Miller FH, Pereles FS, Yaghmai V, Berlin JW. Helical CT in the evaluation of the acute abdomen. *AJR Am J Roentgenol.* 2000;174:901-13.

Kumar S, Kamath PS. Acute superior mesenteric venous thrombosis: one disease or two? *Am J Gastroenterol.* 2003;98:1299-1304.

Rhee RY, Gloviczki P, Mendonca CT, et al. Mesenteric venous thrombosis: still a lethal disease in the 1990s. *J Vasc Surg.* 1994;20:688-697.

Tsushima Y, Yamada S, Aoki J, Motojima T, Endo K. Effect of contrast-enhanced computed tomography on diagnosis and management of acute abdomen in adults. *Clin Radiol.* 2002;57:507-513.

case 72

Candace Y. Williams, BS, and Gilbert R. Upchurch, Jr., MD

Presentation

A 33-year-old grand multiparous woman with a past medical history significant for acute cholecystitis treated by laparoscopic cholecystectomy 3 years ago, and 7 previous vaginal deliveries, presented to the emergency department with non-productive cough and shortness of breath. She has no prior history of pulmonary disorders. Social history was negative for tobacco and alcohol use. On physical examination, lung fields were clear to auscultation bilaterally. Review of systems was negative for any other pathology. She received a pregnancy test, which was negative, and a chest radiograph, which showed no acute cardiopulmonary disease. She was sent home and given symptomatic treatment for a viral upper respiratory infection. She now presents to your office 2 weeks later for evaluation of additional findings on chest radiograph suggestive of additional pathology.

▨ Chest X-Ray

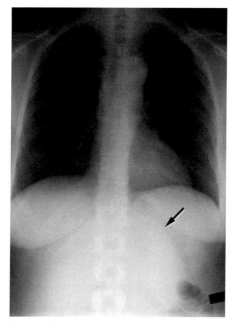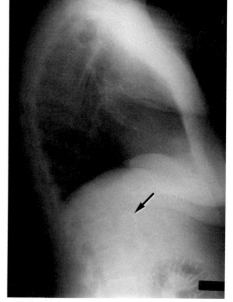

Figure 72-1

Chest X-Ray Report

Posteroanterior (PA) and lateral chest x-ray demonstrating no acute cardiopulmonary disease. Cholecystectomy clips in right upper quadrant. A 2.5-cm calcification is noted in left upper quadrant (*arrow*) (Fig. 72-1).

Differential Diagnosis

The differential diagnosis for left upper quadrant calcifications include (1) calcifications due to splenic artery aneurysm (SAA), (2) opportunistic infections, such as cytomegalovirus, *Pneumocystis carinii*, or *Mycobacterium avium-intracellulare*, (3) hemoglobinopathies, such as beta-thalassemia and sickle cell anemia, or (4) lymphoma. Mesenteric lymph node calcifications would suggest lymphoma. Given the patient's multiparous history without signs of lymphoma or risk for opportunistic infections, the most likely diagnosis is a SAA.

Discussion

The incidence of SAA is approximately 0.78% in the United States. Because the splenic artery likely has inherent structural abnormalities along with discontinuity of the internal elastic lamina at branching points, aneurysms of the splenic artery constitute 60% of all splanchnic artery aneurysms. Unlike other aneurysms, which occur more often in men, SAA has a 4:1 female:male ratio, probably associated with its main risk factors applying to women. The 3 main risk factors for SAA are (1) medial fibrodysplasia (4% of these patients develop SAA), (2) grand multiparity (45% of SAA patients are grand multiparous women), and (3) portal hypertension with splenomegaly (10% of these patients develop SAA). In medial fibrodysplasia, the mechanism is likely medial degeneration with fibrotic and atherosclerotic changes resulting in mural outpouchings in the vessel. Patients with this disorder have 6 times the normal risk of developing SAA. Grand multiparity (average of 4.5 pregnancies, often more than 6) poses a risk due to increased splenic blood flow during pregnancy, as well as high levels of gonadal hormones that alter the integrity of the extracellular matrix. In portal hypertension with splenomegaly, increased production of hormones, such as estrogen, with cirrhosis and increased blood flow through splenic circulation, leads to SAA development. Other risk factors for developing SAA include inflammatory vessel changes that occur in the setting of chronic pancreatitis and pseudocyst formation or gastric ulcers, trauma to the splenic artery, systemic vasculitic disorders, such as polyarteritis nodosa, congenital anomalies of foregut arterial circulation, and mycotic infections.

The main symptoms of intact SAA include nausea, vomiting, and vague left upper quadrant abdominal pain or epigastic discomfort that radiates to the left scapular area. This pain can become considerably worse with acute expansion of the aneurysm. Abdominal tenderness on physical examination may be noted. Rarely, an abdominal bruit may be heard or a pulsatile mass felt if the aneurysm is larger than 2 cm. Despite these symptoms, SAA often goes unnoticed because epigastric symptoms may mimic gastroesophageal reflux disease, peptic ulcer disease, gastritis, pancreatitis, or cholecystic disorders. In addition, most cases of SAA are asymptomatic and are discovered incidentally on radiographic studies done for other purposes. On abdominal x-rays, left upper quadrant signet-ring calcifications are a nonspecific sign suggestive of SAA. Computed tomography (CT) scans, magnetic resonance imaging, and ultrasound (US) can often identify aneurysms and detect whether the lesions are actively bleeding. US with color Doppler can also be useful to differentiate cystic and solid lesions from aneurysms. Despite the usefulness of these other studies, selective celiac arteriography is necessary to confirm the diagnosis.

Recommendations

Given the likelihood that the patient has SAA, a selective celiac arteriogram is indicated. In addition, although improbable without evidence of constitutional symptoms or signs of infection, obtaining a complete blood count with differential is indicated to rule out infection or lymphoma as a cause of the calcifications.

Case Continued

The patient had a complete blood count that was within normal limits, and the following CT scan and arteriogram.

▉ CT Scan

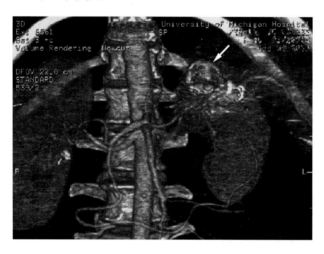

Figure 72-2

CT Scan Report

Calcified SAA measuring 2.8 × 3.1 cm located distal to pancreatic tail (*arrow*) (Fig. 72-2).

Arteriogram

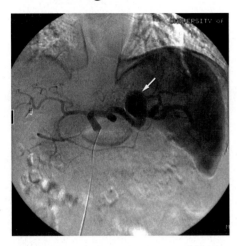

Figure 72-3

Arteriogram Report

Calcified 2.8-cm SAA, which originates distal to the pancreatic tail without involvement of the splenic hilum (Fig. 72-3).

Diagnosis

Splenic artery aneurysm

Discussion

With the diagnosis of asymptomatic SAA, decisions must be made regarding treatment. The purpose of treatment is to prevent the deadly consequences of rupture. Risk of rupture includes aneurysms larger than 2 cm, pregnant patients (95% of those recognized during pregnancy have ruptured), and patients who have had orthotopic liver transplants. As previously suggested, however, rupture risk is not associated with age, hypertension, or the absence of calcifications in the aneurysm. Therefore, it is recommended that all symptomatic aneurysms be repaired because the risk of rupture is greatest in those patients. In addition, asymptomatic pregnant patients as well as patients of childbearing age should undergo aneurysm repair to avoid the risk of rupture during pregnancy. This is especially crucial because the maternal mortality following rupture is 75% and fetal mortality is 95%. In all other patients, data suggest that the risk of rupture in the general population is only 2%, and that the nonpregnant operative mortality is less than 25%. Therefore, the patient's past medical history and risk associated with undergoing operation must be weighed against the risk of rupture. In patients who have a high operative mortality risk, close follow-up with US or CT scans can be initiated. In addition, transcatheter embolization of the aneurysm also offers an option for repair in some patients at high operative risk.

Recommendations

Given that the patient is asymptomatic and of childbearing age, an elective repair is scheduled at a time convenient for the patient.

About 2 weeks prior to scheduled SAA repair, the patient develops acute onset of left upper quadrant abdominal pain that radiates to her left scapular area, along with nausea and vomiting. Upon presentation to the emergency department, she was hypotensive and tachycardic initially, but then quickly stabilized following 2 liters of IV fluid.

Discussion

The most probable cause of the patient's new onset of symptoms is an acute rupture of the preexisting SAA. This is demonstrated by symptoms suggestive of acute expansion of the aneurysm, as well as hypotension and tachycardia suggesting hemorrhage. The patient's stabilization in the setting of rupture is likely due to what is deemed the "double rupture" sign. In SAA, patients initially rupture into the lesser sac and experience brief tachycardia and hypotension. While the blood is contained in the lesser sac, it serves to tamponade the vessel and stop bleeding. With time, however, the blood will escape out of the lesser sac through the foramen of Winslow, and flow freely into the peritoneum. At this point, patients lose massive amounts of blood and experience hypovolemic shock and cardiovascular collapse. Urgent operative therapy is indicated for hemostatic control and is critical at this point for the patient's survival.

Other manifestations of rupture can occur in the setting of SAA associated with portal hypertension and inflammatory conditions, such as pancreatitis and gastric ulcers. In the case of portal hypertension, an arteriovenous fistula can occur between the aneurysm and the splenic vein. In the case of inflammatory disorders, patients can experience gastrointestinal bleeding instead of peritoneal bleeding, with an arterioenteric fistula between the SAA and gastric ulcer. In addition, pancreatic duct bleeding may occur in the setting of chronic pancreatitis and SAA with arterio-pseudocyst-fistula formation.

Recommendations

Based on the likelihood that the patient has experienced an initial SAA rupture now contained in the lesser sac, it is critical to repair the ruptured aneurysm immediately to prevent further bleeding. Therefore, it is recommended that the patient undergo emergent exploratory laparotomy for ruptured SAA repair.

Surgical Approach

Splenic artery aneurysms can be repaired through open or laparoscopic approaches. If an open procedure is selected, incisions may be made vertical midline, left subcostal, extended right subcostal, bilateral subcostal, or transverse epigastric. Depending on the location of the SAA, several different procedures are indicated for the repair. If the aneurysm involves the proximal vessel, the typical procedure involves gaining exposure through the lesser sac by excising the gastrohepatic ligament, excising all entering and exiting vessels to the aneurysm, and then ligating or excising the aneurysm without reconstruction. This can be performed because the spleen has multiple collaterals for blood supply. If the aneurysm is located in the midsplenic artery area, it is likely associated with pancreatitis and erosion of a pseudocyst into the splenic artery. In this situation, exposure is gained through a Kocher maneuver to gain a retroperitoneal view. Then, proximal arterial ligation is achieved by going through the aneurysmal sac. The use of monofilament suture in the setting of pancreatic infection is necessary to avoid spreading infection. The pseudocyst is then incised and left to drain. If the pseudocyst and aneurysm involve the distal body or tail of the pancreas, a distal pancreatectomy and splenectomy may be performed. Finally, and most importantly for the case presented, aneurysms occurring at the hilum of the spleen are repaired in two ways. The first involves excision via splenectomy. More commonly, after splenic mobilization, suture obliteration of aneurysms or excision of distal aneurysms is performed to reduce the immunocompromise associated with splenectomy. However, this surgery can be complicated by segmental splenic infarction.

Case Continued

The patient is taken to the operating room is taken operating room for exploratory laparotomy and repair of SAA. A ruptured distal splenic artery aneurysm was noted. In the operating room, due to anatomic difficulties, a splenectomy was performed as part of the repair.

Discussion

The spleen is an important organ in the immune system. Following splenectomy, due to decreased ability to opsonize encapsulated organisms and subnormal levels of antibodies, patients are at increased risk for postoperative infections and postsplenectomy sepsis within the first 2 years, especially if they have preexisting hematologic abnormalities. In the current patient, given a negative hematologic history, her risk of serious postsplenectomy sepsis is less than 1% over 2 years. Although the patient has a low risk, she should be given *Pneumococcal* and *Haemophilus influenza* vaccines. With these measures, it is unlikely that the patient will experience serious complications from splenectomy.

Case Continued

The patient recovered well from surgery and remained in the hospital for 7 days without signs or symptoms of infection. She was followed regularly for 2 years without complications.

Suggested Readings

Angelakis EJ, Bair WE, Barone JE, et al. Splenic artery aneurysm rupture during pregnancy. *Obstet Gynecol Surv*. 1993;48:145-148.

McDermott VG, Shlansky-Goldberg R, Cope C, et al. Endovascular management of splenic artery aneurysms and pseudo aneurysms. *Cardiovasc Intervent Radiol*. 1994;17:179-184.

Pulli R, Innocenti AA, Barbanti E, et al. Early and long-term results of surgical treatment of splenic artery aneurysms. *Am J Surg*. 2001;182:520-523.

Stanley JC. Treatment of renal, splenic, and hepatic artery aneurysms. In: Fischer JE, Baker RJ, eds. *Mastery of Surgery*. 4th ed. Philadelphia: Lippincott Williams & Wilkins; 2001: 1993-2000.

Stanley JC, Fry WJ. Pathogenesis and clinical significance of splenic artery aneurysms. *Surgery*. 1974;76:898-908.

Zelenock GB, Stanley JC. Splanchnic artery aneurysms. In: Rutherford RB, ed. *Vascular Surgery*. Philadelphia: WB Saunders; 2000: 1369-1382.

case 73

Omar Araïm, MD, and Seth W. Wolk, MD

Presentation

A 68-year-old woman with a long-standing history of hypertension, apparently well controlled until 3 months ago, is admitted to the hospital with worsening renal function. Her blood pressure is 193/72 mm Hg. She is compliant with her four-drug antihypertensive regimen. Her physical examination is unremarkable. She has a serum creatinine level of 3.0 mg/dL.

Differential Diagnosis

The most common cause of elevated blood pressure despite previously well-controlled hypertension is progressive vascular disease and noncompliance with medications. The differential diagnosis for surgical causes of hypertension includes renovascular hypertension, pheochromocytoma, Conn's syndrome (aldosterone-secreting adenoma), Cushing syndrome, and coarctation of the aorta.

Discussion

Renovascular hypertension (RVH) is believed to account for 2% to 10% of all hypertensive patients. The prevalence of RVH is increased in certain subgroups that merit further investigation. RVH should be suspected in patients with hypertension that is severe, refractory to multidrug therapy, or associated with renal dysfunction. Hypertension that presents at the extremes of age should be suspected of having a renovascular origin.

On examination, an abdominal or flank bruit may be heard. Other potential findings include retinopathy, unexplained hypokalemia, or a history of congestive heart failure or pulmonary edema. No single feature or test is diagnostic for RVH. However, in those patients with the above findings, a noninvasive assessment of the renal vasculature is warranted.

Renal duplex ultrasonography has emerged as a screening tool for renal artery stenosis (RAS). Renal artery peak systolic velocities (RA-PSV) correlate with the degree of RAS found on angiography. A focal RA-PSV less than 2.0 m/s is associated with stenosis less than 60% on angiography. In contrast, a focal RA-PSV greater than 2.0 m/s is associated with stenosis greater than 60% on angiography.

Renal Duplex Sonography Results

Renal duplex sonography of the patient's left renal artery demonstrates RA-PSV of 3.77 m/s proximal, 0.74 m/s mid, and 0.25 m/s in the distal renal artery. Right renal artery is occluded. Left kidney measures 12.0 cm in length, and the right kidney measures 5.5 cm in length.

Discussion

In some centers, renal arteriography is used routinely as an initial screening modality for hypertensive individuals who are clinically suspected of having RAS. In this patient with renal dysfunction, sonography was chosen as the initial imaging modality. Depending on available expertise, other modalities are used in the diagnostic evaluation of RAS, such as renal scintigraphy, magnetic resonance angiography, and spiral computed tomographic (CT) angiography. The presence of a hemodynamically significant lesion on ultrasound mandates the use of renal arteriography to fully evaluate the lesion.

■ Renal Arteriography

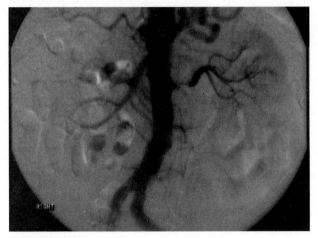

Figure 73-1

Renal Arteriography Report

Selective renal artery catheterization with arteriography shows a left renal artery stenosis greater than 95%. An occlusion of the right renal artery without evidence of reconstitution is demonstrated.

Discussion

In patients with hypertension and RAS diagnosed by angiography, the decision to proceed with surgical intervention is based on multiple factors: age, severity of hypertension, medical comorbidities, and presence of ischemic nephropathy. In certain cases, functional studies may be useful in determining the physiologic significance of RAS. Renal vein renin assays (RVRA) can be used to evaluate the functional significance of lesions found by arteriography, but are not routinely available. The physiologic basis for RVRA is as follows: Patients with RVH and unilateral RAS demonstrate hypersecretion of renin from the ischemic kidney and suppression of renin from the normal kidney. Almost 90% of these patients can be predicted to benefit from renal revascularization. However, many patients have bilateral lesions, and in those cases the diagnostic value of RVRA is limited. As many as 50% of patients with nonlateralizing RVRA have been shown to benefit from revascularization. Thus, patients who could potentially benefit may be excluded from consideration for treatment.

Diagnosis and Recommendations

The options for renal revascularization include percutaneous angioplasty or surgical revascularization in patients with RAS and RVH refractory to medical management. In this patient, the decision is made to proceed with surgical revascularization of the left kidney and concomitant right nephrectomy. An aorto-left renal bypass using 6-mm Dacron is performed to revascularize the left kidney.

▥ Surgical Approach

Multiple surgical options are available to revascularize the kidney, including aortorenal bypass, extra-anatomic bypass, endarterectomy, and reimplantation. A transperitoneal approach utilizing either left or right medial visceral rotation provides adequate exposure of the appropriate renal hilum.

Aortorenal Bypass

Aortorenal bypass using autogenous saphenous vein graft (SVG) is the most common surgical method of treatment for RVH in adults. This technique provides an anatomic reconstruction of renal arterial flow. Alternate choices for conduit include both polytetrafluoroethylene (PTFE) and Dacron. In pediatric patients, hypogastric artery or prosthetic conduits are routinely used, because saphenous vein conduits may undergo aneurysmal degeneration. In patients with atherosclerosis of the abdominal aorta, aortorenal bypass is technically difficult and has a risk of embolic complications.

Extra-anatomic Bypass

The hepatic, splenic, and iliac arteries, as well as the thoracic aorta, can be used as bypass conduits to revascularize the renal arteries. Nonanatomic renal artery bypasses are used to avoid cross clamping the aorta in the presence of significant abdominal aortic or systemic disease. When using one of its tributaries, the patency of the celiac artery must be confirmed by the preoperative arteriogram. A common hepatic artery to right renal artery bypass may be constructed using SVG; however, in patients with left RAS, a direct splenic artery to left renal artery anastomosis is used.

Thromboendarterectomy

This technique is limited to patients with atherosclerotic RAS. Thromboendarterectomy is often combined with operative treatment for aortic aneurysm or aortoiliac occlusive disease. Thromboendarterectomy is frequently performed via an axial aortotomy extending from the superior mesenteric artery to the infrarenal aorta. This approach is often used because it enables the treatment of bilateral renal artery lesions simultaneously, as well as allowing for access to the superior mesenteric and celiac arteries.

Nephrectomy

In a minority of patients with RVH, the affected kidney has non-reconstructible vessels and contributes only minimally to excretory function. In those patients, nephrectomy is a reasonable option because it can benefit the patient in controlling hypertension, while not significantly affecting excretory function over-all. The general reluctance to use this approach is based on the fact that about one of three patients with RAS secondary to atherosclerosis will develop lesions in the contralateral kidney. Nephrectomy should not be done in patients with a reasonably sized kidney in lieu of renal artery exploration for bypass.

Case Continued

The patient does well in the initial postoperative period with marked improve-ment in her blood pressure parameters. However, on postoperative day 3, the patient develops severe hypertension, with normal urine output. Her serum cre-atinine is 1.9 mg/dL.

Renal Arteriography

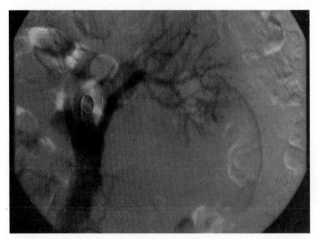

Figure 73-2

Renal Arteriography Results

Aortogram demonstrates a patent aortorenal bypass graft, with widely patent proximal and distal anastomoses. No nephrogram is visualized on the right con-sistent with a nephrectomy.

Diagnosis

The patient has essential hypertension.

Recommendation

The patient is started on oral antihypertensive medication. She is sent home on a two-drug antihypertensive regimen, with blood pressure of 138/72 mm Hg at discharge, and a serum creatinine of 2.2 mg/dL.

Discussion

The large majority of hypertensive individuals in the United States have essential hypertension. However, RVH accounts for a higher percentage of patients with severe hypertension.

The concerns regarding surgical treatment of RVH are based on the operative risk, technical difficulties, and the rate of "unfavorable" blood pressure response after the operation. Several studies report a favorable blood pressure response in 85% to 90% of patients operated on for renovascular hypertension. However, studies have also shown a mortality rate with surgically treated atherosclerotic RAS of 20% to 25% at 5 years. The most common causes of death are myocardial infarction, stroke, and malignancy. The increased long-term mortality rate reflects the multiple comorbidities of patients with atherosclerotic RAS. However, it also reinforces the need for careful selection of patients for renal revascularization.

Because of the prevalence of essential hypertension and its coexistence with RAS, some patients should be expected to remain hypertensive after renal revascularization. In those patients, the definitive diagnosis is made only after operation. Patients with underlying significant essential hypertension should not expect a cure after renal revascularization. In patients with coexisting RVH and essential hypertension, improvement in hypertension, rather than its complete elimination, is the goal. The health risks of hypertension are directly related to its severity. As such, if the ultimate result is better blood pressure control after surgery than before (with or without medication), the patient should be expected to derive a clinical benefit from the operation, as well as have a potentially more protected renal mass, which may not have been the case without revascularization.

Suggested Readings

Hansen KJ, Dean RH. Renovascular disease. In: Moore WS, ed. *Vascular Surgery: A Comprehensive Review*. 6th ed. Philadelphia: WB Saunders; 2002:548-569.

Novick AC. Long-term results of surgical revascularization for renal artery disease. *Urol Clin North Am.* 2001;28:827-831.

Olin JW. Atherosclerotic renal artery disease. *Cardiol Clin.* 2002;20:547-562.

Safian RD, Textor SC. Medical progress: renal artery stenosis. *N Engl J Med.* 2001;344:431-442.

Stanley JC. Surgical treatment of renovascular hypertension. *Am J Surg.* 1997;174:102-110.

Majid Tayyarah, MD, and W. Anthony Lee, MD

Presentation

A 65-year-old man with a history of coronary artery disease and a previous left carotid endarterectomy now presents with a blood pressure of 200/110 mm Hg. He has a 90 pack-year history of tobacco use. He did not have problems with his blood pressure until about two 2 months ago. His primary care physician started him on a moderate dose of a beta-blocker and a diuretic. An angiotensin-converting enzyme (ACE) inhibitor was later added, and his creatinine increased from 1.0 to 1.7 mg/dL. A renal artery duplex scan is obtained.

Duplex Scan Results

Aortic peak systolic velocity (PSV): 51 cm/s; right renal artery PSV: 516 cm/s; left renal artery: 75 cm/s; aortic PSV/right renal artery PSV ratio: 10. Interpretation: greater than 60% right renal artery stenosis, less than 60% left renal artery stenosis.

Differential Diagnosis

Essential hypertension is the cause of hypertension in more than 95% of cases. However, in patients with recent-onset severe (greater than 200 mm Hg systolic and/or greater than 100 mm Hg diastolic) hypertension, a renovascular or surgical etiology should be suspected. In the current case, this diagnosis is supported by the patient's significant past history of peripheral and coronary artery disease and acute deterioration of renal function after administration of an ACE inhibitor.

Discussion

Renovascular hypertension is due to atherosclerosis in more than 90% of cases. Fibromuscular dysplasia (FMD) and other vascular pathologies account for the remainder. Atherosclerotic plaque occurs mostly at the ostium and within the proximal 1 cm of the renal artery, and represents aortic plaque spillover.

Renal artery stenosis can be detected using duplex ultrasound. A renal artery PSV to aortic PSV ratio greater than 3.5 is 95% sensitive for stenosis greater than 60%. Gadolinium-enhanced magnetic resonance angiography (MRA) can also be used to detect RAS, but is dependent on operator technique, and at times may overestimate the degree of stenosis (sensitivity 93% to 100%, specificity 88% to 95%; for stenosis greater than 50%). Conventional contrast angiography remains the gold standard. A stenosis greater than 75% diameter is usually considered clinically significant. During angiography, a pressure gradient across the stenosis can be measured and therapeutic interventions performed at the time of the diagnosis.

Recommendation

Endovascular therapy for renovascular hypertension.

Discussion

Predictors for success after endovascular therapy for renal artery stenosis are similar to those after surgical revascularization. They include (1) recent-onset hypertension or deterioration of previously well-controlled hypertension in the setting of unilateral renal artery stenosis; and (2) renal insufficiency with concomitant severe hypertension and bilateral renal artery stenosis.

Renal artery intervention for patients with anatomic stenosis but well-controlled hypertension with less than three drugs is without clinical benefit. In general, after a technically successful renal artery intervention, 10% of patients will be "cured" (normal blood pressure on no medications), 60% will improve (require either fewer medications, reduced doses, or have better blood pressure control), and 30% will remain unchanged. This rate is similar to open surgical series.

Renal artery stenting is better than angioplasty alone for the treatment of orificial atherosclerotic RAS. Technical success (residual stenosis less than 10%) is greater than 95% with restenosis rates of 10% to 20% at 1 year. Percutaneous transluminal angioplasty (PTA) alone has a lower technical success rate and higher restenosis rates (60% at 1 year). However, PTA is preferred in patients with FMD and non-ostial lesions where selective stenting can be performed for PTA failures, such as recoil and dissection. For FMD, PTA alone enjoys technical success rates greater than 90% and long-term cure rates greater than 50%. For both types of interventions, complications are mostly related to the puncture site, such as hematomas and pseudoaneurysms, and occur in 2% to 12% of patients. Other complications include renal artery dissections, parenchymal perforations, and contrast nephropathy.

Renal Artery Stenting for Ischemic Nephropathy

There have been reports of hemodialysis-dependent patients with RAS recovering their renal function after renal artery intervention. This is distinctly unusual. Several uncontrolled studies have evaluated patients with renal insufficiency after renal artery stenting performed for ischemic nephropathy. As in renovascular hypertension, only 15% to 25% showed any clinical improvement in their renal function and most either remained the same or continue to worsen. Predictors of clinical improvement after renal intervention for ischemic nephropathy include: (1) bilateral renal artery stenosis or unilateral stenosis in a solitary or lone-functioning kidney (greater than 8 cm in length by ultrasound); (2) rapid and recent (within 6 months) deterioration in renal function; (3) severe hypertension; and (4) low parenchymal arteriolar resistance by duplex assessment.

Conversely, those without significant hypertension, with unilateral renal artery stenosis and a patent contralateral renal artery, or long-standing renal dysfunction are unlikely to benefit from any intervention, because they probably have parenchymal arteriolar disease.

▓ Surgical Approach

Although renal artery interventions may be performed from either the femoral or brachial approach, the femoral approach is preferred in most situations. Retrograde femoral access is obtained using a micropuncture needle (21 gauge) and

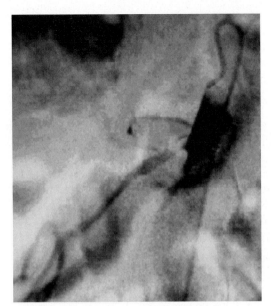

Figure 74-1. Flush aortogram using a Sos Omni angiographic catheter demonstrates an 80% right renal artery stenosis.

a Seldinger technique, and a short 6F introducer sheath is inserted over a 0.035-inch guide wire. An angiographic catheter is advanced to the L1 vertebral body and a flush aortogram is performed (Fig. 74-1). After confirmation of a culprit lesion, intravenous heparin bolus (5000 IU) is given. A variety of selective catheter options are available. You select a shepherd's hook or Cobra-type catheter, and engage the renal artery orifice. A guide wire is used carefully to cross the lesion, and the selective catheter is exchanged for a guide catheter, which is advanced to the renal artery origin. A selective arteriogram is performed (Fig. 74-2) and the lesion predilated with a 4 × 20-mm balloon. The guide catheter is advanced over the balloon beyond the stenosis, and a 6- or 5.5-mm (diameter) × 15- or 18-mm (length) balloon-expandable stent is delivered to the site of the stenosis through the guide catheter; the guide catheter is retracted, and the stent is deployed. A completion angiogram is performed (Fig. 74-3).

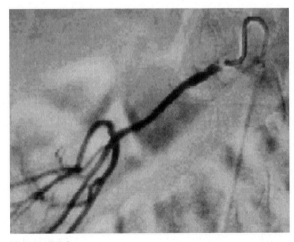

Figure 74-2.

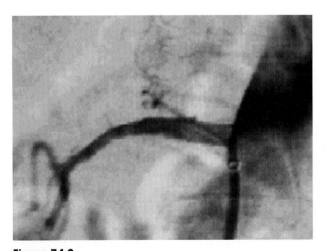

Figure 74-3.

Selective right renal arteriogram Selective catherization of right renal artery orifice (Fig. 74-2). Completion angiogram after right renal artery stent deployment (Fig. 74-3).

Discussion

The renal arteries are usually located at the L1-L2 disk space, and it is best to perform an initial aortogram to identify accessory renals or aortic disease that may affect the intervention. A guide catheter is a relatively large-lumen catheter that has several preformed shapes, and serves to lend support to wires, facilitate delivery of balloons and stents, and enable interval angiograms during an intervention.

Renal interventions can be difficult because of the proximity of the end organ to the lesion, which limits the length of wire "purchase" into the artery. Constant vigilance and meticulous technique is required to prevent inadvertent loss of guidewire access across the lesion during multiple catheter exchanges. Conversely, if the wire is pushed too far distally, it can cause arterial and parenchymal perforation and lead to massive subcapsular or retroperitoneal hemorrhage, and even to loss of the kidney.

Case Continued

The patient is admitted for overnight observation and gentle hydration and to monitor his blood pressure and urine output following renal artery stent placement. Antiplatelet therapy is started immediately in the recovery room with clopidogrel (Plavix) 150 mg orally, which is adjusted the following day to 75 mg/d for 30 days; the patient is later switched to aspirin 325 mg/d.

The patient's serum creatinine returns to baseline the next morning and his systolic blood pressure decreases to 120 to 140 mm Hg. The patient is discharged with instructions to maintain a diary of his blood pressure at home twice a day and consult his primary care physician regarding adjustments to his antihypertensive regimen. He is followed up at 1 month for a review of his serial blood pressures recorded over the previous month, a repeat serum creatinine, and a renal artery duplex scan. Lifelong outpatient follow-up with a renal duplex scan is repeated at 6-month intervals to look for early signs of restenosis.

Discussion

Clinical signs of restenosis include recurrent hypertension, rising creatinine, and elevated renal artery velocities on duplex scan. Endovascular therapy for recurrent stenosis is technically similar to treatment of *de novo* stenosis, with repeat stenting performed only selectively for angioplasty failures. Although controversial, after 2 re-interventions for recurrent stenosis, the patient should be considered for a surgical revascularization. This can be technically challenging in the setting of a stented renal artery.

Suggested Readings

Burket MW, et al. Renal artery angioplasty and stent placement: predictors of a favorable outcome. *Am Heart J.* 2000;139:64-71.

Bush RL, et al. Endovascular revascularization of renal artery stenosis: technical and clinical results. *J Vasc Surg.* 2001;33: 1041-1049.

Henry M, et al. Stents in the treatment of renal artery stenosis: long-term follow-up. *J Endovasc Surg.* 1999;6:42-51.

Leertouwer TC, et al. Stent placement for renal arterial stenosis: where do we stand? A meta-analysis. *Radiology* 2000;216:78–85.

Schneider PA. *Endovascular Skills: Guidewire and Catheter Skills for Endovascular Surgery.* 2nd ed. New York: Marcel Dekker; 2003.

Taylor DC, et al. Duplex ultrasound in the diagnosis of renal artery stenosis: a prospective evaluation. *J Vasc Surg.* 1988;7:363-369.

Kamran Indrees, MD, and Charles J. Shanley, MD FACS

Presentation

A 66-year-old man presents for evaluation of an abdominal aortic aneurysm (AAA) noted incidentally on routine computed tomography (CT) of the abdomen. His past medical history is remarkable for hypercholesterolemia, poorly controlled hypertension, and renal insufficiency (serum creatinine 1.9 gm/dL). The patient denies abdominal or back pain and has no history of coronary artery disease, peripheral arterial occlusive disease, diabetes mellitus, or chronic obstructive pulmonary disease. He admits to a 25 pack-year history of cigarette smoking. His medications include a recently prescribed angiotensin-converting enzyme (ACE) inhibitor in addition to the calcium channel blocker and beta-blocker that he has taken chronically for hypertension. On physical examination, his blood pressure is 170/95 mm Hg in both upper extremities. Heart rhythm is regular at 72 beats per minute. Cardiac examination is remarkable only for a faint S4 gallop. Lungs are clear to auscultation bilaterally. The abdomen is soft with an expansile epigastric mass. Peripheral pulses are easily palpable and symmetric in the upper and lower extremities bilaterally.

CT Scan

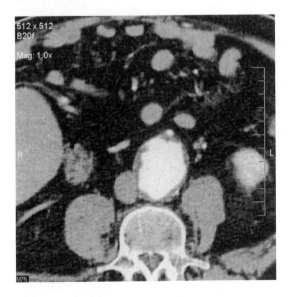

Figure 75-1

CT Scan Report

CT scan reveals a 5.7 × 4.9 cm infrarenal AAA. No other abnormalities are found.

Differential Diagnosis

The differential diagnosis for accelerated or poorly controlled hypertension in older adults is quite extensive. In addition to essential hypertension (the most common cause), a variety of endocrinopathies (pheochromocytoma, hyperaldosteronism, and hypercortisolism) should be considered and excluded with appropriate imaging studies and biochemical testing.

Clearly, in this patient with a history of AAA, hypercholesterolemia, and long-standing tobacco use, it is important to exclude hemodynamically significant atherosclerotic renal artery occlusive disease as a causative or aggravating factor for his poorly controlled hypertension and renal insufficiency.

Discussion

The optimal management of concomitant renal artery occlusive disease in patients undergoing elective aortic reconstruction remains a challenge. The prevalence of renovascular hypertension in the general population is approximately 3%, but the prevalence increases to approximately 50% in severely hypertensive adults over 60 years of age, and is even higher (greater than 70%) in patients with documented renal insufficiency. The vascular surgeon must maintain a high index of suspicion for concomitant renal artery occlusive disease in any elderly patient presenting with aortic aneurysm or occlusive disease.

In "good risk" patients, there appears to be reasonable consensus that staged or concomitant renal revascularization should be considered for patients with uncontrolled or poorly controlled hypertension, especially in the context of progressive deterioration in renal excretory function. In contrast, the optimal management of concomitant asymptomatic renal artery occlusive disease in patients with "reasonably well-controlled" hypertension and "relatively normal renal function" continues to be as controversial as it is common. This controversy promises to continue (if not escalate) in the coming decade with the advent of increasingly sophisticated catheter-based approaches to renal artery atherosclerotic disease.

Currently, little prospective evidence exists upon which to base decision-making in patients undergoing aortic reconstruction with concomitant renal artery stenoses. Most published series suggest that experienced vascular surgeons can perform combined procedures safely in selected patients. The more important question from the standpoint of the individual patient is whether a significant benefit can be expected in exchange for the incremental risk associated with a procedure of greater magnitude.

In patients undergoing arteriography for aortic atherosclerosis, the incidence of renal artery stenoses greater than 50% (ie, hemodynamically significant) ranges from 30% to 40%. Moreover, natural history studies suggest that anatomic progression occurs in up to 50% of untreated stenoses with a significant incidence of occlusion at 5 years. Interestingly, available data does not support a clear association between anatomic progression and either worsening hypertension or accelerated functional deterioration. A possible exception may be patients with bilateral disease and documented reduction in renal size. In these patients, progression appears to correlate with longitudinal worsening of renal function.

Screening studies to document the presence of hemodynamically significant renal artery stenoses can be either functional or anatomic. Functional screening studies include renal venous renin sampling and Captopril renography. After sodium restriction and removal of beta-blockers, a positive study is indicated by a renal vein renin ratio at or greater than 1.5. Despite favorable reported results in selected patients (sensitivity: 100%, specificity: 90%), these tests are expensive, time consuming, and require considerable experience for accurate interpretation. In addition, they are often less accurate in the presence of bilateral disease or in patients with documented renal insufficiency.

Noninvasive screening to document the presence of significant renal artery occlusive disease includes duplex ultrasonography and gadolinium-enhanced magnetic resonance angiography (MRA). Until relatively recently, the mainstay of vascular imaging and diagnosis was conventional arteriography, with the attendant risks of iatrogenic vascular injury and contrast-induced renal insufficiency. Duplex ultrasound is rapidly becoming the initial diagnostic modality of choice owing to its availability, cost effectiveness, and safety when compared to contrast arteriography. B-mode ultrasound provides important anatomic information about aneurysm and kidney morphology as well as renal arterial anatomy and plaque morphology. Spectral Doppler is used to detect turbulent (nonlaminar) flow at sites of significant stenosis. In addition, peak systolic and end-diastolic velocity determinations in conjunction with spectral waveform analysis help to localize and determine the hemodynamic significance of obstructive lesions. Peak velocity measurements are obtained in the aorta as well as the renal artery at the site of the stenosis, and are highly predictive of hemodynamically significant stenoses.

Recommendation

Renal duplex ultrasonography.

Ultrasonography

Table 75-1. Comparison of right and left kidneys on renal duplex ultrasonography.

	Right Kidney	Left Kidney
Size (cm)	9.1	8.2
PSV (cm/sec)	514	472
RAR	9.2	8.4

Abbreviations: PSV, Peak systolic velocity; RAR, renal/aortic ratio
The PSV associated with significant renal artery stenosis increases relative to aortic PSV; therefore, the ratio of velocities in the renal artery and aorta can be used as an index of severity of a renal artery stenosis. A PSV greater than or equal to 180 cm/s and RAR greater than or equal to 3.5 is indicative of greater than 60% stenosis of the renal artery.

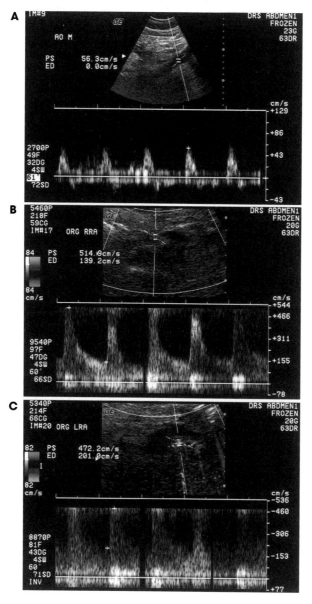

Figure 75-2

Ultrasound Report

Normal renal arteries typically show peak systolic velocity (PSV) values of less than 180 cm/s. (Fig. 75-2) (*A*) Doppler of the proximal native aorta with PSV of 56 cm/s. (*B*) Doppler at origin of the right renal artery with PSV of 514 cm/s and end-diastolic velocity (EDV) of 139 cm/s. (*C*) Doppler at origin of the left renal artery with PSV of 492 cm/s and EDV of 201 cm/s.

Diagnosis

Infrarenal AAA with severe bilateral renal artery occlusive disease.

Discussion

The risk of fatal rupture in patients with infrarenal abdominal aortic aneurysm increases exponentially as aneurysm size increases. Currently, elective repair should be considered to prevent fatal rupture in all patients with an infrarenal AAA exceeding 5.5 cm in maximal diameter. The presence of poorly controlled hypertension and renal insufficiency with duplex evidence of bilateral renal artery occlusive disease suggests that consideration be given to concomitant renal revascularization in this patient, assuming acceptable medical risk. In patients with no history or noninvasive evidence of peripheral, visceral, or renal artery occlusive disease, it is probably reasonable to proceed directly to operative repair of a large aortic aneurysm on the basis of CT scan alone without further vascular imaging. In contrast, detailed anatomic imaging is imperative for preoperative planning of complex aortic reconstructions in combination with renal or visceral revascularization.

MRA provides high-resolution, 3-dimensional vascular imaging in a relatively short time with a high degree of sensitivity and specificity. MRA with gadolinium enhancement can be used as a single imaging modality in surgical management of renovascular disease in selected patients with significant azotemia and/or pulmonary edema. As with MRA in other anatomic locations, one must be cautious because renal MRA has the tendency to overestimate the degree of stenosis. Limitations to MRA relate primarily to its expense and confounding artifacts (ie, signal drop-out due to turbulence, motion, surgical clips, stents, and vascular prostheses).

Contrast arteriography is still considered the "gold standard" of vascular imaging owing to its superb anatomic detail. Limitations include cost, invasiveness, and the need for administration of both ionizing radiation and iodinated contrast. Serious complications occur in less than 1% of patients. Contrast-induced nephrotoxicity occurs in up to 11% of patients and increases in patients with underlying renal insufficiency and diabetes. Efforts to reduce contrast loads and ensure adequate hydration help to minimize this risk. In addition, peri-procedural administration of N-acetyl cysteine (Mucomyst) has also been shown to reduce the risks of contrast-induced nephropathy. Alternative contrast agents, including intravenous gadolinium and CO_2, minimize contrast-related nephrotoxicity and allergic reactions at the expense of cost and reduced anatomic detail.

Recommendation

Abdominal aortography with bilateral selective renal arteriography.

Abdominal Aortography

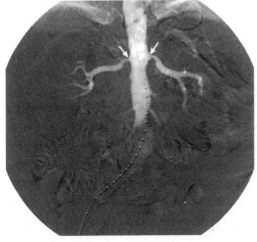

Figure 75-3

Aortography Report

Aortogram showing high-grade osteal stenosis (*arrows*) of both renal arteries, the left more severe than the right.

Discussion

In this patient, anatomic considerations preclude endovascular repair, and therefore open repair is indicated. Options for management of the renal artery stenoses include angioplasty with or without stent insertion, aortorenal or extra-anatomic bypass, and endarterectomy.

A detailed discussion of catheter-based approaches to renal artery atherosclerotic disease is beyond the scope of this case. In general, when compared to the results for fibromuscular disease in young adults, angioplasty for atherosclerotic renal artery occlusive disease responds less favorably, has less durable long-term results, and has higher rates of restenosis as compared to surgical renal artery reconstruction. However, if the patient were a candidate for an endovascular stent graft, then percutaneous transluminal angioplasty and stenting of the renal artery would be adjunctive to the endovascular procedure.

The most common approach to concomitant renal revascularization during aortic surgery is aorto-renal bypass employing either autogenous vein or prosthetic graft conduits originating from the aortic prosthesis. Occasionally, in patients with highly redundant renal arteries, it may be possible to re-implant the renal arteries into the aortic prosthesis in end-to-side fashion. Renal endarterectomy has been used with excellent results in patients with aortoiliac occlusive disease, but should be avoided in patients undergoing aortic aneurysm repair owing to the frequently degenerated nature of the peri-renal aorta in these patients. Extra-anatomic bypasses (hepatorenal and splenorenal) are most commonly used in patients with isolated renovascular hypertension for whom aortic cross clamping is either contraindicated or impossible.

For experienced vascular surgeons, the mortality risk for repair of an infrarenal abdominal aortic aneurysm with concomitant renal revascularization should be less than 5%. Other complications include a 10% incidence of renal failure, although this risk increases substantially in patients with underlying renal insufficiency. Of patients that develop postoperative renal failure, approximately 50% will require dialysis. Assuming there are no complications, 70% to 80% of patients will experience improved control of their hypertension with fewer medications.

Recommendation

Aortic interposition graft repair of abdominal aortic aneurysm with bilateral aorto-renal bypasses.

▓ Surgical Approach

Given the magnitude of the surgical undertaking, patients undergoing concomitant aortic and renal revascularization should undergo complete preoperative cardiac evaluation. Intraoperative transesophageal echocardiography has also proven useful in selected high-risk patients with decreased left ventricular function. Intravenous mannitol is routinely administered prior to aortic cross clamping as both an osmotic diuretic and free radical scavenger. In the senior author's experience, cold perfusion is only necessary if prolonged renal ischemia is anticipated.

Case Continued

The patient underwent transabdominal exploration via a transverse supraumbilical laparotomy incision. This incision provides maximal exposure when bilateral renal revascularization is contemplated. The abdominal aorta was exposed from the base of the superior mesenteric artery to the iliac bifurcations. The aneurysm extended to the origins of the renal arteries, precluding clamp placement below the renal arteries. To minimize warm renal ischemia, 6-mm expanded polytetrafluoroethylene side grafts were sutured in end-to-side fashion to the body of the aortic prosthesis prior to cross clamping. The iliac vessels, renal arteries, and suprarenal aorta were controlled.

To minimize renal ischemia, a sequential clamping technique was used. First, the proximal aortic anastomosis was constructed in end-to-end fashion at the level of the renal arteries. Next, the proximal left main renal artery was suture ligated and divided, and a spatulated end-to-end distal anastomosis was constructed to the distal left main renal artery. At this point, flow was restored to the left kidney. Subsequently, the proximal right main renal artery was similarly ligated and divided, and a spatulated end-to-end distal anastomosis constructed to the right main renal artery. Flow was then restored to the right kidney. Using this technique, total warm ischemia time was 24 minutes for left kidney and 36 minutes for the right kidney. Adequate flow to both renal arteries was confirmed using a continuous-wave hand-held Doppler. Finally, the distal aortic anastomosis was performed in end-to-end fashion and flow was restored to the lower extremities. The retroperitoneum and abdomen were closed after ensuring hemostasis.

Postoperatively, the patient was monitored initially in the surgical intensive care unit and begun on an antiplatelet agent. All antihypertensive medicines were discontinued with the exception of a low-dose beta-blocker. Serum creatinine rose transiently to 2.1 mg/dL on postoperative day 2, and then gradually decreased over the course of the next week to a new baseline of 1.4 mg/dL. The patient was discharged on postoperative day 7. At his 6-month follow-up appointment, surveillance duplex ultrasound revealed bilateral patent aorto-renal bypass grafts with no evidence of hemodynamically significant stenoses. The patient's blood pressure was 135/76 mm Hg and serum creatinine remains stable. He continues on a low-dose beta-blocker and antiplatelet agent.

Suggested Readings

Cambria RP, Brewster DC, L'Italien G, et al. Simultaneous aortic and renal artery reconstruction: evolution of an 18-year experience. *J Vasc Surg.* 1995;21:916-924; discussion 925.

Chaikof EL, Smith RB 3rd, Salam AA, et al. Ischemic nephropathy and concomitant aortic disease: a 10-year experience. *J Vasc Surg.* 1994;19:135-148.

Dean RH, Benjamin ME, Hansen KJ. Surgical management of renovascular hypertension. *Curr Probl Surg.* 1997;34:209-308.

Hansen KJ, Starr SM, Sands RE, et al. Contemporary surgical management of renovascular disease. *J Vasc Surg.* 1992;16:319-330; discussion 330-331.

Hansen KJ, Tribble RW, Reavis SW, et al. Renal duplex sonography: evaluation of clinical utility. *J Vasc Surg.* 1990;12:227-236.

McNeil JW, String ST, Pfeiffer RB Jr. Concomitant renal endarterectomy and aortic reconstruction. *J Vasc Surg.* 1994;20:331-337.

Olin JW, Melia M, Young JR, et al. Prevalence of atherosclerotic renal artery stenosis in patients with atherosclerosis elsewhere. *Am J Med.* 1990; 88:46N-51N.

case 76

Peter K. Henke, MD

Presentation

A 45-year-old woman, G6/P5, is evaluated for vague right upper quadrant pain. Past medical history includes hypertension controlled with two medications, including an angiotensin-converting enzyme (ACE) inhibitor and a diuretic. The patient denies any history of tobacco use, diabetes, and hyperlipidemia, and there is no family history of any aneurysmal or other major vascular disease. She is perimenopausal.

CT Scan

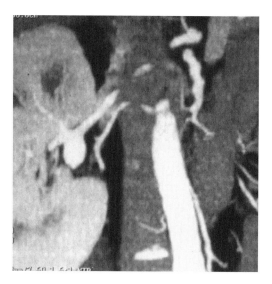

Figure 76-1

CT Scan Report

A computed tomographic (CT) scan shows no evidence of gallbladder or liver pathology, but there is an incidental finding of a right renal artery aneurysm (RAA) approximately 2.5 cm in size, not noted on a prior right upper quadrant ultrasound (Fig. 76-1), and other mesenteric aneurysms are identified.

Further Diagnostic Work-up

No hematuria is detected on urinalysis and serum creatinine is normal. An arteriogram should be obtained in these patients to delineate the renal anatomy with dedicated catheter injections and multiple projections of both renal arteries.

▧ Arteriogram

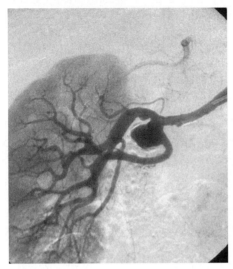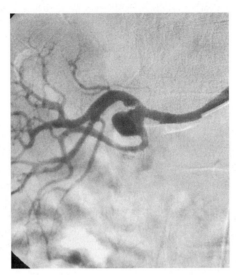

Figure 76-2

Arteriogram Report

A large right RAA at the bifurcation of the main renal artery, and a smaller left RAA in a first-order branch (Fig. 76-2). No other intra-aortic pathology is identified.

Treatment Considerations

Because this patient is just beyond childbearing age, indications for repair are slightly less compelling than if premenopausal, where repair is definitely indicated. The main risk with RAA is rupture. If this occurs, mortality ranges between 10% and 15%. Rupture risk is higher in premenopausal women and kidney loss is high in the setting of rupture, ranging between 50% and 100%. Although endovascular repairs have been documented, this does not seem appropriate for most RAA, because they are often fusiform and not amenable to coil embolization. A technical mishap may cause total kidney infarction. The patient's RAA is a size that is suitable for repair, given that she otherwise has few cardiovascular risk factors. Various methods for repairing these lesions have been described including *ex vivo* reconstruction with kidney autotransplantation, but it is the author's practice to perform the repair *in situ*, using aneurysm resection, primary repair, and/or bypass as the individual anatomy dictates.

▧ Surgical Approach

At operation, a lumbar roll is placed to create a lumbar lordosis. A transverse supraumbilical incision allows for excellent exposure of the kidneys. An extensive Kocher maneuver is used to expose the right kidney and renal vasculature. Care must be taken to fully dissect the RAA from surrounding renal venous and hilar structures. A right RAA resection with primary repair is performed. The patient's postoperative course is unremarkable, with normal renal function and a technically adequate repair confirmed on arteriogram at postoperative day 7 (Fig. 76-3). Postoperatively, she requires only one antihypertensive agent. Careful postoperative laboratory follow-up of her creatinine is important as well as blood pressure monitoring. Perioperative intermittent increases in diastolic blood pressure can be a sign for renal arterial stenosis and may signal repair failure.

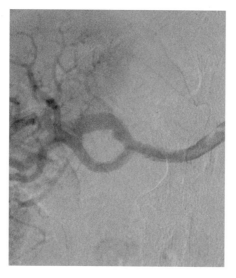

Figure 76-3

Long-Term Follow-Up

The patient should undergo close blood pressure evaluation, but screening invasive arteriography is rarely indicated. MRA scanning and/or CT scanning with 3D reconfiguration may be useful as well for following any change in the left RAA size. At this point, the patient has opted to observe the left side, for which the overall rupture risk with RAA less than 2.0 cm is quite low. However, if the left RAA grows in size, an approach similar to the one used on the right side can be performed, though it does necessitate reoperative surgery. Overall, the durability of repair is excellent, with clinical patency at least 95% at 8 years follow-up. Unplanned nephrectomy rates in the settings of repair are very low; however, in one large series, no late dialysis was required in patients who did require an unplanned nephrectomy. Interestingly, hypertension is often improved after RAA repair, though the distinct mechanisms responsible for this observation are not certain.

Suggested Readings

Henke PK, Cardneau JD, Welling TH, et al. Renal artery aneurysms: a 35-year clinical experience with 252 aneurysms in 168 patients. *Ann Surg.* 2001;234:454-463.

Karkos CD, D'Souza SP, Thompson GJ, Chomal A, Matanhelia SS. Renal artery aneurysm: endovascular treatment by coil embolization with preservation of renal blood flow. *Eur J Vasc Endovasc Surg.* 2000;19:214-216.

Prince MR, Narasimham DL, Stanley JC, et al. Breath-hold gadolinium-enhanced MR angiography of the abdominal aorta and its major branches. *Radiology.* 1994;197:785.

Schorn B, Valk V, Dalichau H, Mohr FW. Kidney salvage in a case of ruptured renal artery aneurysm: case report and literature review. *Cardiovasc Surg.* 1997;5:134.

Stanley JC, Messina LM, Wakefield TW, et al. Renal artery reconstruction. In: Bergan JJ, Yao JST, eds. *Techniques in Arterial Surgery.* Philadelphia: WB Saunders; 1990:247.

Tham G, Ekelund L, Herrlin K, et al. Renal artery aneurysms: natural history and prognosis. *Ann Surg.* 1983;197:348.

Mark W. Sebastian, MD

Presentation

A 42-year-old man with no significant past medical history presents to your office after he was referred by his primary medical doctor for unilateral lower extremity swelling. He is referred after being followed by both his primary care physician and a wound care clinic for this condition. The symptoms initially manifested in adulthood as swelling from the foot to an area superior to the inguinal ligament. He had been treated with manual decompressive physiotherapy, nonelastic compressive dressings, custom clothing, and meticulous skin care. The patient has complained of progressive lack of response to this conservative therapy targeted at volume reduction and preservation of skin integrity. He also states that his skin has lost its elasticity, becoming flaccid and painful in areas. He states that areas of hardening of the skin and subcutaneous tissue have appeared recently. He has also noted some reddening of these areas, but denies fever, chills, or skin breakdown.

On physical examination the patient is a well-developed male, anxious, and in mild distress. He has gross asymmetry of the lower extremities, with the affected limb showing redundant skin folds at the ankle, edema of the skin, and subcutaneous tissue with areas of induration and generalized loss of skin tone and altered skin turgor. The femoral pulses are palpable bilaterally, and distal perfusion is intact, with triphasic Doppler signals audible in the affected limb, and palpable distal pulses in the contralateral lower extremity (Fig. 77-1).

Differential Diagnosis

The differential diagnosis for swollen leg includes systemic conditions: congestive heart failure, renal failure, liver failure (hypoalbuminemia), malnutrition, protein loss nephropathy, cellulitis, infection, and parasitic infestation.

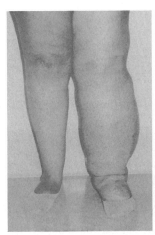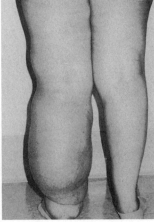

Figure 77-1

The differential diagnoses for unilateral lower extremity swelling includes the following:

1) Chronic venous insufficiency
   A) Intrinsic valvular insufficiency
   B) Obstructions
2) Extrinsic compression
   A) Anatomic
   B) Pathologic
2) Postphlebitic syndrome
3) Myxedema
4) Lipedema
5) Lymphedema
   A) Primary
      i) Congenital: present at birth, or by age 2
      ii) Praecox: puberty to third decade
      iii) Tarda: after age 35
      iv) Familial: Milroy's disease
   B) Secondary
      i) Surgery
      ii) Radiation

Case Continued

Based on the age at presentation, lack of inciting factors, progression of symptoms, physical manifestations, and failure of conservative therapy, isotopic lymphoscintigraphy is performed.

▨ Isotopic Lymphoscintigraphy

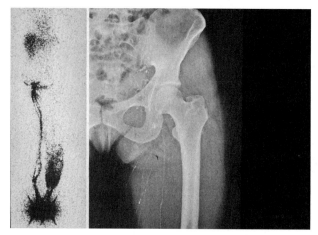

Figure 77-2

Isotopic Lymphoscintigraphy Report

Radiolabeled sulphur colloid is administered via the subcutaneous route, into the subdermal interdigit region of the affected extremity. A gamma camera captures the isotope progression up the affected limb.

Diagnosis

Primary lymphedema tarda.

Interpretation

Lymphatic obstruction identified with pooling of radiocontrast in left groin area.

Case Continued

With the results of the test (Fig. 77-2) the progression of the pathologic process, the severe lifestyle limitations, and the patient's request, surgical therapy is offered. Based on the extent of the skin and subcutaneous tissue changes, excisional debulking and plastic surgical coverage is offered. Due to the advanced stage of the skin and soft tissue changes, lymphatic reconstruction is not indicated.

Surgical Approach

The patient is brought to the operating room and placed in the supine position. After adequate induction of general orotracheal anesthesia, the affected extremity and the tissue donor site on the contralateral extremity are prepped with chlorhexidine solution and draped as a sterile field. The medial and lateral aspects of the affected limb are incised and the skin, subcutaneous tissue, and deep fascia are completely excised (Fig. 77-3).

The affected and the non-affected tissue are completely excised. After adequate hemostasis is obtained, full-thickness skin grafting is applied to the muscle beds of the affected extremity. Standard plastic surgery dressings are applied. The patient is extubated in the operating room and taken to the postanesthesia care room in stable condition, having tolerated the procedure well.

Discussion

Lymphedema is the medical term used for generalized swelling of an affected area caused by the accumulation of protein-rich fluid that is unable to drain via the

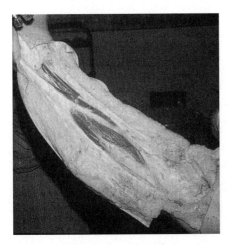

Figure 77-3

normal process of lymphatic drainage. Although it is seen in the lower extremity in the vast majority of cases (70% to 80%), it can affect any part of the body where normal lymphatic drainage is compromised. The affected area is prone to acute and chronic changes, including swelling, sclerosis, skin breakdown, infection, and neoplastic changes. The diagnosis is one of exclusion followed by confirmation. The differential diagnosis includes systemic diagnoses, such as congestive heart failure, renal failure, liver failure (hypoalbuminemia), malnutrition, protein loss nephropathy, cellulitis, infection, and parasitic infestation. Unilateral or local conditions include deep venous thrombosis, chronic venous insufficiency, anatomic obstruction of the iliac vein by the iliac artery, myxedema, lipedema, postphlebitic syndrome, malignancy, and primary and secondary lymphedema.

A thorough history and physical examination is critical to narrowing the focus of the differential diagnosis and tailoring diagnostic testing. Typically, important components of a medical history with a chief complaint of swollen extremity include cardiac, renal, hepatic, dermatologic, infectious, and malignant possibilities. Tailored history includes age at onset, location of onset, pattern of spread, and pattern of progression. Any surgical and radiation therapy must be documented. The physical examination centers on both the affected extremity and the contralateral limb, including limb circumference, skin turgor, skin condition, integumentary structures, trophic changes of hair and nails, lymph node status, skin temperature, and proximal and distal arterial perfusion.

Basic laboratory examination includes blood work to assess renal and hepatic function, and urinalysis to assess sediment and presence or absence of protein.

Diagnostic tests of unilateral limb edema include an array of radiologic tests, including lymphangiogram, lymphoscintigram, ultrasound, duplex ultrasound, computed tomography (CT), and magnetic resonance imaging (MRI). Lymphangiogram is limited to intraoperative assessment of lymphatic bypass. Lymphoscintigraphy is the gold standard of diagnostic assessment, although duplex ultrasound is useful as an adjunct. CT scanning may be used to monitor effects of treatment. CT scan findings in lymphedema include thickened skin of the calf, enlarged subcutaneous compartment, tissue stranding, increased fat density, and thickened perimuscular aponeurosis. MRI findings in lymphedema are similar to those found on CT scan.

Lymphedema predisposes to disabling changes in the affected extremity. It also predisposes to infection and malignancy. Therefore, conservative, consistent, and longitudinal multidisciplinary therapy is critical. Manual decongestive therapy followed by compressive dressings is the mainstay of conservative therapy. Limb elevation is not useful in lymphedema. Meticulous skin care and physical therapy are equally important in the long-term conservative care of patients with lymphedema. Benzopyrones as pharmacologic adjuncts reduce protein accumulation by enhancing macrophage presence in the affected extremity. This reduces edema and minimizes the infectious potential in the affected area. Their use is limited by hepatotoxicity.

Surgical therapy is indicated for refractory and progressive lymphedema that does not respond to decongestive and physical therapy. The two categories of surgical intervention are reconstructive, or lymphatic bypass, and surgical debulking. The bypass approach is described in the literature as end-to-side lymphovenous bypass, and adipolymphaticovenous transfer, in which autologous saphenous vein, together with its lymphatic-containing adipose tissue, is transposed into the affected area. Free omental transfer has also been reported, with satisfactory results reported in one series. Debulking excisional surgery involves excision of the entire affected limb either in a one- or a two-stage procedure with complete coverage with skin grafting. Complete excisional therapy of the affected limb, including both affected and non-affected regions, leads to a superior cosmetic and functional outcome when compared with excisional therapy of only affected areas of the extremity. Prophylactic surgery is reserved for cases in which extensive pelvic and inguinal lymph node dissection and extirpation are employed. The most commonly cited technique of prophylactic surgery is omentoplasty. The consensus within the literature advocates coordinated multidisciplinary conservative therapy for lymphedema with surgical intervention reserved for cases refractory to aggressive nonoperative therapy. When surgical therapy is recommended for refractory cases of lymphedema, excision of the entire skin, soft tissue, and fascial complex of the affected and non-affected regions of the extremity is indicated. Staged and immediate skin grafting is subsequently employed. Though an uncommon condition, lymphedema requires a measured and coordinated therapeutic strategy.

Suggested Readings

Bland KL, Percyzk R, Du W, et al. Can a practicing surgeon detect early lymphedema reliably? *Am J Surg.* 2003;186:509-513.

Hinrichs CS, Gibbs JF, Driscoll D, et al. The effectiveness of complete decongestive physiotherapy for the treatment of lymphedema following groin dissection for melanoma. *J Surg Oncol.* 2004;85:187-192.

Kim DI, Huh SH, Hwang JH, et al. Excisional surgery for chronic advanced lymphedema. *Surg Today.* 2004;34:134-137.

Kim DI, Huh S, Lee SJ, et al. Excision of subcutaneous tissue and deep muscle fascia for advanced lymphedema. *Lymphology.* 1998;31:190-194.

Rockson SG. Lymphedema. *Am J Med.* 2002;110:288-295.

Ruocco V, Schwartz RA, Ruocco E. Lymphedema: an immunologically vulnerable site for development of neoplasms. *J Am Acad Dermatol.* 2002;47:124-127.

Tiwari A, Koon-Sung C, Button M, et al. Differential diagnosis, investigation, and current treatment of lower limb lymphedema. *Arch Surg.* 2003;138:152-161.

Note: Page numbers followed by *f* indicate figures